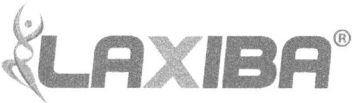

# The Nutrition Navigator

## M.Sc. Henry S. Grant

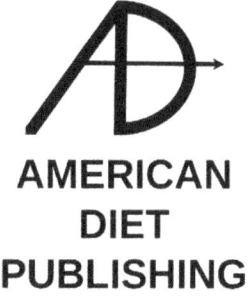

**AMERICAN DIET PUBLISHING**

Koblenz and Wilmington

ADP American Diet Publishing GmbH
Copyright © 2014 by Henry S. Grant. All Rights Reserved.
Library of Congress Control Number 2014957224
ISBN 978-1-941978-14-6
Front cover design by Mahmood Ali
Interior design by Rose Hristova
E-Mail of the author: Grant@AmericanDietPublishing.com

ADP American Diet Publishing GmbH

| | |
|---|---|
| Johannes Mueller-Strasse 12 | 913 N Market Street |
| 56068 Koblenz | Wilmington, DE, 19801 |
| Germany | United States of America |

**For organizations and corporations:** Interested in a bulk order? Visit us at www.AmericanDietPublishing.com/discounts.php

All rights reserved. No part of this book may be used or reproduced in any manner whatsoever. Without written permission of the author, reprints, translations, taking values or illustrations, saving it in data systems or on electronic devices as well as providing parts of the book online or on other communication services is liable to prosecution. Avoid being a cheat and only read the book, if you obtained it in a legal way.

The data set for the algorithmic ordained statements concerning fructose, lactose and sugar alcohols is from the University of Minnesota Nutrition Coordination Center 2014 Food and Nutrient Database. The database license has been acquired for this book due to its high quality and scope based on international research. Statements regarding fructans and galactans have been drawn from four cited international studies. Those regarding fructans and galactans have been drawn from six different sources that are indicated in the tables. Nevertheless, the contents of the book bear no guarantee. Neither the author, publisher, any cited scientist nor the University of Minnesota is liable for personal injuries or physical or financial damage. Please note that the quantities of critical ingredients in the mentioned products, which are the foundation for the stated portion sizes, are relative and in part based on derivations. Portion sizes the reader is expected to tolerate are based on approximations of various details. The precise tolerable portion size of any product varies depending on its processing, country-specific composition, degree of maturity and cultivation.

# ACKNOWLEDGMENTS

*Special thanks to M. Thor and the nutritional research team of the University of Minnesota, J. S. Barrett, J. R. Biesiekierski, P. R. Gibson, K. Liels, J. G. Muir, S. J. Shepherd, R. Rose and O. Rosella as well as the rest of the gastroenterology research team of the Monash University, all other cited scientists for their research, B. Hartmann of the Bundesministerium für Ernährung, Landwirtschaft und Verbraucherschutz, G.-W. von Rymon Lipinski of the Goethe Universität, and H. Zorn of the Justus Liebig-Universität, for copyediting L. Gomes Domingues, F. Lang, L. Popielinski and M. Vastolo, as well as my mother, sister and friends, especially C. Schlick and all other contributors who enabled me to write this book in first place.*

*To my daughter—Paula Anna*

# Contents

Preface .................................................................................................. 11

## 1. Information ........................................................................................ 1
- 1.1     Why you deserve this book ............................................................ 1
- 1.2     Prehistoric monsters take vengeance… ........................................ 4
- 1.3     Diagnostic check ............................................................................. 7
- 1.4     Background of the disease ........................................................... 10
- 1.5     The bricks and how your belly is fighting ................................... 11
  - 1.5.1    Brick number one: Lactose ................................................ 13
  - 1.5.2    Brick number two: Fructose .............................................. 17
  - 1.5.3    Brick number three: Fructans ........................................... 21
  - 1.5.4    Brick number four: Galactans ........................................... 23
  - 1.5.5    Brick number five: Sorbitol and others ............................. 25
  - 1.5.6    Abdominal discomfort in children .................................... 27
- 1.6     Summary of Part 1 ....................................................................... 28

## 2. Strategy ........................................................................................... 29
- 2.1     Mission planning ......................................................................... 29
  - 2.1.1    Roadmap ............................................................................ 30
  - 2.1.2    Symptom test sheet ........................................................... 34
  - 2.1.3    Test result calculation table ............................................... 35
  - 2.1.4    Keeping your balance ........................................................ 37
- 2.2     Your individual strategy .............................................................. 45
  - 2.2.1    It depends on the total load .............................................. 47
  - 2.2.2    Prevalence of the intolerance types .................................. 48
  - 2.2.3    Substitute test .................................................................... 49
  - 2.2.4    Level test ............................................................................ 51
  - 2.2.5    Symptom based test process ............................................. 69
  - 2.2.6    Alternative strategies ........................................................ 73
- 2.3     General diet hints ........................................................................ 75
  - 2.3.1    Good reasons for your persistence ................................... 75
  - 2.3.2    Mealtimes ........................................................................... 79

| | | |
|---|---|---|
| 2.3.3 | Reasons for using the bricks | 79 |
| 2.3.4 | Eating out | 79 |
| 2.3.5 | Convenience foods | 80 |
| 2.3.6 | Medicine and oral hygiene | 80 |
| 2.3.7 | Nutritional supplements | 81 |
| 2.3.8 | Positive aspects of the diet | 82 |
| 2.3.9 | Testing yourself | 82 |
| 2.3.10 | Protein shakes—nutrition for athletes | 82 |
| 2.3.11 | Sweeteners | 82 |
| 2.3.12 | Fish and meat | 82 |
| 2.3.13 | These actions lead to lasting change | 83 |
| 2.4 | The leaflets | 84 |
| 2.4.1 | Fructose and sugar alcohols | 89 |
| 2.4.2 | Fructans, galactans and lactose | 91 |
| 2.4.3 | The safe products list | 93 |
| 2.5 | For hosts | 95 |
| 2.6 | Stress management | 96 |
| 2.7 | General summary | 99 |

**3. FOOD TABLES** ............ 103

| | | |
|---|---|---|
| 3.1 | Introduction to the tables | 103 |
| 3.1.1 | Your personal tolerance levels | 104 |
| 3.1.2 | Explanation of the abbreviations | 105 |
| 3.1.3 | Level multipliers | 112 |

**TABLES BY CATEGORY** ............ 113

| | | |
|---|---|---|
| 3.2 | Athletes | 114 |
| 3.3 | Beverages | 116 |
| 3.3.1 | Alcoholic | 116 |
| 3.3.2 | Hot beverages | 121 |
| 3.3.3 | Juices | 124 |
| 3.3.4 | Other beverages | 126 |
| 3.4 | Cold dishes | 129 |
| 3.4.1 | Bread | 129 |
| 3.4.2 | Cereals | 131 |
| 3.4.3 | Cold cut | 134 |

- 3.4.4 Dairy products ........................................................................ 137
- 3.4.5 Nuts and snacks ..................................................................... 141
- 3.4.6 Sweet pastries ........................................................................ 144
- 3.4.7 Sweets .................................................................................... 149
- 3.5 Warm dishes ................................................................................ 154
  - 3.5.1 Meals ..................................................................................... 154
  - 3.5.2 Meat and fish ......................................................................... 159
  - 3.5.3 Lactose hideouts ................................................................... 161
  - 3.5.4 Sauces and spices ................................................................. 162
  - 3.5.5 Side dishes ............................................................................ 167
- 3.6 Fast food chains .......................................................................... 169
  - 3.6.1 Burger King® ........................................................................ 169
  - 3.6.2 KFC® ..................................................................................... 171
  - 3.6.3 McDonald's® ......................................................................... 172
  - 3.6.4 Subway® ................................................................................ 174
- 3.7 Fruit and vegetables ................................................................... 176
  - 3.7.1 Fruit ....................................................................................... 176
  - 3.7.2 Vegetables ............................................................................. 180
- 3.8 Ice cream ..................................................................................... 186
- 3.9 Ingredients .................................................................................. 189

**SUGGESTIONS** ................................................................................ 190

**KEYWORD INDEX** ........................................................................... 192

**GLOSSARY** ...................................................................................... 256

**SOURCES** ........................................................................................ 258

# Preface

This book shows you ways to find relief from abdominal discomfort due to any of the covered intolerances or from irritable bowel syndrome. With this book you will be able to identify those ingredients that lead to symptoms, enabling you to control your intake for a healthier and more worry-free life!

The book's information is drawn from intensive research and interviews with professors. The portions indicated in the food lists are based on results of laboratory research. An analysis of the US database has allowed us to produce practical recommendations regarding the portion sizes that your stomach can handle. Moreover, you will learn about the background and consequences of the ailments discussed. This book provides you with a broad spectrum of insights: removable key facts lists for your purchases, strategies to determine the amounts of critical foods you can stomach and even a discussion on the topic of stress management.

Nevertheless, only your doctor is qualified to make any mandatory nutritional recommendations. All those made in the book are non-binding. It is not possible to guarantee recovery, and there are other triggers of abdominal symptoms that may be relevant (see Chapter 2.2.6). This book should not be the sole basis for any decisions you make. Talk about any diet with your doctor before you begin in order to limit discomfort. You are responsible for your personal health, including how you choose to interpret data and specialists' advice.

As a long time sufferer, I know about the need for clarity and practical advice. The focuses of the strategy discussed in this book are quality and suitability for daily use. I wholeheartedly wish you ongoing success on your way to greater abdominal comfort!

Your author,

*Henry S. Grant*

Henry S. Grant

# 1

# INFORMATION

## 1.1 Why you deserve this book

You have courage. You took the initiative. By buying this book you have shown your will to overcome your discomfort. Many suffer due to such discomfort, yet only a few act, and you are one of them! You know that you and those around you will gain more from your life if you regain comfort in your belly. Hence, I welcome you to the mission of developing a successful nutritional routine.

If you bought the book so you could learn to adapt to those in your life suffering from intolerances, you will learn how in Chapter 2.5. This shows a consideration for others that would make anyone glad to be a guest at your table. Furthermore, you will find generally useful hints regarding healthy nutrition in Chapter 2.1.4, and in Chapter 2.6 you will learn to reduce stress in your everyday life and improve your decision-making skills.

If your employer or educational institution has given you this book as a gift, it is an expression of their appreciation of you and trust in your willingness to take action. The book has been written with the intention of enabling you to live more of a free life, by improving your digestive well-being. It will help you to change your life so you can stop losing happiness due to abdominal discomfort.

Before we begin, realize that starting soon after your birth, your mother ensured your adequate nutrition by giving you only baby food. Unlike creatures in the wild, we usually do not face natural restrictions concerning what we eat when. You, as an adult, choose what you want to eat. That being so, is it any wonder that finding a nutritional plan that fits your needs is a factor in your health? With this book, you benefit from a comprehensible description of current scientific research and probably the most useable food table on the market for countering food intolerance.

In this first part of the book you will find out which diagnostic procedures you should go through with your doctor before changing your diet. Moreover, the causes and effects of irritable bowel syndrome [IBS] will be explained, and you will discover the elements of foods that can cause abdominal discomfort. These are easily fermentable carbohydrates. We will call these comprehensive *bricks*, as a brick sits heavily in one's stomach. Some of these, like fructose and lactose, may already be familiar to you. Others are less well known and form one reason as to why discomfort persists for those who live on a "brick diet." Whether you have an intolerance or IBS, knowing about these triggers will help you improve your dietary health. After the triggers are discussed, the second part of the book will acquaint you with the nutrition navigator strategy. You can find out which bricks you can stomach well and how much you can eat of those that are problematic for you. Furthermore, you will read about the basic principles of a healthy diet. What's more, you learn how to stick to the diet in your everyday life, along with how you can reduce stress, which is also a factor that can upset your stomach. These are the aims of the nutrition navigator:

You **improve** your **quality of life** by gaining back **comfort** in your **stomach** while **maintaining** a **healthy diet**.

In order to help you achieve a healthy diet, the book guides you to choose portion sizes you are able to stomach with regard to fructose, lactose, sugar alcohols and other bricks in athletic products, beverages, cold and warm dishes, fast food chain products, fruits and vegetables and many other products and ingredients. The food table contains numerous brand-name products and enables you to reduce limitations on your choices as much as possible. If your doctor has made a diagnosis based upon nutrition diaries, he or she might choose to retest you after considering the data from this book. For example, the amount of sugar alcohols in some fruits and vegetables or the amount of free fructose in cereals is hard to discern from the currently available literature. Your doctor may thus be able to finally discover and accurately diagnose a specific intolerance. Additionally, you get two practical lists for your wallet, to make it easier for you to make smart purchases for yourself.

Only if you know which bricks you are able to stomach, along with the portion sizes of products that contain problematic ingredients, will you be able to eat in a way that suits your profile and helps you avoid losing quality of life. Your mission is a challenging one. Bricks can hide everywhere—even in oral hygiene products and medicine. Please read this book's recommendations carefully and act accordingly. The consequences of being negligent about having an intolerance are harsh, as you will learn later. An unknown malabsorbtion of an ingredient can lead to depression and much more unpleasantness. The "brick-eating dragons" presented in the following chapter are a fictive symbol of potential discomfort, while the "interception shield" is a symbol of the body's usual metabolism. The effects described, however, are real.

# 1.2 Prehistoric monsters take vengeance…

How do brick-eating dragons steal drive, fun and lust from you? Dragons were believed to have been stamped out in the Middle Ages—but some small ones persevered, and now they are back and are seeking revenge. Yet, we did not do them any harm. People had good reasons for hunting them in the Middle Ages for their extreme aggression. These so-called brick dragons are carrying out their vendetta by making themselves invisible and smuggling themselves into bellies. Even women and children are targeted. Anyone can be affected. They are called brick dragons here because they can only do harm if we eat too many of certain bricks. These bricks exist naturally in some foods and are usually used by our bodies to provide us with energy. However, as a brick dragon enters our stomach, it damages our stomach's engine or "brick interception shield," letting more bricks enter the dragon's lair, the bowel. There are different types of bricks. The penetrability of the interception shield can only be determined via tests that will be introduced later. Remember for now that for the dragons any means will do—revenge at any price—even if they themselves have to put themselves into a very uncomfortable place for their attacks. Some people may show no symptoms but still test positive for intolerance. They have an intolerance without having irritable bowel symptoms, suggesting that their shield is damaged for reasons other than a brick dragon.

## How brick-eating dragons irritate us:

Some dragons build walls, and this leads to constipation. Others try to burn the bricks. The body is forced to extinguish the fire, leading to diarrhoea. Still others eat the bricks, and when they have collected enough energy, they blow up the stomach, resulting in flatulence and bloating.

# Attack of the brick-eating dragons! Losses are suffered by…

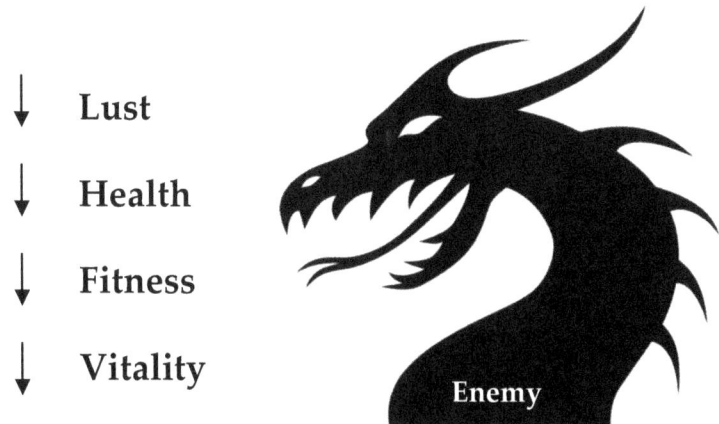

↓ Lust
↓ Health
↓ Fitness
↓ Vitality

Brick-eating dragons are associated with extensive limitations to one's quality of life. Those who are affected are worse off with regard to their fitness, the frequency of their bodily pains, their vigilance, their vitality and their overall physical and mental health. Analogously, it is harder for them to discharge their social roles and enjoy emotional fulfilment. As if that were not enough, those concerned are more likely to have sexual dysfunctions, such as reduced libido.

It is not surprising that these symptoms leave their mark on absenteeism at work. A study in the USA and one in the Netherlands found that people with an untreated brick-eating dragon, i.e., an irritable bowel, miss school or work about twice as often as the general population. On average, this amounts to over five sick days per year. Increasing discomfort leads to a noticeable worsening of work efficiency, physical fitness, ability to fulfil social obligations, vitality, mental fitness and general health; sick days stack up. Up to a certain point, the body is able to intercept bricks before they can reach the dragon. Those that are intercepted are used as usual to generate energy. When consumed in tolerable amounts bricks are good for the energy supply and gut flora and thus one's well-being. If you eat more than your body can handle, however, your brick dragon rejoices and may affect your social and professional success as well as your love life. Luckily, you can and should fight back. Comprehensive studies show that the majority of those affected can substantially reduce their symptoms by adopting an appropriately low-brick diet. With such a diet, they ideally only target those bricks that their shield cannot effectively handle. This is the book's aim. Still, before we get into strategy, you will learn about the diagnostic check.

## Summary

Bricks are parts of foods. Your bowel has an interception shield. This shield can catch a certain amount of bricks and transform them into energy. This amount will be determined below. If you take in more bricks than your shield can intercept, however, then the result is discomfort, if you have an irritable bowel. By eating consciously, you can make sure that you take in only as many bricks as your shield can handle.

# 1.3 Diagnostic check

If you suffer from abdominal pains, bloating, constipation, flatulence or diarrhoea, do not accept your discomfort any longer; be the person who acts. You can expect the whole procedure to take about half a year, but it will pay off: you are likely going to get your symptoms under control and minimize the limitations you face in your diet. The first step—before the book's actual diagnostic procedure begins—is to ask your doctor to refer you to a gastroenterologist in order to **avoid false diagnosis**.

The diagnosis will include a stool analysis, an ultrasonic check and some camera shots inside your stomach in order to reject other causes. These tests will allow the specialist to check whether there is an abnormal bacterial colonization of the small intestine. This may lead to false positives in uncovering an intolerance to a brick type. The next test looks for intolerance to gluten, an ingredient in grains, an intolerance to which is called celiac disease. In people who have untreated celiac disease the tolerance test for the brick sorbitol is often positive, even if they are able to stomach it. Following this, a genetic test regarding hereditary fructose intolerance should be administered. Hereditary fructose intolerance is rare, but it is serious: the fructose test itself can be lethal to those with this disease.

After other diseases have been ruled out, what follows are checks regarding three of the mentioned brick types. For the breath test, you will take a high dose containing fructose, lactose or sorbitol on different days. If bricks pass your shield and arrive at a brick-eating dragon, gases emerge from your intestine. These can and will then be measured in your breath. If the breath test is negative for fructose and sorbitol separately, please ask whether you can also do a combined test of fructose and sorbitol. The combined test is only comparable if the added amount of sorbitol is deducted from the amount of fructose. That is, if 5g of sorbitol is added to the fructose dilution, and the dilution of the previous fructose breath test contained 25g of fructose, then it should now contain only 20g of fructose in addition to the 5g of sorbitol. When the amount of gas in your breath reaches a certain level, the diagnosis is an intolerance towards the respective brick. Having an intolerance means that your shield's ability to intercept that brick is currently small, and bricks of that kind will be able to easily pass through to arrive at the brick dragon.

The threshold for a positive diagnosis for a fructose dilution (typically containing 25–50g) is usually 20ppm (parts per million, a concentration measure). This threshold also applies for lactose and sorbitol.

The recommended breath test, however, is not available everywhere. In Chapter 2.2.3 you will learn about a substitute test, in case you have no access to the breath test. In general, do not accept a diagnosis without a test. If none of the tests comes to a conclusive result, your irritable bowel syndrome is at least—for now—undefined.

For some people the breath test will give a positive result even if none of the usual symptoms are exhibited. The general diagnosis for people who do suffer from symptoms is a functional gastrointestinal disorder. Irritable bowel syndrome belongs in this category. Irritable means that your stomach reacts sensitively to stimuli like air in the stomach—more on that in the next chapter. The bowel is the final segment of your alimentary canal and the dragon's lair.

In a study regarding the intensity of symptoms and intolerance to bricks, no differences were found between people diagnosed with "functional disorder of the bowel (by an intolerance)" and those diagnosed with irritable bowel syndrome. Thus, to simplify matters, remember that people who do suffer from the mentioned symptoms suffer from irritable bowel discomfort. It makes sense to differentiate between a defined irritable bowel syndrome, for which it is clear what bricks one is intolerant towards, and an undefined irritable bowel syndrome, where either no intolerance exists towards one of the three bricks or no test has been conducted yet. Having an intolerance without this leading to discomfort is thus defined as having an intolerance without having an irritable bowel. Nevertheless, your doctor will tell you whether you have an intolerance or whether you have an—in this case undefined—irritable bowel syndrome.

Irritable bowel symptoms are similar regardless of whether the irritable bowel syndrome is defined or not because most of the bricks' effects are independent of the type of brick, as they result from osmotic effects and fermentation and each brick can induce these. Bricks that pass your interception shield, i.e. are not metabolized by your body, lead to an accumulation of water and fermentation. Incidentally, for up to 90% of patients with an irritable bowel, the syndrome can be defined in terms of an intolerance to one or more of the three bricks.

If you suffer from irritable bowel symptoms, you are not alone: **20–30%** of Europeans have an intolerance, i.e., their bowel shield is too weak for one or more of the three bricks for which a breath test is usually conducted. Worldwide, 10–15% of all people suffer from undefined abdominal discomfort. About 20% of Americans, 9% of the Dutch, 22% of the English, 25% of the Japanese and 44% of West Africans are affected.

## Summary

If you regularly suffer from abdominal discomfort, visit a specialist. Checks can take up to half a year. Many others share your fate, but you are holding in your hands the key to fighting the symptoms!

# 1.4 Background of the disease

Irritable bowel syndrome is a common disease. The symptoms can usually be clearly differentiated from those caused by an allergic reaction by using approved methods such as the breath test diagnostic procedure. The symptoms exhibit themselves as an oversensitivity—not in the strength of your character, but related to your intestine. The exact causes are unknown. In some cases, infections and emotions may be an issue. The influence on emotions results from the close connection between the brain and the gut. On the one hand, a bad mood can cause your belly to grumble; on the other hand, a grumbling belly can adversely affect your mood. This link is useful to know to save us from foods we do not stomach well and to find a potential cause when we're having trouble with stress (see Chapter 2.6). You can imagine the diagnosis as a signal disturbance between head and stomach. The bad news is that this sensitivity appears in about 70% of those affected over the long term. The good news is that it does not cause cancer, and the ramifications can be reduced considerably in most cases. Due to the chronic nature of the disease, adjusting your diet as appropriate to your needs can supersede medical treatment. Most medicine has side effects, and a diet is often cheaper.

## Summary

An irritable bowel usually accompanies you for a long time. It is an oversensitivity of the digestive system. Anxiety coincides with grumbling in the belly. An irritable bowel is not a cause of cancer. By following an appropriate diet most affected people are able to overcome most of their symptoms. An effective diet can be better than medical treatment. A sensitive bowel is not a sign of weakness of character, but failing to adapt one's lifestyle to it may be interpreted as such!

# 1.5 The bricks and how your belly is fighting

**B**ricks are carbohydrates that can either be absorbed by your body to be changed into energy or pass by your shield, in which case you have a dragon behind your barriers, gobbling bricks and breeding symptoms. Your body's brick interception shield works similarly to the toddler game in which the child pushes differently shaped blocks through openings in a box. If a brick fits through, it is intercepted and metabolized. What is tricky is that each human can stomach different amounts of the different bricks (has a different kind of shield). Some of the bricks cannot be efficiently intercepted by anyone's shield, but this is not an issue for people who do not have a brick-eating dragon. The following drawing illustrates that some bricks cannot be intercepted by the shield by the no entry-sign on the shield's round brick.

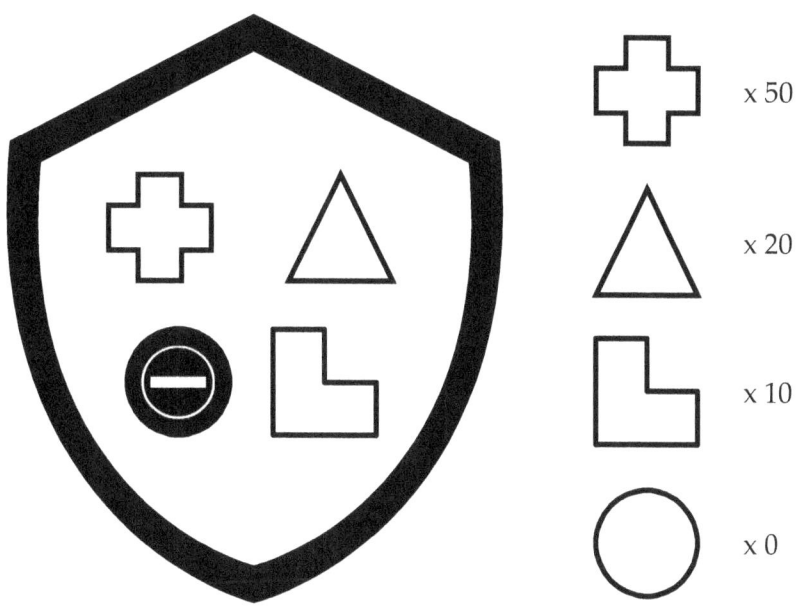

The depicted bowel shield can absorb cross-bricks very well with a capacity of over 50 pieces. Unfortunately, however, it offers no protection against round bricks. A round brick passes directly by to the affected person's dragon, which then reacts, e.g., by blowing up her belly or trying to spit fire. In such a case, the stomach reacts in the same way a dry sponge reacts when you put it in water. It sucks itself full and expands—the quenched water accumulates. Air and/or water lead to discomfort. Therefore, if bricks enter the intestine it means:

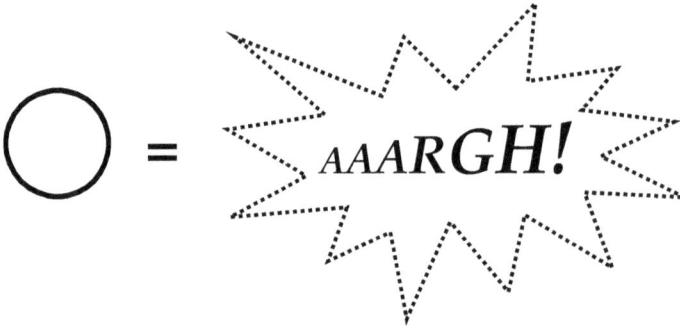

## It depends on your shield

Did your breath test show that your shield's capacity for fructose, lactose and/or sorbitol is great? That is one-to-nothing for you against the dragon. You can continue eating those products that contain bricks your shield intercepts well—i.e., that you tolerate—without having to think about them. The others you have to avoid, more or less. But what are these mysterious bricks? In the following, you will find their profiles.

# 1.5.1 Brick number one: Lactose

## In brief

Lactose is primarily contained in milk and other dairy products and is therefore also known as milk sugar. All toddlers need lactose and are able to stomach it. A lactose intolerance evolves after the fifth birthday at the earliest. About 5–17% of the light-skinned and 50–100% of the remaining world population have a lactose intolerance. Even so, not all of those with lactose intolerance also have an irritable bowel. What is more, those who are affected are usually able to stomach—that is to intercept—small amounts of lactose.

**Basic tolerance level (BTL): 1.5g per meal (as defined in the glossary)**.

There are four tolerance levels ranging from zero to three. These tolerance levels [TL] are used to determine one's tolerable portion sizes in the third part of this book. Applying the basic tolerance level [BTL], i.e. TL 0, you will be able to determine the portion sizes with which you can avoid symptoms induced by the respective bricks independent of your shield strength. The BTL portion sizes are the lowest for the respective brick. In order to find your TL, you will conduct a level test, as per Chapter 2.2.4. Observe the BTL during the implementation diet, unless your breath test shows that you tolerate the respective brick. You can find the portion tables in Chapter 3.

In one study, the symptoms appeared for those affected at 1.5g (though a 3g dose was not given for contrast). The authors were surprised that symptoms also appeared from lactose-free milk used for comparison. The reason for this may be the prevalence of other easily fermentable carbohydrates that were contained in the test milk. These have a positive effect on the gut flora but can also trigger discomforts depending on the amount consumed. The ingredients to which these symptoms can be attributed are galactans, which will be discussed later. The amount of galactans in milk depends on the breed, race and lactation month of dairy cattle. The highest average amounts are to be found in cow milk with 0.137g/100ml, followed by goat milk with 0.117g/100ml. As 100mL of milk contains about 5g lactose and 0.137g galactans, about 0.03g will be added to the galactans for each gram of lactose. The BTL of galactans is thus crossed at 350mL of milk. In combination with other foods such as cereals, however, it can play a role regarding discomfort.

The tolerance threshold of pure lactose in cases of intolerance is likely to be 10g per day and thus about 3g per meal.[1] Thus you should be able to stomach the amount of lactose that is used in some medicine you take orally, as long as you avoid other products that contain lactose during the days of your treatment. The BTL has been chosen as half of the recommended 3g per meal, as some affected nevertheless either completely avoid lactose or still feel that their tolerance threshold is lower.

## Influence of fructans

For most people suffering from a lactose intolerance combined with an irritable bowel, simply reducing the consumed amount of lactose only partially leads to the symptoms' disappearance. Even though this may already be enough, it indicates that intolerances regarding other bricks play a role and may be worth considering in the nutrition plan. Some lactose intolerant people suffer irritation from the brick fructans, which will be introduced in Chapter 1.5.3, more than by lactose.

---

[1] Milk acid bacteria, which are being used to produce cheese, are able to break down these galactans. For that reason their share in cheese is perhaps lower. However, more specific data is not available yet.

# Calcium

When you reduce the amount of dairy products you consume, it is important to increase your supply of calcium from other sources. An adult under 50 years of age should take in about 1,000mg (1,300mg for teenagers), and a woman over 50 (or a man over 60) should take in 1,200mg. You can take in calcium through some lactose-free milk (replacement) products, some protein powders (1,200mg/100g), cheddar cheese (721mg/100g), almonds (236mg/100g), salmon and sardines (240mg/100g), spinach (210mg/100g) and figs (162mg/100g) or by taking calcium tablets. Please only choose tablets that do not contain (critical amounts of) other bricks that are problematic for you, if possible.

# Depression

In a study of randomly chosen participants who were suffering from depressed moods, a breath test showed that over 70% of them had a brick intolerance, while the average percentage among people from the same region suffering from a brick intolerance was only 15%. This does not indicate that many who have an intolerance are depressed but that many people with depression have an intolerance. Thus, in further research, tests were conducted to work out how many randomly selected people with an intolerance showed signs of depression. For 28.5% of the test group—a number significantly greater than the general population—the scores denoted depression.

Serotonin, a neurotransmitter that elevates one's mood is produced by the body from tryptophan, which is contained in food. Presumably at least some of the bricks that pass the interception shield merge with tryptophan to form a non-absorbable substance. This reaction reduces the amount of available tryptophan and causes the body to produce less serotonin. Hence, the bricks that arrive at the dragon's lair hinder the body's ability to let positive feelings emerge. In an experiment in which fructose and sorbitol consumption was reduced, depression scores normalized for most participants. Keeping within the tolerance levels that apply to you when choosing your portion sizes can therefore improve your mood (your serotonin metabolism) because fewer bricks arrive at the dragon's lair. Extra discipline is required to maintain the portion thresholds in cases of depression, however: a lack of high spirits (tryptophan) can foster a hunger for sweets. Now, sweets often contain bricks. If an intolerance is present, the intake of the respective bricks further lowers one's mood, creating a vicious circle. You can find the amount of bricks contained in sweets in the lists in Part 3. Even if you are not depressed, please remember that in the presence of a dysfunctional metabolism, depression can result from consuming too much of foods that contain problematic bricks. Affected people should always seek help rather than trying to counter these effects through sheer willpower.

## Enzyme capsules

Assuming your body can metabolize 3g lactose by itself, taking enzyme capsules pays off once you are past the 3g tolerance level number 1 with your meal. Please make sure the enzyme capsules are free of other bricks that are problematic for you; for example, some contain sorbitol and mannitol. In order to be effective, the lactose enzymes not only have to arrive at the small intestine without being destroyed by acid before they get there, but they need to do so at the same time as the lactose. For this purpose, stomach acid-resistant capsules seem most appropriate. One study found that the most effective capsule was only able to break down 2.7g of lactose. At least four capsules would thus be required to take in a 250mL glass of lactose-free milk, which makes up for 12.5g of lactose after subtracting the 3g from that amount. You can find the required amount of capsules in the K-column of the food tables contained in the third part of the book.

## Which foods contain this brick?

All (mammal) milk products contain milk sugar, as do many processed foods and consumable products such as breads, bologna, sauces and medicine (although the amount in medicine is often unproblematic if no additional products containing lactose are consumed). Raw milk tends to contain the highest amount of lactose, while some sorts of dry cheese, like cheddar, are nearly free of it. Luckily, you can intercept and metabolize at least some limited amounts of lactose, and there are enzyme capsules as well as numerous milk replacement and lactose-free products available, including rice milk. But be mindful that soymilk contains other bricks, fructans and galactans, while rice milk is free of them.

# 1.5.2 Brick number two: Fructose

## In brief

Fruit naturally contains fructose, and it is therefore known as fruit sugar. For 39% of those affected by unexplained regular abdominal discomfort, symptoms arise after the consumption of 15g fructose; for 70%, they appear after a dose of 30g. People around the globe consume between 11 and 54g per day, or 4–18g per meal. Accordingly, fructose triggers discomforts for many people who have an irritable bowel. As with the other bricks, the tolerable amount varies individually. If you do not have a fructose intolerance, there is no need to watch your fructose intake; the fructose TLs only apply to those with a fructose intolerance or a currently undefined irritable bowel syndrome.

**BTL:** (Glucose balanced fructose 5g per 100g)[2]
Glucose-free fructose 0.5g per meal[3]

If you are restricted in your ability to stomach fructose, please get acquainted with the following factors that affect your body's fructose assimilation:

## Influence of glucose

Imagine your interception shield (see Chapter 1.5) is being carried by a giant guard. Fructose is like a brick with the characteristics of a fly, and catching it is usually a challenge for the guard, especially when numerous fructose units appear at once. It is another game when glucose, a drop of sugar juice with the reaction time of a slug, enters the stage. Like any fly, fructose loves to come to rest on glucose, so the guard will have no trouble intercepting it. At times, however, sorbitol appears on the scene, as well, like a buzzing mosquito. Sorbitol is especially hard to catch and distracts the guard from the fructose. Hence, when sorbitol is present, more of the brick fructose gets through to arrive at the dragon.

This means that when quantities of glucose equal or exceed those of fructose, fructose interception is strongly improved. Therefore, let us differentiate between glucose-balanced and glucose-free—or just "free" fructose. You can

---

[2] The food contains fructose and glucose in equal amounts. Thereby, fructose is absorbed much better.
[3] The amount of fructose that exceeds the amount of glucose in the food.

stomach much more fructose if it is balanced with glucose. According to the amount of gas measured during breath tests, glucose-balanced fructose is intercepted ten times more easily than free fructose. For foods where the relationship leans more towards fructose than glucose, you can create balance artificially by eating foods that contain a lot of excess glucose. A note regarding the tolerance level (TL) of glucose-balanced fructose: different studies show that people who are intolerant towards fructose are nevertheless able to stomach up to 50g of glucose-balanced fructose. The limitation for glucose-balanced fructose has only been mentioned due to an ambiguous study result. Despite the apparently optimal assimilation rate in a balanced glucose relationship, at a dose of 17g per day, 0.4g arrived at the intestine. When the test was repeated with 98g of balanced glucose, the amount was still just slightly higher at 0.56g; however, due to the study setup, bacterial decomposition prior to the analysis may have distorted the result. Balanced fructose is disregarded in the food list because of the dubiousness of the test results. You can, however, adjust your consumption according to the sugar amount per 100g as shown in the ingredients, if you want, because sugar consists of one part glucose and one part fructose. At the same time, you can determine your adequate portion size with regard to free fructose in this book's food tables. If you want to limit your sugar consumption, and a beverage contains too much of it, you can dilute it with a suitable amount of water. It is good to reduce sugar consumption in general (see Chapter 2.1.4).

## Influence of sorbitol

If you have a fructose intolerance, you should try to avoid sorbitol as much as possible. Sorbitol inhibits the assimilation of fructose and is itself poorly absorbed by many people; thus, it is the dragon's best friend. Unfortunately, no hint for an adequate BTL could be found. Still, you can determine your own TL as part of the tolerance level strategy upon finishing the three-week introductory diet (see Chapter 2.2.4).

## Hereditary fructose intolerance

If you have been diagnosed with a rare and unfortunately not yet curable hereditary fructose intolerance, consuming fructose can be lethal. Please seek your doctor's advice. You can use the food table in this book to determine foods that are free of fructose.

## Folic acid deficiency

A fructose intolerance often negatively affects folic acid absorption. As a folic acid deficiency increases risk of cardiovascular disease, it would be sensible to take suitable supplements. Otherwise, folic acid is contained in Kellogg's® Corn flakes (323µg/100g), some protein powders (280µg/100g) and short-grain rice (225µg/100g), for example. The recommended daily dose is 300µg for men, 250µg for most women and 400µg for expectant mothers.

## Depression

Please see page 15.

## Enzyme capsules

Xylose isomerase is available on the market. The author is aware of only one study that aimed to prove its efficiency, and it showed symptoms improving by about 41%. Whether this justifies the current high sales price remains for you to decide.

## Foods with excess glucose

Few foods have an excess of glucose while being free of other bricks. When you eat one of the following foods together with a food that is restricted due to its amount of free fructose, you may be able to multiply your TL-adjusted portion size of the restricted food by the factor that applies to your TL. If you are interested, just test it out for yourself. Your multiplier is shown in one of the last four columns of the next table.

| Foods | Portion weight | Free glucose | BTL x | TL 1 x | TL 2 x | TL 3 x |
|---|---|---|---|---|---|---|
| Avocado (Florida) | 37.5g | 0.72g | 2.25 | 1.5 | 1.25 | 1.25 |
| Maple syrup | 30g | 0.32g | 1.5 | 1.25 | 1 | 1 |
| Mozzarella | 28g | 0.16g | 1.25 | 1 | 1 | 1 |
| Sweet corn | 82g | 1.22g | 3.25 | 2 | 1.75 | 1.5 |
| Thin slice of pineapple | 56.3g | 0.68g | 2.25 | 1.5 | 1.5 | 1.25 |

You can also purchase pure glucose as a powder online, though high sugar consumption should be avoided due to potential health implications (see Chapter 2.1.4).

## Which foods contain this brick?

Nowadays, fructose is the cause of the sweet taste of many foods. It is added in the form of honey, gelling sugars and corn syrup. In the absence of an intolerance, humans can smoothly break down fructose. The way you mainly take in fructose depends on your nutritional habits. In the USA, about two thirds are taken in as soft drinks and enriched convenience foods and about one third as fruit. In Finland, the relationship is reversed.

# 1.5.3 Brick number three: Fructans

## In brief

Fructose evolves while fructans metabolize, hence the similarity of their names. It has been discovered that during the exploitation (fermentation) of **short-chain** fructans by brick-eating dragons (bacteria), gas emerges. However, that is not all; our body barely uses fructans. Up to 89% of them—more than of any other brick—are dished up for the bacteria in the colon. What makes matters worse is that other bricks like fructose are digested much less effectively when more fructans are consumed. For some lactose intolerant people, the discomforts induced by fructans are worse than those triggered by lactose itself. As with holds for the other bricks, people without an irritable bowel are hardly bothered by them. If symptoms persist and are not reduced satisfactorily by limiting consumption of fructose, lactose and/or sorbitol, try reducing the amount of fructans and galactans (to be presented later in the book) in your meals.

**BTL of the sum of fructans and galactans: 0.5g per meal.**

## Which foods contain this brick?

We primarily take in fructans when eating the following (tolerable amounts for the BTL in parentheses): garlic (one clove), onions (15g), artichoke (17g), cereals (21–45g) and noodles (147g), as well as pastries like bread, cake, cookies and pizza. Grain products contain far fewer fructans than vegetables, but the quantities in which we eat them makes them a primary source of fructans. Onions hold second place. There is no relation between fructans and gluten. Even gluten-free bread often contains fructans, albeit about one third less than common bread. Rice bread is free from fructans as the dough is commonly made without wheat, in contrast to potato or cornbread. In addition, spelt bread is especially well tolerated (250g) compared to rye or wheat bread (one slice each). Fructans are also contained in some fruits. Limit yourself, for example, to three fourths of a banana, half a nectarine and two slices of pineapple. The high amount of fructans contained in chicory or in Jerusalem and regular artichokes calls for avoidance.

In tolerable amounts, fructans have positive effects, so they are added to various foods as inulin. For example, some beverages, brands of butter, candies, cereals, chocolates, ice creams and yogurts contain inulin. The added amounts of inulin are not always certain, aside from the derivations mentioned in the food table of this book. And so, to be on the safe side, you can avoid products that list inulin in their ingredients, use similar products in the food table of this book as a reference for the consumable amount according to your fructan TL or make a single-product test using the amount you can tolerate as a guideline (see Chapter 2.2.6). Some people are also allergic to inulin.

You can even meet the 0.5g-per-meal BTL for fructans with little adaptation to your diet. Fructan-containing products are often consumed with other foods. When reviewing the portion sizes in Part 3 of the book, consider that when you combine fructan-containing foods, the respective single portion sizes decrease. In order to combine a fructan-containing product with another product that contains fructans or galactans you can, for example, bisect both portion sizes.

## Influence on the nutrient supply

A reduction in fructans can require you to plan your intake of proteins, short-chain fatty acids and fibre. You can find compensation strategies from Chapter 2 onward.

# 1.5.4 Brick number four: Galactans

## In brief

Short-chain galactans, like short-chain fructans, are poorly absorbed by the body and arrive at the intestine in large chunks. As fructans and galactans are similar oligosaccharides, they share a BTL of 0.5g in sum.

**BTL of the sum of fructans and galactans: 0.5g per meal**.

## Buy prebiotics?

The European Food Safety Authority (EFSA) has repeatedly disregarded the claim that prebiotics and probiotics have a positive effect on the gut due to lack of solid proof. It regards them as at best potentially helpful. Prebiotics producers ascribe artificial galactans a contribution to improved gut flora. A study set up by in collaboration of an employee of a prebiotics producer suggested that 3.5g of a special kind of artificial galactans improved the gut flora and thereby led to an average improvement of 37% regarding symptoms like abdominal pain, bloating, constipation, diarrhoea and flatulence. Health claims are also associated with short-chain fatty acids that emerge during the breakdown of galactans by bacteria. Some artificially produced galactans produce less gas when they are assimilated by bacteria than those that occur naturally. However, as stated before, the EFSA refuses to support prebiotics beyond their statement regarding their potential. Over 80% of participants in a study who followed this book's approach and consistently limited their consumption of fructose and fructans according to the BTLs listed experienced relief from their symptoms by about 70%. Moreover, reducing the amount of bricks that arrive at the colon might a have favorable effect on mood (see page 15). These findings support the principles underlying this diet.

## Enzyme capsules

There are special enzyme capsules available that may help you to avoid symptoms that may otherwise be induced by galactans, though their effectiveness is disputed. They contain the enzyme alpha-galactosidase and are made from the mildew aspergillus niger, though packages may not fully reflect this information; they also contain the brick mannitol, a sugar alcohol, prevalent in mushrooms, to which some people exhibit allergies. You should be careful with these enzyme capsules if you have a fructose intolerance, as the galactans are metabolized into fructose by the enzymes. Unless your body immediately intercepts the fructose, it arrives at the intestine. There, gas-producing bacteria rejoice, since you have done some of their work for them. So, you actually gained nothing. These enzyme capsules can only be helpful if you tolerate fructose and sorbitol and do not have an allergy to aspergillus niger.

## Which foods contain this brick?

Beans and bloating go hand in hand for some—critical amounts of galactans combined with fructans (BTL portion size in parentheses) can be found in beans (1 tbsp., 15g), peas (1 tbsp., 15g), chickpeas (9 tbsp., 135g) and soybeans (3 tbsp., 45g). Vegetarians should pay particular attention to these. Considerable amounts are also contained in oat flakes (5 tbsp., 75g), lentils (5 tbsp., 75g) and wheat or rye bread (one slice, 42g). Moreover, short-chain galactans are also contained in milk. Agar and carrageenan also contain galactans, but those they contain are longer and are not fully broken down by gut bacteria. At times people suffering from an irritable bowel are suspicious towards these. Due to a lack of solid evidence, these are not considered in this book. Still, if you have doubts about them, you can explore their impact yourself by adopting an alternative diet (see Chapter 2.2.6).

# 1.5.5 Brick number five: Sorbitol and others

Some fruits and vegetables naturally contain sugar alcohols like sorbitol. Furthermore, they are used as sweeteners and as carriers for some medicines. Often sugar alcohols are only mentioned in code on packages. In Chapter 2.4 you will learn how to identify the relevant information on labels.

**BTL for the nine sugar alcohols being considered, including sorbitol: 0g.**

Foods containing sorbitol often trigger abdominal discomforts. Sorbitol is unproblematic if a breath test or substitute test indicates you can tolerate it, and that you can tolerate fructose as well. If you only have a fructose intolerance but not a sorbitol intolerance, you can use the sorbitol-adjusted portion sizes for fructose as indicated in the tables of Part 3 of this book. If you have a sorbitol intolerance, it makes sense to determine your personal TL (see Chapter 2.2.4) due to the radical BTL of 0g. There are three reasons in favor of this BTL:

1. The breath test for sorbitol shows an intolerance present at 5g in **58%** of those experiencing abdominal discomfort due to an irritable bowel and **53%** of healthy participants (based on a combination of studies with a total of 564 participants).
2. If you have a fructose intolerance, sorbitol will aggravate your symptoms. Fructose emerges when sorbitol gets broken down. Meanwhile, sorbitol hinders already-present fructose from being intercepted because fructose and sorbitol share a transportation mechanism where sorbitol is preferred.
3. Sugar alcohols are incompletely absorbed by many and can sometimes even lead to a water aggregation in the small intestine, reducing the intestine's ability to metabolize nutrients. On average, 25–40% of consumed sugar alcohols arrive at the colon. Even small amounts of sorbitol can trigger discomforts.

## Influence on symptoms

In a Dutch study in 1993 high amounts of glucose were added to apple juice, reducing symptoms caused by apple juice by 80%. However, the added glucose also bound the released fructose from sorbitol degradation. Assuming that one third of symptoms caused by sorbitol arise due to non-degraded sorbitol, another third by the free fructose emerging from sorbitol that has been broken down and the remaining third due to fructose whose interception was hindered by sorbitol, sorbitol causes 30% of the discomfort resulting from apple juice. Considering the average amount of sorbitol contained in an apple (about 0.56g sorbitol and 4g of free fructose), 1g of sorbitol combined with free fructose causes about three times as many symptoms as 1g of free fructose alone, and 1g of sorbitol alone causes about twice as many symptoms as 1g of free fructose. This relationship is taken into account in the amount recommended for foods that contain both fructose and sorbitol.

## Which foods contain this brick?

Sugar alcohols occur naturally in different fruits and vegetables (fresh as well as dried). Moreover, they are added as sugar replacements in a large number of products, including beverages, candies, convenience foods, diabetic products like jelly (up to 57g/100g) and chocolate (up to 40g/100g), breaded fish and meat, ice cream, juices, medicine, oral hygiene products, sauces, sugar-free chewing gum (up to 2.5g/piece), sugar-free mints (up to 2g/piece) and even sausage. As you can see, some diabetic products contain more than 20g of sorbitol. In one study, 84% of the 39 healthy participants had a sorbitol malabsorption for a 20g dose. Consumption of these products therefore deserves caution.

# 1.5.6 Abdominal discomfort in children

Children ages 14 to 58 months were administered 250mL of apple juice in a study. Afterward, all children who suffered from chronic diarrhoea, as well as 65.5% of the healthy children, tested positive for malabsorption. Avoiding apple juice led to recovery for **all** of the children. This result corresponds with other research that shows that many children suffer from diarrhoea and abdominal pain if they drink too much fruit juice. Juices that contain high levels of sorbitol have commonly been identified as triggers. Generally speaking, you should give your child a maximum of 10mL juice per kilogram of body weight. Moreover, you should avoid giving them fruit juices that contain sorbitol or high amounts of free fructose, like apple or peach juice.

# 1.6 Summary of Part 1

Your stomach is able to intercept some bricks and metabolize them into energy. However, the capacity for doing so differs from human to human. Lactose is primarily contained in milk products. Sufferers of an intolerance can usually tolerate small amounts well. When reducing the amount of lactose one consumes, it is important to make up for the simultaneous reduction in calcium intake. Fructose is most common in fruits, soft drinks and cereals. Combined with sorbitol, it is absorbed more poorly; combined with glucose, it is absorbed better. The most common dietary sources of fructans include grain products like bread, cereals and noodles, as well as garlic and onions, and they are not broken down well by the body. Galactans, which are predominantly found in beans, lentils and grains, are similarly poorly absorbed. The strictest BTL is associated with sorbitol, which should be avoided for the most part. Sorbitol is mainly found in many diabetic and light products, some fruits and vegetables and sauces and breadings. Stevia, by the way, is free of sorbitol.

## Basic tolerance levels (BTLs)

The following table contains all of the BTLs previously introduced. Use it as a guide to the bricks you are intolerant to, at least during the three weeks of the introductory diet, and partially afterward during the level tests. Whether it is for the next wedding, project presentation or sailing trip, there are occasions when you especially want everything to run smoothly regarding your digestion. You can feel more secure on days like these if you manage your meals according to the BTLs for those bricks that you have an intolerance to. The BTLs are:

| | |
|---:|:---|
| Glucose-free fructose | 0.5g/meal |
| Glucose-balanced fructose | 5g/100g |
| Lactose | 1.5g/meal |
| Sorbitol and other sugar alcohols | 0g/meal |
| Sum of fructans and galactans | 0.5g/meal |

As you adjust your diet according to the BTLs that are relevant for you, you can avoid those carbohydrates that cause discomfort as best as is practicable.

# 2

# STRATEGY

## 2.1 Mission planning

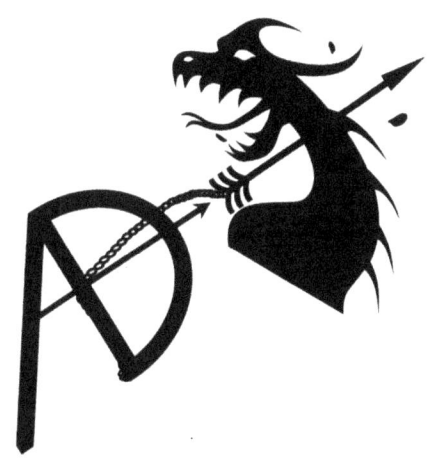

Stop letting brick-eating dragons attack and tempt you. Get ready for the dragon hunt. With positivity and discipline, chances are that we will chain your dragon. As the dragon is invisible, the best strategy is to feed it as few bricks as possible. Meanwhile, if you stay on your guard and wield your interception shield by eating portions close to the recommended maximum for your TL, the dragon will have a tough time. You can thereby reduce to tolerable amounts the consumption of those bricks that induce your symptoms to tolerable amounts. In order not to restrict yourself unnecessarily by avoiding foods that you love, you can **determine your personal tolerance thresholds for the bricks by taking a level test (Chapter 2.2.4).** See a qualified doctor to authorize this process, especially if the person with the intolerance is a child.

# 2.1.1 Roadmap

In the following strategy table, you will find the five major steps, their urgency, their titles, their durations and their purposes.

| | | |
|---|---|---|
| 1) Required | **Symptom test (sheet)**<br>Duration: four days | Determining your status quo: Which symptoms do you have, and how severe are they? |
| 2) Optional | **Breath test from a specialist**<br>Duration: six days | Identifying the bricks you absorb with difficulty. The target is to reduce your effort in Step 3. |
| "quick-exit option" after positive breath test | **Keep the BTL for those bricks towards which you have an intolerance.**<br>Fill out the following symptom test sheet once more after two weeks for four days and evaluate your diet's success.<br>Duration: At least three weeks, depending on your satisfaction; see column on the right. | A) You are satisfied. Do you want to reduce your limitations to the extent possible? Perform the level test (see Step 5).<br><br>B) You are unsatisfied. First perform Step 3 and then at least the substitute test for fructans and galactans. If no improvement occurs, test the alternatives shown in Chapter 2.2.6. |
| 3) Required | **Introductory diet and symptom test (sheet)**<br>during the last four days.<br>Duration: three weeks | Did the diet according to the BTLs lead to the expected reduction of symptoms? If no, see Chapter 2.2.6. |
| 4) Optional: Instead of Step 2 | **Substitute test (for the breath test)**<br>Duration: five weeks for all bricks | Uncovering the discomfort triggers for which no breath test is offered. Moreover, reducing the effort for Step 5. |
| 5) Optional | **Level test**<br>Duration:<br>1 brick  ~½ month<br>2 bricks  ~1½ months<br>3 bricks  ~2½ months<br>4 bricks  ~5 months | Enabling you a diet that is as varied as possible while taking your intolerance(s) into account by determining your TLs. |

The broad strategy is to determine your shield's interception capacities. The first step is checking your status quo. To do so, note down your symptoms on the following test sheet. It is important to choose days on which neither drugs nor sickness nor stress might influence your symptoms. If you aren't sure if you have produced contaminated results on a given day due to any of these factors, cross out the day and fill out the next one you consider unaffected. **Important: This also holds true for all of the subsequent tests. If you are in doubt as to whether the day was "normal," on which no uncommon circumstances distorted the symptoms, repeat the test to get a more reliable result.** On days where you track your symptoms, carry a copy of the symptom test sheet with you. Ideally, you should fill it out immediately after your main meals, e.g., at 7am, 1pm and 7pm. After the four days of your status quo check, you should also classify the type of stool you usually have. Depending on whether you have constipation, diarrhoea or a mix of both, you are type IBS-C, IBS-D or IBS-M. If you are spared constipation and diarrhoea, your IBS type is un**classified**. Take that information with you when you visit the doctor.

After tracking your symptoms for four days, you can take a breath test to determine malabsorbtions. To do so, please ask your doctor to refer you to a gastroenterology specialist. If this type of test is not offered in your area, you can take a substitute test after following the introductory diet (see Chapter 2.2.3). To follow the introductory diet, read on to Chapter 2.2.2. This also holds for the "quick-exit option." You can disregard those bricks towards which the breath or substitute test does not indicate malabsorbtion. **Even if malabsorbtion is detected, you may be able to stomach more than the BTL portions.** You can therefore determine your personal TL with a level test (see Chapter 2.2.4) if the introductory diet reduced your symptoms. This is to save you from unnecessarily harsh restrictions on foods you enjoy. For example, if you have a lactose intolerance and like cheese, you can determine the highest tolerable amount of cheese per meal in Step 5. Be prepared to spend at least half a month on the level test (see page 30). You can be sure afterward that you are neither straining your body too much nor excessively restraining your consumption of foods you enjoy. Only an individual level test can lead you to that result.

In the quick-exit option, you skip the introductory diet (at least at first) but try to determine whether adhering to the BTLs for those bricks you don't absorb well according to the breath test has enough of a positive effect for you to just consider those bricks. If your symptoms don't improve to your satisfaction, go back and follow the introductory diet and conduct at least a substitute test for fructans and galactans. If this does not lead to satisfying results, read Chapter 2.2.6.

During the introductory diet, you keep those BTLs that are relevant for you (see Chapter 2.2). Exception: If the breath test comes out negative for fructose, lactose and sorbitol, the BTLs apply to all bricks. If symptoms improve while you are on the diet, continue with the substitute test for fructans and galactans. To be on the safe side, you can also do the substitute test for the remaining bricks, in order to exclude potential interdependencies like between sorbitol and fructose, which can be found together in apple juice, for example, as a cause. Otherwise, you will find alternative strategies in Chapter 2.2.6. If you have not done the breath test, all BTLs apply.

After two weeks of the quick-exit option or after the introductory diet, make an efficiency check by filling out the symptom test sheet again for four days. To evaluate the effect, compare the status quo check symptom test sheet with the efficiency check symptom test sheet. If you have fewer symptoms at the end of the diet—that is, if your evaluations for the efficiency check are clearly lower than those for the status quo check—the diet was a success. You can learn how to mathematically determine the diet's success in Chapter 2.1.3. **Put your symptom test sheets into a folder.** The most important one is the final test of **your introductory diet,** as you can use it as a **reference for all of your further tests.**

# Stool types after Bristol

| |  |  |
|---|---|---|
| | Separate hard lumps, like nuts (hard to pass) | **Type** A: Constipation <br><br> **Value** 4 |
| | Sausage-shaped but lumpy | **Type** B: Constipation <br><br> **Value** 2 |
| | Like a sausage but with cracks on the surface | **Type** C: normal <br><br> **Value** 1 |
| | Like a sausage or snake, smooth and soft | **Type** D: normal <br><br> **Value** 1 |
| | Soft blobs with clear-cut edges | **Type** E: Diarrhoea <br><br> **Value** 2 |
| | Fluffy pieces with ragged edges, a mushy stool | **Type** F: Diarrhoea <br><br> **Value** 4 |
| | Watery, no solid pieces; **entirely liquid** | **Type** G: Diarrhoea <br><br> **Value** 5 |

Types 3 and 4 are normal. The farther away your type is from these two, the worse your ailments.

## 2.1.2 Symptom test sheet

Test:_____ End date:_____

For each test, you need two copies of this page!

| | Type/ Value | Defecation count | | Stool grade | Bloating grade | Pain grade | |
|---|---|---|---|---|---|---|---|
| **Day 1 prior** 🐓 | | x | = | | | | **TEST DAY** |
| ☀ | | x | = | | | | |
| ☾ | | x | = | | | | |
| | | Total | | | | | |
| **Day 2 prior** 🐓 | | x | = | | | | **Day 1 after** |
| ☀ | | x | = | | | | |
| ☾ | | x | = | | | | |
| | | Total | | | | | |
| **Day 3 prior** 🐓 | | x | = | | | | **Day 2 after** |
| ☀ | | x | = | | | | |
| ☾ | | x | = | | | | |
| | | Total | | | | | |
| **(Day 4 prior)** 🐓 | | x | = | | | | **Day 3 after** |
| ☀ | | x | = | | | | |
| ☾ | | x | = | | | | |
| | | Total | | | | | |

Note down your stool type in the morning 🐓, afternoon ☀ and evening ☾ and your stool value from 1 to 5 (see page 33) as well as the number of times you visited the toilet and multiply the stool value with the number of toilet uses to estimate the stool grade. In addition, evaluate bloating and pain from 1 to 5 according to the following scale:

1   No discomfort, like someone without symptoms
2   Hardly any discomfort relative to someone without symptoms
3   Medium discomfort relative to someone without symptoms
4   Severe discomfort relative to someone without symptoms
5   Very severe discomfort relative to someone without symptoms

# 2.1.3 Test result calculation table

You can probably trust your gut in evaluating your symptoms. If you prefer numbers, you can use the following two convenient procedures.[4] For the first application, you need the symptom test sheets from the status quo check[5] and the efficiency check.[6] You have the following two calculation options (please use a copy of the following table and a pencil); Option A is easier. With Option B, you save yourself calculation work for all the following tests and receive a statement regarding your tolerance.

**A)** Use the following table and calculate your results for all days up row B. A1 to A4 are the efficiency check days and A5 to A8 the status quo check days or, for the surrogate or level test, the test day and its three subsequent days. **A-grade calculation**: A1 = Stool total grade (grade in the morning plus grade in the afternoon plus grade in the evening) on Day 1. Note down the result in the cell with a cursive A1. Proceed likewise with all other A-numbers. Afterward, determine the **B-grades**: B1 = A1 plus total bloating grade on Day 1 plus total pain grade on Day 1. Then calculate B2 acording to the Day 2 grades and so on. Now determine C2 and D2, i.e., the average of the status quo check days or, for the surrogate or level test, the average of the test and its three subsequent days. For the evaluation, compare D2 with the highest day grade from the efficiency check days. This is the largest grade of the grades B1 to B4. The further D2 is above the highest grade of that group, the more likely the introductory diet has worked or, if you took any other test, the more likely it is that you have an intolerance.

**B)** Calculate A1 to A8 as well as B1 to B8 with Option A. Then calculate C1 and D1 and proceed by calculating the further calculation steps in the table until L. To determine the efficiency of the introductory diet, also calculate C2 and D2. In an efficiency check of the introductory diet, compare D2 instead of L, the **lid grade**,[7] with K, the **K.O. threshold grade**,[8] for the interpretation. If D2 is greater than or equal to the K-grade, this points to an effective introductory diet. For the surrogate or level test, compare the K- with the L-grade, as explained in the following table.

*Spare yourself time: Acquire the printer-friendly Excel version on www.Laxiba.co.uk/trc.*

---

[4] From a statistical point of view the survey is slim and the result vague.
[5] Symptom test sheet filled out before starting the introductory diet.
[6] Symptom test sheet filled out at the end of the introductory diet.
[7] L = the day with the most severe symptoms following a live test.
[8] K = If the L-grade reaches this K. O. threshold, there is an intolerance.

|   | Efficiency check day | | | | | Status quo check day<br>day-after test | | |
|---|---|---|---|---|---|---|---|---|
|   | 1: | 2: | 3: | 4: | 1: or Test day: | 2: / 1: | 3: / 2: | 4: / 3: |
| A | A1 | A3 | A3 | A4 | A5 | A6 | A7 | A8 |
| B | B1 | B2 | B3 | B4 | B5 | B6 | B7 | B8 |
| C | C1 | \multicolumn{5}{l}{C1 = B1 + B2 + B3 + B4<br>Add up the results of the cells B1 to B4.<br>C2 = B5 + B6 + B7 + B8<br>Add up the results of the cells B5 to B8.} | | C2 | |
| D | D1 | \multicolumn{5}{l}{D1 = C1 ÷ 4  Divide your result in cell C1 by 4.<br>D2 = C2 ÷ 4  Divide your result in cell C2 by 4.} | | D2 | |
| E | E1 | E2 | E3 | E4 | \multicolumn{4}{l}{E1 = B1 - D1, E2 = B2 - D1 and so on. To calculate E1, subtract D1 from B1. Negative results are allowed.} | | |
| F | F1 | F2 | F3 | F4 | \multicolumn{4}{l}{F1 = E1 × E1, F2 = E2 × E2 and so on. To calculate F1, multiply E1 with itself. A negative times a negative equals a positive. Thus, each result must be positive.} | | |
| G | G | \multicolumn{7}{l}{G = F1 + F2 + F3 + F4<br>Add up the results of the cells F1 to F4.} |
| H | H | \multicolumn{7}{l}{H = G ÷ 4<br>Divide G by 4.} |
| I | I | \multicolumn{7}{l}{I = Take the square root of your result in cell H. On your calculator, the symbol for square root is: √.} |
| J | J | \multicolumn{7}{l}{J = I × 2<br>Multiply I by 2.} |
| K | K | \multicolumn{7}{l}{K = J + C1  Add the result in cell J to the result in cell C1.<br>The **K**-grade is called **K.O.** threshold grade, as a D2 (used for checking the introductory diet's success) or L-grade that is greater than or equal to K suggests an intolerance.} |
| L | L | \multicolumn{7}{l}{L = The biggest grade of the group B5, B6, B7 and B8. This group contains either the daily results of the status quo check (in that case D2 replaces L) or the results of the test day (B5) and its three subsequent days (B6 to B8). The L-grade is called lid grade, as it is used to evaluate the strength of the symptoms caused by an ongoing surrogate or level test.<br>Analysis:<br>L ≥ K indicates an intolerance, L< K a tolerance.<br>An **L**-grade that is below the **K**-grade indicates a tolerance. A lid grade that is greater than or equal to the **K.O.**-threshold grade indicates an intolerance.} |

# 2.1.4 Keeping your balance

## Fundamental recommendations

| | | |
|---|---|---|
| 1 | Eat a rich variety of foods, i.e., something different each day and with lots of natural ingredients. Eat with a relaxed posture. | 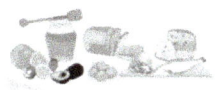 |
| 2 | Take care of your supply of fiber, e.g., by eating potatoes, flaxseeds, lentils, nuts. |  |
| 3 | Ingest five portions of vegetables (ideally dark green, red or orange) and fruit. | 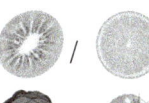 5/day |
| 4 | Have some reduced-fat milk products like reduced-fat milk, yogurt or cheese every day. |  ,  |
| 5 | One or two times a week, eat fish and eggs, as well as 300–600g of low-fat meat, ideally poultry. |  |
| 6 | Use vegetable oils if possible, like canola oil, and fats. |  |
| 7 | Reduce your consumption of salt and sugar. |  |
| 8 | Drink at least 1.5 liters of non-alcoholic drinks per day. Best are unsweetened beverages and water. Drink alcohol minimally to moderately. |  |
| 9 | Preferably, cook fresh and at lower temperatures to reduce nutrient leaching. |  |
| + | Stay fit: exercise regularly. |  |

*This page has been intentionally left blank.*

# 2.1.4 Keeping your balance

## Compensation needs due to your diet

If you reduce the fructans and galactans in your meals, you might have to compensate for the resulting loss of proteins, short-chain fatty acids and fibre. These three elements belong to a balanced diet. You usually ingest a large portion through fructan- and galactan-rich wheat products like bread, cereals and noodles, which you may be consuming less of. A regular intake of 20 to 38g of fibre, along with getting moderate exercise, can actually help to alleviate constipation. As a guideline for your nutrition, find the recommended daily amounts in the following examples.

**Proteins**
0,66g/kg

One needs 0.66g of protein per kilogram of body weight per day. You can ensure your protein supply by consuming the following products. The rough amount of proteins per portion is shown in parentheses: 85g meat (28g protein), 85g fish (26g), 150mL instant coffee with or without caffeine (18g, but normal espresso contains only 0.3g), 200mL whole milk with added vitamin D (15g), 200mL whole milk or fat-free milk without additives (6g), 85g corn or wild rice (12g), 90g kidney beans (18g), 140g pasta (15g), 90g soy beans (14g), a medium-sized egg (7.5g), 90g lentils (8g), 110g potatoes (4g), 25g nuts, especially peanuts, peanut butter and almonds (5g), a slice of whole grain bread (5g), 25g cheese (4g), a slice of rice bread (3.5g), 30g cereal (3g), 24g rice bran (3g), 25g dark chocolate (2g) and 50g couscous (1.5g). You may notice that maintaining a supply of protein is rather easy. Vegetarians, however, should plan their protein intake consciously.

**S. c. fatty acids**
**1.2/1.3g/day**

Short-chain fatty acids emerge as bacteria break down bricks, especially fructans. These are then partially absorbed by the intestine, as they are important sources of energy. They have a chain length of up to six carbon atoms, which is the basis for the following list.

Foods that are particularly rich in short-chain fatty acids include (fatty acids per portion without triglycerides in parentheses): 10g butter (0.5g), 25g goat's cheese (0.5g), 25g gouda, Swiss cheese, cheddar or Roquefort (0.4g), 50g mozzarella (0.3g), 47g M&M's® (0.3g), 25g blue cheese (0.25g), 20mL coconut oil (0.2g), 50g coconut meat (0.18g), 150g French fries (0.13g) or 20mL palm kernel oil (0.08g). Even if your change in diet does not lead to a deficiency in short-chain fatty acids, daily consumption of dairy products is recommended. As short-chain fatty acids ought to amount to 1/60 of the daily amount of consumed fats, which ought to be 70g for women and 80g for men, the required minimum dairy intake is 1.2g per day for women and 1.3g for men. Even if you have a lactose intolerance, you can usually consume small amounts of lactose and thus reach the target, for example, by eating three slices of cheddar. If you are a vegan, reaching the target is a challenge.

## Omega 3 fatty acids

Another important food component is short-chain omega 3 fatty acids, although they are hardly affected by your diet. Women should take in 6.1g of the omega 3 fatty acid known as alpha-Linolenic acid, or ALA, while men should take in 7g. Alternatively, maintaining a 2:1 proportion of omega 6 to omega 3 will lead to an intake of up to 9.6g per day for women and 11g for men. ALA fatty acids have a positive effect on your cardiovascular system. The following foods contain high levels (rough ALA amount per portion in parentheses): 200g fish (4g), 20mL linseed oil (10.5g) for which the consumed amount should be below 100mL per day (linseeds themselves contain 25% oil and thus 24g of linseeds, see page 54, at least 3g; however, during pregnancy you should avoid both), 20mL canola oil (1.8g), 20mL mayonnaise (1g), 20mL soy oil (0.8g), 100g wheat crackers (0.8g), 70g French fries (0.3g), 16g peanut butter with omega 3 (0.5g), 25g walnuts (0.5g), 10g butter (0.3g) and 10g margarine (0.3g). The data sheds a positive light on the fibre Strategy A as described in the following. You can reach the target amount of 7g for men just by consuming 1 tbsp. linseed oil per day. Alternatively, you can arrive at 6g, for example, by eating three portions of salad with 20mL of canola oil each and a slice of bread with omega 3 peanut butter. Apart from ALA, EPA (eicosapentaenoic acid) and DHA (docosahexaenoic acid) are also important. Your daily intake of EPA should be 250mg and of DHA, 500mg. If you eat fish at any time during the week, you will usually have covered your need. Krill or fish oil capsules containing these amounts are an alternative.

**Fibre**
**20-38g/day**

The following products are rich in fibre (fibre per portion in parentheses): 90g lentils (27.9g), 90g kidney beans (22.5g), 25g almonds (12g), 110g potatoes (8.7g), 30g bran cereals (up to 8.7g for Kellog's® All-Bran®), 24g linseeds (6.5g), 100g wild rice (6.2g), 24g rice bran (5g), one 42g slice of rye bread (5g), 30g wheat cereals (3.3g), 25g hazelnuts or pine nuts (2.7g), 25g dark chocolate (2.7g), 25g pistachio or pecans (2.5g), 60g (2.4g), 25g walnuts (1.7g), 25g chestnuts or butternuts (1g), 25g peanuts, coconuts or macadamia nuts (0.4g). Fruits and vegetables contain about 1 to 5g per portion, e.g., avocado (1.7g), banana (3g), blackberries (4.4g), cauliflower (1.2g), salad (0.8g), olives (1.2g), orange (2.4g), spinach (7g), tomatoes (1.4g). As fibre may be sort of a challenge, two different compensation strategies follow.

# Strategy A: Linseeds

Linseeds contain a high amount of fibre and many omega 3 fatty acids. They are good at reducing constipation and can also help a little against pain and bloating. The downside of this all-around effect is that linseeds contain fructans and galactans. If you apply this book's strategy, the BTL portions you take in for fructans and galactans will be reduced to 28% (Level 1: 64%, 2 or 3: 86%) of their former quantity. As you take in linseeds at three different times of the day, the amount per meal is 24g at most. This way the linseeds account for 6.5g of fibre at the highest daily stage. In order for your body to get acquainted with linseeds, start off in the first two weeks with one tablespoon combined with at least 75mL of water at breakfast. In the following weeks, you can then increase the intake amount according to the following table. The amount printed in normal type relates to the linseeds, and the amount in italics to the required minimum amount of water you should drink with it as a dilutor:

| Week | 3–4 | 5–6 | 7–8 | 9–10 | 11–12 | 13–14 | 15–16 | 17f |
|---|---|---|---|---|---|---|---|---|
| Break-fast | 1 tsp<br><br>*75 mL* | 1 tsp<br><br>*75 mL* | 1 tbsp<br><br>*150 mL* | 1 tbsp<br><br>*150 mL* | 1 tbsp<br><br>*150 mL* | 1 tbsp<br>1 tsp<br>*225 mL* | 1 tbsp<br>1 tsp<br>*225 mL* | 1 tbsp<br>1 tsp<br>*225 mL* |
| Lunch | 1 tsp<br><br>*75 mL* | 1 tsp<br><br>*75 mL* | 1 tsp<br><br>*75 mL* | 1 tbsp<br><br>*150 mL* | 1 tbsp<br><br>*150 mL* | 1 tbsp<br><br>*150 mL* | 1 tbsp<br>1 tsp<br>*225 mL* | 1 tbsp<br>1 tsp<br>*225 mL* |
| Dinner | - | 1 tsp<br><br>*75 mL* | 1 tsp<br><br>*75 mL* | 1 tsp<br><br>*75 mL* | 1 tbsp<br><br>*150 mL* | 1 tbsp<br><br>*150 mL* | 1 tbsp<br><br>*150 mL* | 1 tbsp<br>1 tsp<br>*150 mL* |

You can also accommodate linseeds in your meals. Whether the linseeds are whole or crushed should not make a difference. Make sure that you buy linseeds instead of psyllium as study results for suggest that psyllium is less effective. Wheat bran as well has not been shown to lead to any improvement. **Warning: Do not eat linseeds during pregnancy or lactation, as these can disturb your hormonal balance and cause premature birth.** With 24g of linseeds you cover 7g of your fibre demand. One portion of fruits or vegetables contains 2.5g of fibre on average. You can reach your ideal daily fibre intake by eating five of them per day and adding wild rice to one of your meals together with the 17th week amount of linseeds as indicated in the last table.

## Strategy B: Brown rice/rice bran

This strategy focuses on rice bran, rather than on linseeds as in Strategy A (page 54). After all, rice bran contains 21g of fibre per 100g and thus accounts for 5g of the daily amount recommended for the plan's optimal stage. The advantage of using rice bran is that your TL of fructans and galactans remain unchanged. Furthermore, rice bran appears to be unproblematic during pregnancy. If for example you eat 30g cereal mixed with rice bran for your breakfast, 25g dark chocolate and 20g almonds, as well as two oranges in between; for lunch a portion of tomato salad with avocado and 45g of potatoes; and for your dinner, 45g rice as a side dish, you will have consumed about 28g of fibre in total. Hence, with a little bit of planning you can maximize your fibre intake and minimize your fructan and galactan intake, while avoiding fibre supplement capsules.

# Summary

Drink at least 1.5L of water per day and get moderate exercise. In order to keep your diet in balance you should focus on consuming the following:

**Proteins**: E.g., by eating fish, meat, eggs, rice or rice bran.

**Short-chain fatty acids**: E.g., by consuming dairy products. In case of a lactose intolerance, cheddar is suitable due to its low lactose content.

**Omega 3:** E.g., by using linseed oil or canola oil or eating fish or meat.

**Fibre**: E.g., by using linseeds or rice bran and eating five servings of fruit and vegetables per day, potatoes, rice, dark chocolate and a handful of nuts.

Please also make a point of enjoying a variety of foods. This especially applies to fruits and vegetables, to ensure that your body is adequately supplied with the vitamins that are important for your health. What follows next is the first step of your LAXIBA strategy, a status quo check. This means you should fill out the symptom test sheet on page 34 for four days. Please also read Chapters 2.2 and 2.3 as you do so. Afterward, you will proceed according to the roadmap (see Chapter 2.1.1).

## 2.2 Your individual strategy

This chapter describes your introductory diet plan depending on your diagnosis. The diet has been well-tried. However, should your symptoms not improve after three weeks of adhering to this diet, you should cease or, better, check whether bricks have been entering your meals after all. One way to determine this is for you to keep a food diary and have a dietician or doctor check it. If no critical bricks have been sneaking in, resign from the brick diet. In Chapter 2.2.6 you will find alternatives.

### Diet code table

|         | FI [+] SI [+] | FI [-] SI [+] | FI [+] SI [-] | FI [-] SI [-] | FI [?=+] SI [?=+] |
|---------|:-:|:-:|:-:|:-:|:-:|
| LI [+]  | 8 | 4 | 7 | 3 | 8 |
| LI [-]  | 5 | 2 | 6 | 1 | 5 |
| LI [?]  | 8 | 4 | 7 | 3 | 8 |

FI[+]=Fructose intolerance, FI[-]=No fructose intolerance,
LI[+]=Lactose intolerance, LI[-]=No lactose intolerance,
SI[+]=Sorbitol intolerance, SI[-]=No sorbitol intolerance.

Use the above table to determine your intolerance code. A [+] means that you have the respective intolerance and a [-], that you are untroubled by it. A [?] means that the diagnosis is uncertain. By using the assigned code, you can then find out for which bricks you should adhere to the basic tolerance levels (BTLs), up to a level test, in the "Diet code classification" table that follows:

## Diet code classification

| | FRUCTOSE | LACTOSE | SORBITOL | FRUCTANS & GALACTANS |
|---|---|---|---|---|
| 1 | ☺ | ☺ | ☺ | ▼ |
| 2 | ☺ | ☺ | ☠ | ▼ |
| 3 | ☺ | ▼ | ☺ | ▼ |
| 4 | ☺ | ▼ | ☠ | ▼ |
| 5 | ▼ | ☺ | ☠ | ▼ |
| 6 | ▼ | ☺ | ★ | ▼ |
| 7 | ▼ | ▼ | ☺ | ▼ |
| 8 | ▼ | ▼ | ☠ | ▼ |

☺ = no restrictions, ▼ = reduce consumption to your TL, ☠ = avoid consumption ★ = consumption of sorbitol is not a problem unless you consume it with fructose. It is recommended to use the sorbitol-adapted fructose column in the food tables.

A consumption limit for fructans and galactans generally holds for the introductory diet. Adhering to the BTL portions for all bricks is only required if the breath test was positive for all three bricks or if you did not take it. If the diet is successful, you should take the level test, described in Chapter 2.2.4, to reduce your restrictions as much as possible.

## Procedure for the "quick-exit" option

Follow these steps if you have a lactose intolerance:
1) Reduce your consumption of lactose for three weeks according to the BTL portions and fill out the symptom test sheet at the end. If your symptoms improve to your satisfaction, continue this reduction in your lactose consumption. You may want to do the level test (Chapter 2.2.4). Otherwise, please continue with Step 2.
2) Follow the introductory diet according to your diet code as described earlier. If your diet is successful, do the substitute test for fructans and galactans afterward; it should come out positive. It will also make sense for you to take the level test (see Chapter 2.2.4), especially for lactose. If you remain unsatisfied, however, continue with Step 3.
3) Perhaps consuming less lactose has reduced your discomfort. Still, other foods could be affecting your symptoms as well. In Chapter 2.2.6 you will find suggestions as to which ones these could be and how you can test them.

## 2.2.1 It depends on the total load

You feel discomfort as soon as a threshold quantity of bricks arrive at the dragon. The more bricks arrive at your intestine the worse your symptoms are. In the food tables in the third part of the book, you will find the portion sizes that fit your TL. Yet, what do you do if you want to combine different foods, e.g., as you prepare to cook a recipe? The solution is to reduce the consumption for one or several of the affected foods far enough to reach your TL threshold. Let us say that you want to combine whole wheat bread and corn flakes, both of which contain fructans and galactans. To go below the BTL, restrict yourself to half a slice of the bread and three quarters of a corn flakes portion (22g). Don't worry if the reduced amounts aren't enough to fill you up: there are replacement products, low in or free of fructans and galactans (for example, rice bread, rice cereals, spelt and gluten free bread). Just look at the food table for similar products whose portions are less restricted.

## 2.2.2 Prevalence of the intolerance types

According to an extensive current study in Switzerland, 27% of people with abdominal discomfort were found to suffer from a fructose intolerance, 17% from a lactose intolerance and a further 33% from both. However, the fructose dose of 35g that the study used is high for European conditions, if a Finnish study from 1987 still applies to contemporary diets, and low for American conditions, wherein the average daily amount consumed is 54g. Another research study using 25g fructose as its base level suggests a 49% average prevalence of fructose intolerance. An analysis of several studies (see Chapter 1.5.5) shows that in general, 58% of those with irritable bowel symptoms have an intolerance of one kind or another. What is surprising is that lactose intolerance is only the second most prevalent intolerance in Europe, after sorbitol, yet the European market has adjusted itself better for those patients affected by lactose intolerance, especially with regard to food labelling. Those affected by a sorbitol intolerance, on the other hand, are forced to memorize technical terms to avoid eating sorbitol-containing products.

## 2.2.3 Substitute test

If no breath test is available but you want to find out which bricks you can stomach, then there is a substitute test. It determines the degree of an intolerance by gauging your symptoms after you have consumed the highest dose of the respective brick as is practical in your daily life. Of course, the test is only beneficial if your symptoms have improved through your consequent adherence to the BTL portion sizes for your problematic bricks.

As symptoms sometimes arise with a delay of up to three days, you have to schedule at least a week for the first brick that you want to test. Three days before the first test day, you must pay attention and always eat close ($\leq$) to the BTL portion sizes of the bricks you are examining so that your pre-test meals do not affect your result. During the test day itself, keep all respective BTL portions, except for the brick that is being tested; on the three subsequent days all BTL portions hold once more. However, do not force yourself to eat more of the bricks than you did before starting the introductory diet, except for on the test day. On the test day, at the latest, as well as on the three subsequent days, fill out the symptom test sheet (see Chapter 2.1.2), unless you have already determined that you have an intolerance towards the tested brick. Use the symptom test sheet for the efficiency check days as a reference. If your symptoms do not worsen, then you are able to stomach the tested brick. If you want to test various bricks, you can spare yourself the three buffer days by testing the next brick on the fourth day after the last test day and proceed likewise with the other bricks you want to test.

Discuss the tests with your doctor beforehand so that he or she can consider the potential effects to and of your medical treatments and pre-existing conditions. For all the tests together, you need: a beaker, a 0.5L bottle, 100g of fructose and 20g of sorbitol, both which you can buy at your local pharmacy, scales and 1L of reduced-fat cow's milk without additives. In case of an intolerance you can use the remaining sugars for a level test later on. Now let us go through the test procedure:

### Lactose test

At breakfast, drink half a liter of the milk, using the 0.5L bottle. Repeat at lunch unless your symptoms after the breakfast dose are so severe that you can already conclude that you have an intolerance. In addition to the milk, eat in accordance with your BTL portion sizes for the other relevant bricks.

## Fructose test

Warning: before doing the test, confirm with your doctor that you do not have a hereditary fructose intolerance. For the test, add 25g (if you are in the USA or drink a lot of soft drinks use 35g) of fructose to a clean 0.5L bottle of water and shake it well. Then drink it completely on the morning of the test. In addition to the fructose, eat according to your BTLs on the test day and the next three days. You do not need a test for glucose-balanced fructose. If you want to pay attention to it, you can determine the amount you can tolerate by multiplying the TL amount of free fructose by ten.

## Sorbitol test

Proceed as for the fructose test, but replace the 25g of fructose with 5g of sorbitol.

## Fructans and galactans test

Eat a generous portion of wheat cereal in the morning, beans with garlic and onions at lunch, brownies and crackers in between and a baguette or porridge dish in the evening.

As soon as you notice symptoms on the test day or the three subsequent days, which you can see mathematically if your **Lid grade** is higher than your K.O.-threshold grade, you know you have an intolerance, and you can stop the test. In order to reduce your abdominal discomfort, drink still mineral water (usually up to three liters per day are salutary) and take a walk.

# 2.2.4 Level test

## Level test task list

| # Tasks | Done when? ✓ |
|---|---|
| 1. You filled out the symptom test sheet for the status quo check. | |
| 2. You asked your doctor to refer you to a specialist in order to do a breath test (if available). | |
| 3. A) You decided to take the ("quick-exit") expedited option and found that your symptoms improved to your satisfaction. | |
| 3. B) You performed the three-week introductory diet according to your diet code (page 45) and found improvement to your symptoms at the efficiency check (otherwise please proceed according to Chapter 2.2.6). If no breath test was available, you performed the substitute test. | |
| 4. You decided which bricks you wanted to do the level test for (see page 54): the bricks that you have an intolerance towards as well as fructans and galactans. | |
| 5. You estimated the time span for the level test: for one brick, it takes four weeks, for two bricks about eight weeks, for three bricks about 12 weeks and for four bricks about 16 weeks. However, the **acceleration option** lets you perform the tests right after one another (see page 54). You can thereby shorten the time span to 2½ weeks for one brick, 4½ weeks for two bricks, 6½ weeks for three bricks and 8½ weeks for four bricks. | |
| 6. You convinced a partner to help you with your tests. They will mix your test liquids and interpret your symptom test sheets. You can count on their credibility and availability. | |
| 7. You finished all of the tests, during which your testing partner adhered to the instructions on page 58, and you acted according to the flowchart on page 69. | |
| 8. Finish: You talked your result over with your testing partner and entered your new combined or single TLs into the table on page 103. | |

*This page has been intentionally left blank.*

Did your breath or substitute test demonstrate the presence of one or more brick intolerances? Then you should find out whether the BTLs fit for you. Each human differs in the amount he or she can stomach of each brick. Even in healthy humans the tolerated amount of fructose, for example, fluctuates between 5g and 50g. Moreover, the amount consumed at once for the breath or substitute test is higher than what you would consume in a typical meal. The advantage of a high test dose is that you are unlikely to have symptoms from the respective brick in your everyday life if you are able to stomach it. However, in the case of an intolerance you should take a closer look, as the only thing that is yet certain is that you are in trouble when you consume an extreme amount. What is interesting is how much of a problematic brick you are able to stomach during normal nutritional consumption. For this purpose, you use the level test, where you increase the consumed amount in small steps, e.g., twice the BTL, to determine your tolerance threshold, while keeping the TLs for the remaining bricks. With every step, you then increase the tested consumption amount. The procedure is shown in the flowchart on page 69. The level test is finished last, after you have determined the levels that cause your symptoms for all tested bricks. If you use the mathematical Option B, this is the case when the lid grade is greater than or equal to the K.O. threshold grade. Take the test twice for each consumed amount to make sure your symptoms weren't caused by something else.

In order to make sure that you are also able to stomach your new single TL in combination with, if applicable, the new single TLs (that is, if your personal TL is above the BTL) of other tested bricks, next test all bricks with a new TL together. Note: there have to be at least three days between the two test days in order to avoid distorting the results.

## Bricks to be tested

|  | Fructose | Lactose | Sorbitol | Fruc/Galactans |
|---|---|---|---|---|
| To be tested? Yes/No |  |  |  |  |
| In which sequence (1, 2, …) |  |  |  |  |
| (My calculated K.O. threshold grade is:) |  |  |  |  |

Now, choose the bricks that you want to determine your level for. Fructans and galactans are tested together. If you want to use the mathematical Option B, also enter your K-grade from the efficiency check. Important: disregard bricks that you can stomach and consume them as usual.

## How a test week is run

| Day 1–3 before the test day | On the test day | Day 1–3 after |
|---|---|---|
| Your brick consumption should surpass your current TLs by as narrow a margin as possible, but don't force yourself to eat more of anything than you want. Regulate only those TLs that have been confirmed by your partner so that you are uninfluenced on the test day, as symptoms can occur with three days' delay. If you do not feel as well on the test morning as you did at the end of the introductory diet, re-schedule the test until you do. | Fill out the symptom test sheet on the test day and its three subsequent days. | |
| | At breakfast, lunch and dinner consume only as much of the tested brick(s) as is part of the test dose and no more. For all other bricks, the current TLs hold as described on the left. | Keep your current TLs for your diet. |

**Acceleration option:** Perform the tests right after one another. Three days after the last test day, begin the next test day and thus save the three days described in the column on the left.

Start your test week three days before the test day, as symptoms may occur as many as three days after you consume the bricks that trigger them, and you want to start the test uninfluenced. On the days before the test, eat according to your current TLs. Your current TLs are those that you tolerated during the test and retest of the combination test described below. Initially, these are the BTLs (see page 103). After you have finished the first level test for all tested bricks, whether you perform a combination test and what it looks like depends on your results. It only makes sense if you do the test for at least two bricks and were able to stomach at least two bricks at the first tolerance level. For the combination test, test the respective bricks together at the higher tolerance level.

You do not have to fill out the symptom test sheet during the days leading up to the test (page 34), as you can use the efficiency check sheet as your reference, but from the day of the test to the third day after it, document your symptoms (unless you determine an intolerance earlier). Your testing partner prepares all test doses except for the fructans (F) and galactans (G). See the level table for F and G below to get a sense of the test quantities. For the test, eat the listed amounts of the following foods at the meals (M) breakfast, lunch and dinner. For the first test, these are the TL 1 amounts:

| Level, amount/M | Portion size | Amount per day |
|---|---|---|
| **Level 1** F: 0.5g, G: 0.5g | 26g peas and 38g couscous | 78g peas and 114g couscous |
| **Level 2** F: 1g, G: 1g | 53g peas and 77g couscous | 159g peas and 231g couscous |
| **Level 3** F: 1.5g, G: 1.5g | 79g peas and 115g couscous | 237g peas and 345g couscous |

By consuming the listed amounts, you double the BTL at Level 1. In the following days, continue eating according to the BTLs. Then repeat the test at TL 1 to cover the result. Tell your testing partner whether your symptoms worsened at the test dose and give her or him the filled out test sheet. Afterward, proceed likewise with the next brick in order of precedence. When you have finished this with all bricks that are to be tested, you can perform a combined test of those bricks you were able to stomach at Level 1, perform a single level test or consider the level tests finished. If you want to test a level between two levels, you can calculate the dose as follows:

$$\text{Lower dose} + [(\text{higher dose} - \text{lower dose}) / 2]$$

If you can tolerate this dose, you should then adapt your multiplier for the food tables (see Chapter 3.1.1) by changing the word "dose" in the above formula with the multiplier. When your testing partner confirms you have an intolerance, the level test for that brick is over. Enter the highest TL for that brick in the table in Chapter 3.1.1. There you will find a differentiation between single TLs and combined TLs. At first, the combined TLs are the BTLs of all bricks you absorb badly. Later these may change if you can stomach a number of these bricks at a higher level when combined. You might also find that you are able to stomach two bricks while keeping the combined TLs of the other tested bricks but cannot tolerate both bricks together at the new level. In that case, enter the highest single level of these bricks into the single TL column. Note: if you determine an intolerance in a combined TL test concerning more than two bricks, it makes sense to repeat the test with only two of the bricks on the respective TL afterward. During this single-brick test, the TL that you were able to tolerate last holds for all other bricks. If you do tolerate one of these pairs at the new TL, note the tested TL as the combined TL for the two bricks. You can find the precise procedure in the flowchart in Section 2.2.5. A level test of balanced fructose is unnecessary; you will get the tolerated amount by just multiplying the level amount of tolerated fructose by 10 (see Chapter 3.1.1).

For procedural reasons, wait until after you have repeated the test before trying to interpret the results. Please show your testing partner the table with the bricks for which you want to perform the level test (page 54). He or she can then adapt the test. Please also hand her or him the remaining sugars and measurement instruments from the substitute test (if taken).

## How to handle symptoms

**After** noting test symptoms that were too severe to allow you to stomach the load, drink water (up to three liters per day) and take a walk to reduce your symptoms.

STOP: The following pages are for only your testing partner to read, as they contain information regarding procedural safety! Your partner's instructions will depend on results pertaining to your reactions; if you know how your partner is assessing you, you may alter your behavior and distort the results. Continue reading on page 69 to learn about the procedure resulting from your partner's tolerance statements. The three pages for your testing partner are preceded and followed by four empty pages. You should flick back from the end of the book to arrive at page 69 without reading them.

The **instructions** for your testing **partner** follow on page **58**. As the **reader** of the book you should leave them **unread**, to **produce** a **more accurate** test **result**. Hence, open a new page that is farther **ahead** and then **flick back** to page **69**.

The **instructions** for your testing **partner** follow on page **58**. As the **reader** of the book you should leave them **unread**, to **produce** a **more accurate** test **result**. Hence, open a new page that is much farther **ahead** and then **flick back** to page **69**.

The **instructions** for your testing **partner** follow on page **58**. As the **reader** of the book you should leave them **unread**, to **produce** a **more accurate** test **result**. Hence, open a new page that is much farther **ahead** and then **flick back** to page **69**.

The **instructions** for your testing **partner** follow on page **58**. As the **reader** of the book you should leave them **unread**, to **produce** a **more accurate** test **result**. Hence, open a new page that is much farther **ahead** and then **flick back** to page **69**.

Your friend wants to find out how much she or he can stomach of certain food ingredients. Unfortunately, a placebo effect is quite common in this test. Your role in this test is very important toward avoiding a false result. You are going to test each ingredient twice, each test taking about a week. On one of the two days, you are going to hand out a placebo mix instead of the real one. Your friend does not know about the placebo. Just say that the double test is required to get valid results, as you also have to keep track of certain behaviors she or he might exhibit. IMPORTANT: Keep quiet about the placebo until **all** tests are done (see page 70) and you have talked the results over. Waiting until the end of that final talk, is important as your friend may want more precise results. Between two test days are three monitoring days and three regeneration days.

Here is what you need: a beaker, a letter scale and three 0.5L bottles. Determine the ingredients to be tested on page 54 and for each of the following bricks being tested, prepare:

**Fructose test:** 0.5kg sugar, 100g fructose, vanilla extraxt and 1L of water.

**Lactose test:** 1L reduced-fat cow milk without additives, 1L of lactose free milk (please use cow milk that has been freed from lactose without a flavor or the label sugar free. Moreover, please do not use soy milk or rice milk for the test), vanilla extraxct.

**Sorbitol test:** 10g sorbitolm, vanilla extraxt and 1L of water.

If your friend has not given you the substances for the test solution, you can order them online or from a pharmacy. You can also ask your pharmacist to weigh the amounts you need.

From test to test, increase the level amounts according to the tables on the following pages. Begin with the TL 1 amounts of the highest ranked ingredient on page 54. Before repeating the test, note whether you first handed out the real or placebo mix and the result. Ideally you should ask for the symptom test sheet and write down L for reaL and A for plAcebo as well as the result. Then, keep all of the info sheets for the final discussion of all tests. If your friend has given you the K-grade, you can calculate the tolerance (see row L on page 35). If the L-grade is greater than or equal to K, this indicates an intolerance. There are three possible cases after each double test:

**Case 1:** Neither the placebo nor the real mix causes the symptoms to worsen, i.e., your friend is able to stomach the amounts of the ingredient, and it can be tested at the next level. Tell her/him that.

**Case 2.** Only the real mix causes the symptoms to worsen, i.e., your friend is intolerant for the amount. The test series for this ingredient is over, and your friend can be told. For a more precise level, you can proceed as per page 55.

**Case 3:** The placebo mix causes symptoms to worsen. Regardless of whether or not the real mix causes symptoms to worsen, as well, repeat the test with the same amount, starting with the placebo mix, but tell her that you reduced the amount to half of the dose. If your friend still reports an intolerance, abort the test and tell her/him (only until the final discussion) that s/he has an intolerance for the amount and the old levels remain current.

After the test and retest of the first level of the ingredient with rank number 1, test the next ingredient in order (if applicable) also at the first level. After finishing all single tests for the stated ingredients at the first level, continue according to the level test flowchart on page 70. What follows may be a combination test:

**Combination tests:** For the lactose/fructose, lactose/sorbitol and lactose/sorbitol/fructose combination tests, use the cow milk and lactose freed cow milk together with vanilla extraxt according to the level amounts for lactose. For the fructose/sorbitol combination test alone, use 200mL of water. All ingredients to be tested are put into the liquids. For each one use the level amounts according to the single tables for the ingredients. After a tolerated combination test, the new combined tolerance levels hold for all further test days. Continue with another round of single tests for those bricks that were stomached well. This time, tell your friend that the new combined tolerance levels hold, and apply the Level 2 amounts for each test.

On the eve of one of the two test days, hand out three bottles with the real mix, and on the other one, three bottles with the placebo mix. At breakfast, lunch and dinner your friend drinks one bottle. Find the mixtures for each level in the following explanations and tables:

In the **left column** find the respective **level** and the **total amount** of substances per day, as it is easier to mix the **daily amount in one load** and **then divide** it among the **three bottles**. In the two columns on the right, find the amounts per bottle for the real/placebo substance.

**Lactose:** Required: 1L reduced-fat milk, 1L lactose free cow milk and vanilla extract. To hide taste differences between the normal and the laxtose free milk, please add a little bit of vanilla extraxt (**v.**) to both.

| Level and lactose amount, sum/day | Real (R) 3 × bottle with | Placebo (P) 3 × bottle with |
| --- | --- | --- |
| Level 1 (3g/meal) per day 180mL milk and ½ tsp. of **v.** | 4 tbsp. (60mL) milk 1 drop of **v.** | 4 tbsp. lactose free milk 1 drop of **v.** |
| Level 2 (6g/meal) per day 360mL milk and ¾ tsp. of **v.** | 120mL milk (100) 2 drops of **v.** | 120mL lactose free milk 2 drops of **v.** |
| Level 3 (9g/meal) per day 540mL milk and 1 tsp. of **v.** | 180mL milk 3 drops of **v.** | 180mL lactose free milk 3 drops of **v.** |

**Fructose:** Required: fructose and common sugar. Mix the following amounts with 200mL water (**w**) and add a little bit of vanilla extract (**v.**). Important: the bottles should not be diluted:

| Level, real/placebo in g per day+600mL **w** | Real (R) 3 × 200mL **w** bottle with | Placebo (P) 3 × 200mL **w** bottle with |
| --- | --- | --- |
| Level 1, 3 R/3.5 P, 1 tsp. **v.** | 1g fructose 3 drops of **v.** | 1.17g sugar 3 drops of **v.** |
| Level 2, 6 R/7 P, 1 tsp. **v.** | 2g fructose 3 drops of **v.** | 2.34g sugar 3 drops of **v.** |
| Level 3, 9 R/10.5 P, 1 tsp. **v.** | 3g fructose 3 drops of **v.** | 3.51g sugar 3 drops of **v.** |

**Sorbitol:** Required: sorbitol and common sugar. Mix the amounts with 200mL of water (**w**) and add a little bit of vanilla extract (**v.**). Important: the bottles should not be diluted:

| Level, real/placebo in g per day+600mL w | Real (R) 3 × 200mL **w** bottle with | Placebo (P) 3 × 200mL **w** bottle with |
| --- | --- | --- |
| Level 1, 0.3 R/0.2 P, 1 tsp. **v.** | 0.1g sorbitol 3 drops of **v.** | 0.06g sugar 3 drops of **v.** |
| Level 2, 1.2 R/0.7 P, 1 tsp. **v.** | 0.4g sorbitol 3 drops of **v.** | 0.24g sugar 3 drops of **v.** |
| Level 3, 3 R/1.26 P, 1 tsp. **v.** | 0.7g sorbitol 3 drops of **v.** | 0.42g sugar 3 drops of **v.** |

The **instructions** for your testing **partner** begin on page **58**. As the **reader** of the book you should leave them **unread**, to **produce** a **more accurate** test **result**. The book resumes on page 69.

The **instructions** for your testing **partner** begin on page **58**. As the **reader** of the book you should leave them **unread**, to **produce** a **more accurate** test **result**. The book resumes on page 69.

The **instructions** for your testing **partner** begin on page **58**. As the **reader** of the book you should leave them **unread**, to **produce** a **more accurate** test **result**. The book resumes on page 69.

The **instructions** for your testing **partner** begin on page **58**. As the **reader** of the book you should leave them **unread**, to **produce** a **more accurate** test **result**.

# 2.2.5 Symptom based test process

## Procedural example with fictive bricks

In order to help you to remain impartial, the bricks are labelledhere after actual building materials: granite, wood and sandstone. Test the brick "granite" (having rank one in the example; see brick choice on page 54), "sandstone" (rank two) and "wood" (rank three). If, according to your testing partner, you could not tolerate "granite" during the first test at Level 1, then continue consuming that brick at the BTL amount. If you were able to tolerate "sandstone" at Level 1, however, that amount should now be considered your new TL for this brick if consumed on its own (not in combination with other bricks). Let's say, moreover, that you were able to stomach "wood" at the first level.

Next, perform a combined test of "sandstone" and "wood," as you were able to stomach the two bricks independently in the single tests. You can see this as you follow the [+] of the first diamond in the following flowchart. For this test, you will consume a mix of the two bricks in your test dilution bottles. While taking this test, eat according to the Level 0 portions for "granite," following the food tables in Part 3 of the book. If you are able to stomach that test load, enter Level 1 of "sandstone" and "wood" together with Level 0 of "granite," as a new combined TL in the table in Chapter 3.1.1.

Afterward, do another round of single level tests, as illustrated by the [+] of the second diamond in the line of the flowchart. Begin with the Level 2 test for "sandstone." The test dilution bottle then contains the Level 2 amount for "sandstone" and the Level 1 amount for "wood." On the test day, keep "granite" at Level 0. On the three days that follow, eat according to the Level 1 portion sizes of "sandstone" and "wood." If you tolerate the Level 2 amount of "sandstone" well, then do the Level 2 test of "wood" in which the test dilution contains the Level 1 amount of "sandstone" and the Level 2 amount of "wood." However, let's say you are intolerant towards that solution. If you follow the [-] at the third diamond in line (on the following page) and at the following diamond the [+], you find out that you would enter Level 2 for "sandstone" for the combined TL. Moreover, you learn that you can also do the Level 3 test for "sandstone." At this test again the Level 1 amount for "wood" is added. If you can stomach it, enter Level 3 for "sandstone" in the combined TL column.

Maybe you are interested in whether you can stomach more of the "wood" brick if you keep the BTLs for the other bricks. In this case, ask your testing partner to repeat the Level 2 test for "wood" with a mix that only contains the Level 2 amount of "wood" and none of the other bricks. During the test days, restrict yourself to the BTL portions of the other bricks. If you can stomach the Level 2 amount of "wood" now, enter Level 2 in the single TL column for wood and note down BTLs, as it only holds when you keep the BTLs of the other bricks.

Warning: you must not surpass any TL portion that holds during a level test, as it can distort the result. If this happens, you unfortunately have to repeat the test. Exception: you already finished the test after learning that you are intolerant towards that brick amount.

## Level test flowchart

Starting with the rectangle in the upper right corner, read off the next step by following the arrows. A diamond means that the next step depends on the statement within the diamond being true [+] or false [-]. If the statement is true, follow the [+]-arrow, and if it is false, follow the [-]-arrow. In the rectangular fields, find a statement about what to do next. In fields that follow a field with a flag attached to it saying PATH 1 or PATH 2, you also find data in brackets or parentheses. These are only relevant if you were asked to follow the respective PATH at the end of the second page of the flowchart. The statements within the parentheses apply if you reach them via PATH 1, and those in square brackets if you were asked to follow PATH 2.

All instructions are based on the assumption that you want to take all level tests to the end, which you do not have to do. It might be enough for you to know that you are able to stomach the TL 1 portions. If this is true, just stop after the combined TL 1 test. The regular procedure ends as you reach a field with rounded corners. Enter the respective new levels into the table in Chapter 3.1.1.

What is the use of the combined test? The development of symptoms depends on how many bricks pass your belly's interception shield. Let's say you tolerate a higher level of various bricks in the single test. Exhausting the new portion sizes for these levels at the same time may still lead to symptoms due to interaction effects. Therefore, you want to check whether you are still able to tolerate the new portion sizes, when they are associated with the level advancements, at your shield's maximum combined exposure.

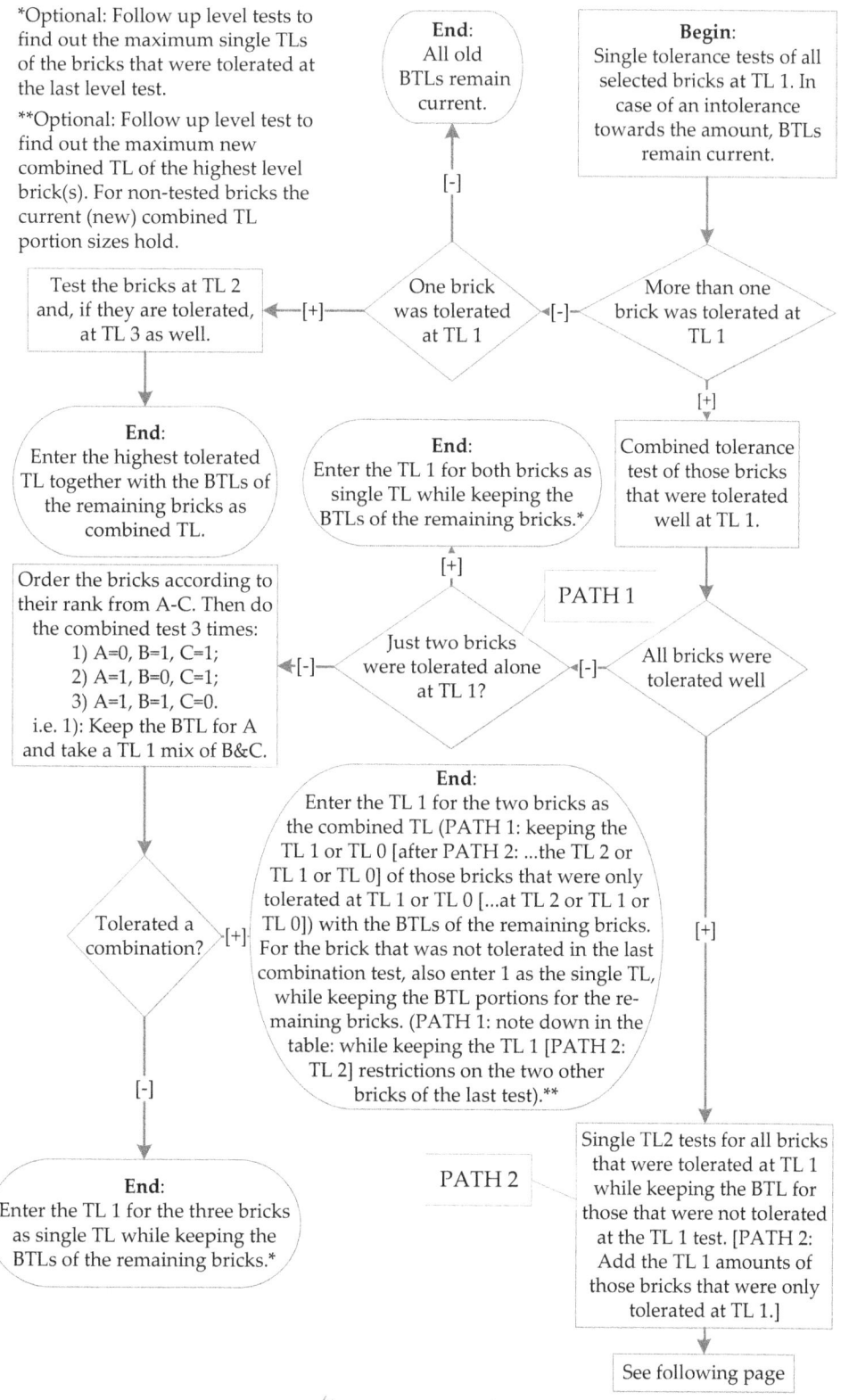

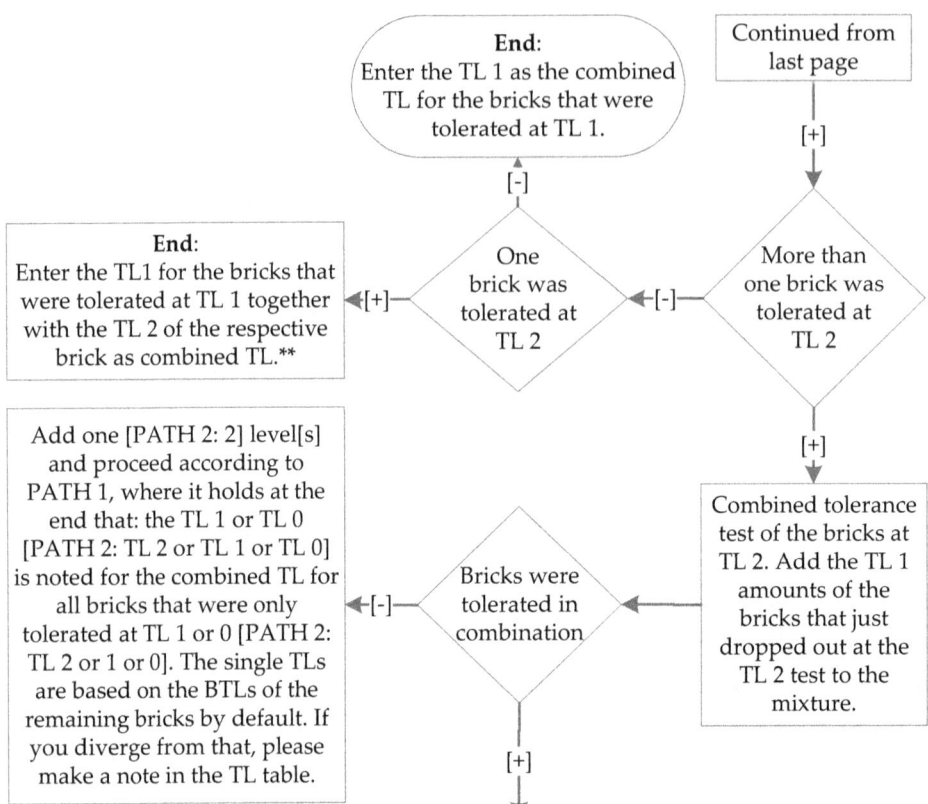

## 2.2.6 Alternative strategies

### General causes of abdominal discomfort

The following triggers have been found most often in an analysis of nutrition diaries. On a subjective scale from 1 (seldom) to 6 (very often): wheat 5, milk 5, coffee 5, eggs 5, potatoes 5, nuts 4, rye 2, barley 2, corn 2, oats 2, banana 2, onions 2, peas 2. The malasorbtions for all of these food products except for coffee, corn, eggs, nuts and potatoes can be explained by the scientific analysis of carbohydrates like fructose, lactose, fructans and galactans. The author was unable to find studies that analyzed the fructan and galactan content of eggs, coffee and nuts.

### Alternative diet strategy

Sometimes a product such as coffee causes discomfort or acts as a trigger for reasons other than the carbohydrates that are the focus of this book. In these cases try adopting an alternative introductory diet. In such a diet, you will abstain from coffee, corn, eggs, nuts and potatoes, as well as up to two to four other products or ingredients that you suspect might be causing you trouble. Before starting the diet take note of the greatest amount you are likely to consume of the affected foods at breakfast, lunch and dinner. You need that sheet later to find out which of the foods, if any, caused you symptoms. Then at the end of the three test weeks, use the symptom test sheet again to determine the efficiency of the diet by comparing it with your former status quo sheet. If you want, you can also employ the mentioned calculation methods, using the final sheet from your alternative diet as your efficiency check sheet. Before starting the diet, discuss potential personal risks with your doctor.

If the diet successfully relieved your symptoms, wait three days and then test the foods that you are abstaining from. Take a look at the notes you made regarding your usual portion sizes of the foods included in the test. Choose one of the foods, and on test day, eat the amounts that are typical for you at the times you usually eat them. On that day and the three that follow, fill out the symptom test sheet (see page 34) and, if you are using math Option B (see page 35), estimate your L-grade. During the test weeks, continue to avoid the foods you are testing as well as those you tested intolerant for. A negative test result indicates that you can safely consume the given food as you did before the alternative introductory diet. With a positive result, you have two options: either you can completely avoid the food or you can determine a tolerable portion size by performing a level test. For the level test, you divide your common portion by four. During the level test weeks, refrain from all symptom-inducing foods you found. On the test day, eat the to-be-tested portion size at the times you normally have your three main meals. Start with one fourth of your normal portion size. If your symptoms do not significantly worsen, repeat the test on the fourth day after your test day with half of your common portion size. If you can stomach this amount, repeat the test with three fourths of your normal portion. If you were not able to stomach one fourth of your normal portion size, you can choose to avoid the food or ingredient or test it further at a reduced test portion size. If symptoms arose at half your usual portion size, then consider your tolerable portion to be one fourth of a full portion; if they arose at three fourths, your tolerable portion is a half-portion. If you could not narrow your symptoms down to a critical food or ingredient, return to your usual diet. Low dosage antidepressants constitute one possible remaining alternative for addressing your symptoms, but consult your doctor to discuss this option further.

## 2.3 General diet hints

## 2.3.1 Good reasons for your persistence

Imagine that one of your best friends goes on a two-week vacation, leaving his beloved Labrador retriever in your care, along with some instructions about the dog's health needs as it has an intolerance towards an ingredient in some dog foods. You run out of dog food after the first week, and while you're on your way out of the house to get more, your partner stops you. "Hold on," s/he says, "There's still the dog food we give your aunt's dog in the pantry." You're tempted to give in and use it, rather than spend an hour driving to the store and back, but you read the ingredient list and know that one of the ingredients is harmful to the dog. Unlike the happy dog image on the package suggests, giving him this food causes him pain, flatulence and lethargy; catching a stick will be out of the question for this poor pooch, and you tell your partner so. "Don't be so worried," s/he argues. "The dogs we had growing up ate it all the time and never had a problem!" But you know that even if your partner's family did it all the time, it doesn't make it right for this dog. Hence, your friend's dog is worth the investment of consideration, money and time for his well-being. for his well-being. The question that you now have to answer yourself is:

do you owe it to yourself, too?

In the end, I call upon you to take responsibility for your nutrition. Show respect to your body. Acquire the necessary courage and discipline. Your body is a part of you. Just as many vegetarians stand by their dietary choices for the duration of their lives, you should stand by your diet and your body. Be yourself. The key is not starting out perfect but starting at all and making small improvements every day. That is something you can do!
Your target should be to change your sustenance day by day, food by food, in such a way as to allow you to lead a largely symptom-free life. All beginnings are difficult, however, and as you leap the initial hurdles, you will find further motivation and discipline in discovering how much your nutritional changes are paying off for you.
   The first step in that direction is to connect that goal with whatever is most important to you in your life. Independent of where your passions lie most

strongly, you will improve on them by gaining more energy and improved wellbeing.

Thus, turn your attention and abilities towards eating in a way that will help you achieve your goals. Overcome any fears of change you might have by imagining that you have already done it. How? Cut out the following card and fold it as indicated. Then put it somewhere you can see it every day. Ideally, you can take a picture of yourself after a particularly successful milestone and put it on the drawing. Then let it encourage you to continue improving your nutrition each day.

Stephen William Hawking has never stopped producing outstanding scientific works despite suffering from amyosthenia. Why? Because he is following his heart and because he has a positive attitude about life. Who seeks excuses when they're passionate about something? When it comes to passion, it is all about the how. It is about doing what is possible and thus it is always all about the solution. There are similar examples in sports. Melissa Stockwell achieves first class athletic performance despite having lost a leg. Her sport is her passion, and she finds ways to excel in it regardless of the circumstances life gave her.

So what is your passion? Write it down. Then make it clear to yourself that a symptom-reducing diet will positively affect your passion. Then get on your way to making this nutrition a part of your life.

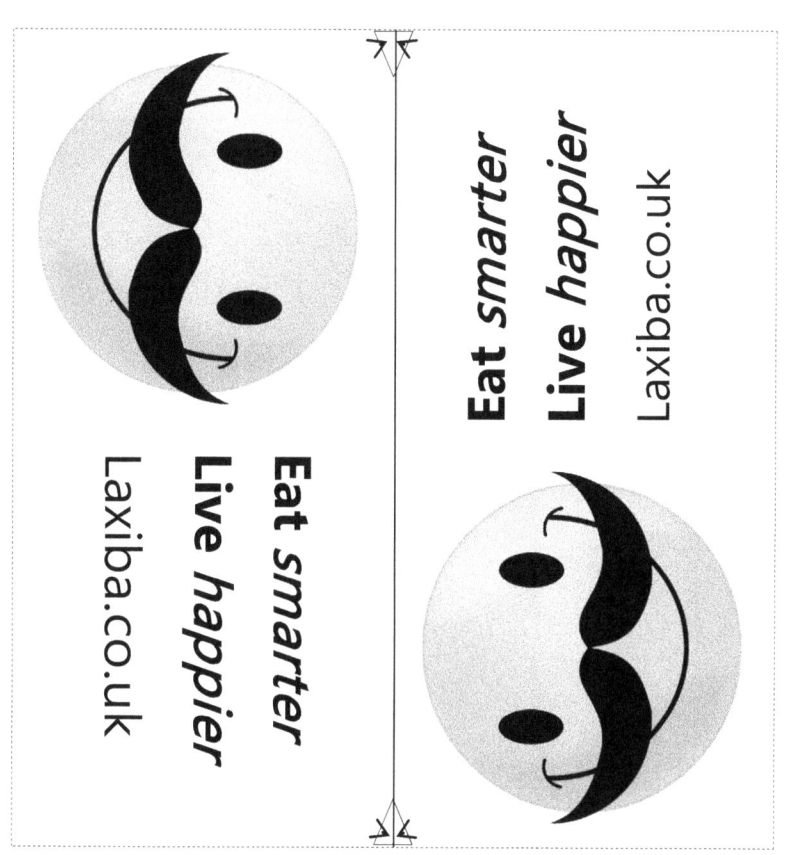

*This page has been intentionally left blank.*

## 2.3.2 Mealtimes

Even when and how often you eat can affect your digestion. Who are the greatest experts on that? People for whom a successful supply of energy is of the utmost importance—that is to say, athletes. An analysis shows that over 97% of elite Canadian athletes eat at least three times a day; 57% of them also take a snack in the morning, 71% in the afternoon and 58% in the evening. Moreover, regular mealtimes have a positive effect on the cardiovascular system. A study of more than 4,500 children showed that the risk of childhood obesity markedly decreases the more often children eat during the day.

## 2.3.3 Reasons for using the bricks

What are bricks doing in medicine, sausage, and all manner of other things you consume on a daily basis? Some reasons bricks get added to products include savings in costs, as well as their use as a flavoring, a preservative, a thickener for meat products or a sugar substitute, e.g., for diabetic. In addition, lactose and sorbitol are used as medicinal carriers. So far, there is no strong lobby against using bricks in foods or making them easier to avoid. Of course, these bricks also occur naturally, but that is not a valid reason to use them instead of the also naturally occurring Stevia in, for example, chewing gums.

## 2.3.4 Eating out

At home, restricting one's consumption of bricks is rather easy, but how about eating out? Some products that are usually safe include eggs, fish or meat without breading or sauce, kiwis, leafy salads dressed with oil, oregano, pepper and salt, oranges, pesto, potatoes, rice, tomatoes, tomato sauce and tortillas. Depending on your intolerances, you have to be careful with diabetics products and prepared sauces, as they often contain bricks like sorbitol. What about menus, however? Have you ever spent time at a restaurant considering what the ideal combination of menu items would be for you? The good thing is that you can often ask for changes to be made to menu items without paying much extra, if you ask the server. You can likewise voice your needs to your hosts when you are invited to a meal. To make it easy, just hand out the safe products list (see Chapter 2.4.3). You can send it out with the following message, for example:

*"Dear [name of the host],*

*I was glad to receive your invitation to [occasion of the invitation], and I am happy to come. If it would not be an inconvenience for you to cook some of the foods that are included in the attached table separately from the other meals, then I would be pleased to take part in the meal, as well. Please tell me whether that will be possible so that I can plan accordingly.*

*Thank you and see you soon!*

*[Your name]"*

The safe products list also makes it easier for a restaurant kitchen to find a suitable meal for you. As fast food chains are not as readily equipped to adapt their menus, you will find many fast food chain products and the portion sizes you can stomach in the third part of this book. You can stay on the safe side by always having your book with you. However, it will hardly be always at hand, unlike a foldable list for your purse or wallet. In Chapter 2.4 you will find two such lists with the tolerable portion sizes of some common products. This list also includes information on brick names and brick-free products.

## 2.3.5 Convenience foods

Unfortunately, fructose, lactose and sorbitol are added to many convenience foods or are naturally contained in the ingredients. However, you will find exceptions, even when shopping on the cheap, including convenience foods that advertise the use of natural ingredients and those that contain tomato sauce. The leaflets (see Chapter 2.4) will inform you of which ingredients on a package are related to bricks.

## 2.3.6 Medicine and oral hygiene

Everything you take into your mouth can cause symptoms if it contains a brick you cannot tolerate. Sorbitol in particular is found in many oral hygiene products. Examples of sorbitol-free toothpastes include Weleda® Calendula Toothpaste. Use dental floss without wax, and find a mouthwash such as TheraBreath® Fresh Breath Oral Rinse.

The search for sorbitol-free medicines may be especially hard, so ask your pharmacist for assistance. Many nasal sprays, eye drops and expectorants contain this additive. However, if you look hard enough, you will usually find alternatives for these as well.

Examples of sorbitol-free pharmaceuticals include: Allerest® PE Allergy & Sinus Relief – Tablets [CONTAINS LACTOSE] (frontal sinusitis), BecoAllergy® 10mg 7 Tablets (allergy) [CONTAINS LACTOSE], Imodium® Capsules classic (diarrhoea) [CONTAINS LACTOSE], Murine® Irritation & Redness Eye Drops (eye irritation), Otex Express® (eardrops), Teva® Loratadine 10mg 30 Tablets (hayfever) [CONTAINS LACTOSE], Venos® Chesty Coughs (expectorant) and Vicks® Sinex Micromist Nasal Spray (frontal sinusitis)

It is good to know that middle-sized capsules contain 0.58g at the most, and the largest, 1.6g per piece, while tablets are usually even a little lighter. For mixtures a teaspoon holds about 5mL/g and a tablespoon 5–15mL/g. Despite your best efforts at researching your own intolerances, you may find yourself unable to stomach a medicine for whatever reason. If you are having symptoms, search for alternatives. If in doubt, use the symptom test sheet. Write down your symptoms while using it and compare it with a record of your diet taken when you were not using the medicine, for example, on your efficiency check sheet. You can use any sheet where you recorded your symptoms after refraining from bricks that you are intolerant towards.

## 2.3.7 Nutritional supplements

If you take vitamin supplements, the following examples are brick-free:

UK: HealthAid® Vitamin B Complex Supreme Capsules, HealthAid® Vitamin B12 1000ug Tablets, Bioglan® Rest and Restore Night Multivitamin For Women Tablets, Bioglan® Rest and Restore Night Multivitamin For Men Capsules.

The use of multivitamin supplements could not be shown in a long-term trial. If you take them, make sure not to take too much of certain vitamins. Vitamins that can be unsafe in excess include B3 and B6, as well as A, D, E and K, which can cause symptoms of poisoning if you overdose. It is thus recommended to discuss your intake with your doctor. One possible approach with these vitamins may be to take them in three-month cycles. That means taking them for three months and then taking the next three months off.

## 2.3.8 Positive aspects of the diet

While you restrict your intake of brick-containing foods, try to think more about what you eat and you will likely find better nutritional balance.

## 2.3.9 Testing yourself

Some of those affected by IBS reportedly struggle to absorb other ingredients like aspartame or maltodextrin. If you have reason to believe that this applies to you, follow the alternative introductory diet outlined in Chapter 2.2.6.

## 2.3.10 Protein shakes—nutrition for athletes

There is a questionable trend among athletes to take special supplements. If you are able to cover your protein demand with the products listed in Chapter 2.1.4, you have no need for protein shakes or the like. Many energy bars and electrolyte products contain sorbitol due to their processed fruit content, but you can find sorbitol-free alternatives in pharmacies. These products have their own category in this book's food tables.

## 2.3.11 Sweeteners

Unlike many other sweeteners, such as those added to "light" products like sugar-free soft drinks, pure Stevia is sorbitol-free.

## 2.3.12 Fish and meat

Breaded fish and meat, processed (such as Bolognese, bratwurst or liverwurst) or with sauce, may contain bricks. Any bricks they contain should be included in the list of ingredients. In the following chapter, you will find leaflets to keep at hand listing bricks and their safe quantities.

## 2.3.13 These actions lead to lasting change

In order to achieve lasting success, it is important that you monitor your own nutrition. If you find yourself starting to ignore the recommended amounts, you should get back on track and restart your commitment as soon as possible. Write down your goal to adapt your nutrition to the stated food and drink portion sizes to reduce abdominal discomfort and improve your quality of life. Stay conscious of the negative consequences of eating "blindly" covered in the first part of this book. Why is it important to change your habits? Reread your goal and then write down your five most important reasons for striving towards it. Moreover, answer this question for yourself: why it is important to act **now**? Inform the people close to you about why changing your nutritional habits is important—ask them to support you. Short-term change is easy. The real challenge is continuing with your dietary commitments in the long run. One way to stay motivated is to write about the positive effects on your quality of life that come from keeping your diet (annotate a calendar or jot down your thoughts daily). It also helps to work with a partner. At our homepage, www.Laxiba.co.uk/coach, you can hire a coach who guides you through the steps in this book and the change process. Furthermore, you can find people in a similar situation to yours, exchange experiences with them and motivate each other at www.Laxiba.co.uk/team

Imagine yourself living with few or no abdominal symptoms. You will have changed your diet in a way that significantly improves your wellbeing through determination and capability. The more vividly and multidimensionally you can picture what your life will be like after you have succeeded, the more likely you are to achieve that success. If you lapse slightly, relax; refocus and sort yourself out for the next day. As you continually adapt your path (like you do when using a compass), you will reach your goal in the end. If you find that this strategy helps you, you can continue to follow it for the long run.

## 2.4 The leaflets

Cut out the two leaflets on the following pages. Please fold them along the thick lines. Start with the dotted line. Then fold each leaflet again at the half-dashed line. You can now keep this important information at hand when you are out and about or shopping.

Front **Flyer for lactose, fructans & galactans**

**Non critical ingredients: lactose intolerance**

| Calcium lactate | Glucono delta-lactone | Sodium lactate |
|---|---|---|
| Lactate | Milk acid | Natriumlactat |
| Potassium lactate | (INS additive numbers: 575, 325-327) | |

**Critical ingredients: lactose intolerance**

| Lactose | Yoghurt | Whey |
|---|---|---|
| Cheese | Kefir, lassi | Milk(-powder) |
| Curd | (Concentrated) butter | Cream |

Asian, Greek, Italian and Spanish meals rather contain little lactose. Asian rice meals also containing few fructans and galactans. Fish, other seafood, meat, black coffee, eggs and oils are also free from lactose. The same holds for fruits and vegetable although some of them contain fructans and galactans.

Only copy with permission. Copyright © 2014 Henry S. Grant

Back **Lactose is often contained in:**
- cereals
- ice cream and sweets like chocolate
- coffee and milk, condensed milk
- dairy products
- breadings, sauces, puréed meat, Tzatziki
- sweet pastries like biscuits, cakes and tarts, cream

**Fructans are primarily contained in:**

artichokes, asparagus, banana, blueberries, bread, Brussels sprouts, cabbage, cauliflower, cereals, chicory root, couscous, garlic, leeks, linseeds, nectarine, noodles, onions, pastries like biscuits and cake, pineapple, pizza, products that inulin has been added to (like some cereals, chocolates and ice creams) raisins, semolina flour, shallots and sunchoke

**Galactans are primarily contained in:**

beans, lentils, linseeds, oat flakes, peas, soy products including tofu, sprouts, wheat and other grains

LAXIBA®

Interior left

## Lactose, fructans & galactans free

Apple
Apricot
Carrots
celery
Chocolate sorbet
Coconut
Drinks without milk, yoghurt etc.
Fish and
Meat
Jelly babies
Ice tea
Ketchup
Kiwi
Lettuce
Oil & vinegar
Oranges
Parmesan
Pear
Peppers
Potatoes
Rice
Spelt flour
Squash

### Lactose poor for normal portion sizes

Butter ☺; 14g
Cheddar 33¼P.; 30g
Fondue sauce ☺; 53g
Margarine 21¾P.; 9g
Nutella ®32¼P.; 37g
Parmesan ☺; 5g
Swiss cheese ☺; 30g

Per strong lactase capsule you take in, you can stomach about 75% more of each shown portion amount:

### Portion unit shown as

| Exemplar | Cup | Glas | Portion | Slice |
|---|---|---|---|---|
| E | C | G | P | S |

☹=avoid; ☹²=1/4 unit at TL2; ☺=contains traces; ☻=is free of it

### Calculation of the remaining TL-portions

| | | | |
|---|---|---|---|
| **Lactose (TL1)** | L0 = ÷2 | L2 = x2 | L3 = x3 |
| **Fru-/Galactans (TL0)** | L1 = x2 | L2 = x4 | L3 = x6 |

Only copy with permission. Copyright © 2014 Henry S. Grant

Interior right

## High amount of lactose

Cacao ¼C.; 150g
Casserole ½P.; 238g
Cheese-sauce ¼P.; 66g
Condensed milk ½P
Creme-soup ½P.; 245g
Kefir ¼P.; 220g
Mashed-potatoe ½P.; 140g
Milk rice ¼P.; 107g 200g
Milk ¼G.; 200g
Mozzarella 9¾P.; 30g
Pan cake ½P.; 187g
Tart ½P.; 87,5g
Yoghurt ¼P.; 250g

## F+G TL 0 portions

Apple strudel ¾ P., 64g
Asparagus ½P., 85g
Baguette 1¾S., 42g
Banana juice ½G., 200g
Granola bar ½P., 27g
Hamburger ½E., 100g
Hot dog ¼E., 199g
Kidney beans ¼P., 90g
Sandwich ☹
Shalot ¼E., 15g

Cake ¼P., 122g
Calzone ¼P., 168g
Cheese cake ☹P., 220g
Chop Suey ¼P., 166g
Cookie ½E., 45g
Corn Flakes 1½P., 30g
Couscous ¼P., 140g
Cracker ¼P., 30g
Crêpe ¾E., 55g
Crispbread ¼S., 42g
Danish pastry ¼E., 125g
Donut ½E., 105g
French toast ¼ P., 131g
Leeks ¼P., 89g
Lentils ¾P., 90g
Muesli ¼P., 55g
Muffin ¼E., 113g
Noodles 1P., 140g
Oat bran 1¼P., 55g
Onion Rings ¼P., 70g
Peas 1¼P., 15g
Pizza ½P., 209g
Plain dumplings ½P., 55g
Ravioli ¼P., 250g
Rye bread ¾S., 42g
Sandwich-cookie 3½E., 14,5g
Snow peas ¾P., 85g
Spring roll ¼P., 140g
Tofu ½P., 85g
Waffles ½P., 95g
White wholegrain wheat bread ¾S., 42g

## Flyer for fructose and sorbitol

### Non problematic ingredients: sorbitol intolerance

| Maltodextrin | Sorbic acid | Barley malt sirup |
|---|---|---|
| Sodium sorbate | Potassium sorbate | Calcium sorbate |
| Sorbitan... | Polyoxyethylene (20) -sorbitan-... | |

(INS add. numbers: 200-203, 432-436, 491-495)

### Problematic ingredients: sorbitol intolerance

| Sorbitol | Mannitol | Xylitol |
|---|---|---|
| Lactitol | (Ethyl-) Maltol | Hexanhexol |
| Glucitol | Maltitol/-Syrup | Inositol |
| Isomalt | Palatinit® | Sionon |
| Erythritol | Pinitol | |

(INS add. numbers: 420-21, 636-37, 953, 965-7)

Only copy with permission. Copyright © 2014 Henry S. Grant

---

## Find further tools at www.Laxiba.co.uk

**Caution... free fructose is contained in:**
- cereals with high fructose corn syrup (HFCS)
- many convenience foods
- jam sugar, honey and corn syrup
- some sweeteners
- many fruit, dry fruit and juices
- many soft drinks and alcoholic beverages

**Sugar alcohols are often contained in:**
- sausages, fish and meat that is puréed, pickled or has a breading
- convenience foods and readymade sauces
- chewing gums and mints, except for those that are only sweetened with Stevia. only traces of sorbitol are contained in: Wrigley's® Spearmint, Doublemint and Juicy Fruit®
- some sugar free, and isotonic beverages
- medicine and mouth hygiene products
- electrolyte products and energy bars
- bars, pralines, sweet pastries, tart, even readymade cream
- diabetic, dietary products

**LAXIBA®**

Interior left

Apple F:☹; S☹²;E 182g
Apricot F:D +¾ P; S¾;E 35g
Bals. vinegar F:D; S23;P 15,94g
Banana F:D +¼ P.; S9¼;E 118g
Beer F50; S10;G 200ml
Big Mac ®F5; S6½;E 215g
Bitter Lemon F☹; S:D;G 200ml
Blackberries F3¾; S:D;P 140g
Blueberry
Muffin F:D;S:D;E113g
Broccoli F3; S:D;P 85g
Cauliflower F:D; S2½;P 85g

Cinnamon Toast
Crunch ®F¼; S:D;P 30g
Coca Cola ®F½; S:D;G 200ml

Corn flakes F:D +1½ P.; S☺, 30g
Cranberries F:D +2¾ P.; S45¼;P 55g
Fiber One Original ®F41½; S:D;P 30g
Garden salad F8¼; S16¾;P85g
Ginger ale F☹; S:D;G 200ml
Lettuce F8¼; S16¾;P 85g
Oat bran F:D; S:D;P 55g
Pears F½; S¼;E 15g

Pickles F4¾; S1;E 85g
Pineapple F¾; S¾;P 140g
Strawberries F½; S¼;P 140g

**Portion unit shown as**

| Exemplar | Cup | Glas | Portion | Slice |
|---|---|---|---|---|
| E | C | G | P | S |

☹=avoid; ☹²=1/4 unit at TL2; ☺=contains traces; ☻=is free of it

**Portion amounts for fructose (F) and sorbitol (S)**

| | | | |
|---|---|---|---|
| **Fructose (TL 0)** | L1 = x2 | L2 = x4 | L3 = x5 |
| **Sorbitol (TL 1)** | L0 = x0 | L2 = x4 | L3 = x10 |

Only copy with permission. Copyright © 2014 Henry S. Grant

Interior right

7UP ®F☹; S:D;G 200ml
Black current F1; S:D;P 140g
Cabbage F:D +¾ P.; S58;P 85g
Champagne F31¼; S¾;G200ml
Cherries F10; S½;L 15g
Chicken, s.n's. F2½; S☺;L 15g
Chocolate F:D; S48; P 25g
Coffee F:D; S:D;T 150g
Granola bar F:D +4¼ P.; S71¼;E 35g

Grapes F¼; S½;P 140g
Honey Smacks ®F:D +12 P.;

S83¼;P 30g

Honey F½; S1¾;L 15g
Ketchup F:D +¼ P.; S3¾;L 15g
Kiwi F1; S:D;E 86g
Lemon F:D; S:D;E 58g
Long island icetea F¾; S16½;G 200ml

M & M's ®F:D; S:D;P 40g
Mango F1; S4;L 15g
Mate-Tee F:D; S:D;G 200ml
Mayo F:D; S:D;P 15g
Melon F1; S14¼;P 140g
Milk F:D; S:D;G 200ml

Mushroom F:D +¼ P.; S¾;L 15g
Nectarine F8¼; S1;L 15g
Noodles F:D +¼ P.; S:D;P 140g
Oranges F2¼; S:D;E 140g
Peach F:D +½ P.; S¼;E 140g
Peppers F½; S:D;E 85g
Pepsi ®F½; S:D;J 200g
Pizza F:D +¾ P.; S¾;E 209g
Plums F:D +¼ P.; S¾;E 15g
Popsicle F:D +1¼ P.; S:D;P52g
Potatoes F:D; S45¼;P 110g
Raspberry F½; S1½;P 140g

Red Bull ®F:D +7¾P.;S:D;G200ml
Rice F:D; S:D;P 140g
Sauerkraut F:D; S¾;L 15g
Squash, bttrnt F:D; S:D;P 130g
Sugar free
Chewinggums F¼; S☹²;E 2g
Sushi F:D; S1½;P 140g
Tomatoes F4½; S1;E 85g
Tonic Water ®F☹; S:D;G 200ml
Wheat bread F¾; S26¼;S 42g
Whopper ®F2¾; S1;E 315g
Winegum F:D+12 P; S:D;P30g
Wine F31¼; S¾;G 200ml

## 2.4.1 Fructose and sugar alcohols

If you have a fructose intolerance, be mindful of fructose and HFCS while reading through ingredient lists. To determine sorbitol-free products, however, you unfortunately have to navigate an unbelievable muddle of identifiers, despite the high prevalence of the condition:[9]

| Noncritical ingredients for sorbitol intolerance[10] | | |
|---|---|---|
| Maltodextrin | Sorbic acid | Barley malt syrup |
| Sodium sorbate | Potassium sorbate | Calcium sorbate |
| Sorbitan... | Polyoxyethylene (20) -sorbitan-... | |

| Critical ingredients for sorbitol intolerance[11] | | |
|---|---|---|
| Sorbitol | Mannitol | Xylitol |
| Lactitol | (Ethyl-) Maltol | Hexanhexol |
| Glucitol | Maltitol/-syrup | Inositol |
| Isomalt | Palatinit® | Sionon |
| Erythritol | Pinitol | |

---

[9] There is an immediate need for simplification here. The declaration "critical in case of a sorbitol intolerance" would spare many efforts.
[10] INS additive (E-)numbers: 200–203, 432–436, 491–495.
[11] INS additive (E-)numbers: 420–21, 636–37, 953, 965–67.

# Caution...

## Free fructose is contained in:

- Unknown quantities in cereals with high fructose corn syrup (HFCS) or isoglucose, glucose-fructose syrup, fructose-glucose syrup and high fructose maize syrup, unless listed in the food tables of this book
- Many convenience foods
- Preserving sugar
- Honey and corn syrup (fructose quantity is unclear)
- Some sweeteners
- Many fruits, dried fruits, juices and alcoholic drinks
- Many soft drinks

## Sugar alcohols like sorbitol are also often contained in:

- Diabetic and dietary products
- Electrolyte products and energy bars
- Convenience foods and prepared sauces
- Chewing gums and mints, except those sweetened only with Stevia, for example. Traces of sorbitol are found in Wrigley's® Spearmint, Doublemint and Juicy Fruit
- Some "light," i.e., sugar free, and isotonic beverages
- Medicine and oral hygiene products
- Bars, pralines, sweet pastries, tarts, prepared cream
- Puréed, pickled or breaded sausages, fish and meat

Moreover, some fruits (like apples, apricots, bananas, cantaloupe, carambola, cherries, cranberries, grapes, guava, lowbush cranberries, mango, nectarine, peach, pear, pinapple, plum, pomegranate, raspberries, strawberries and watermelon) and vegetables (artichoke, asparagus, beets, cabbage, carrots, cauliflower, celeriac, celery, chestnuts, chicory, coleslaw, cucumber, eggplant, endive, fennel bulb, garbanzo beans (chickpeas), kale, kohlrabi, leeks, lettuce (boston), lettuce (green leaf), lettuce (iceberg), lettuce (red leaf), lettuce (romaine), mushrooms, olives, onions, pickled beets, radish, sauerkraut, sour pickles, soybean sprouts, spinach, tempeh, tomatoes and turnip), including juices contain sorbitol. Many alcoholic beverages do, as well, but brandy, gin, rum and whiskey for example, are often sorbitol-free.

## 2.4.2 Fructans, galactans and lactose[12]

| Noncritical ingredients for lactose intolerance | | |
|---|---|---|
| Calcium lactate | Glucono delta-lactone | Sodium lactate |
| Lactate | Lactic acid | Potassium lactate |
| **Critical ingredients for lactose intolerance** | | |
| Lactose | Yogurt | Whey |
| Cheese | Kefir, lassi | Milk (-powder) |
| Curd | (Concentrated) butter | Cream |

Asian, Greek, Italian and Spanish meals tend not to contain much lactose. Asian rice-based dishes are also low in fructans and galactans. Fish and seafood, meat, black coffee, eggs and oils are also lactose-free, as are fruits and vegetables, although some contain fructans and galactans.

## Caution…:

## Lactose is also contained in:

- Coffee with milk or condensed milk
- Cream
- Many cereals
- Many types of ice cream, chocolate and other candy
- Some breads and sauces
- Some sausages
- Sweet pastries like biscuits, cakes and tarts
- Tzatziki

---

[12] INS additive (E-)numbers: 575, 325-327.

## High amounts of fructans are found in:

- Artichokes
- Asparagus
- Bananas
- Blueberries
- Brussels sprouts
- Cabbage
- Cauliflower
- Cereals
- Chicory root
- Couscous
- Linseeds
- Garlic
- Jerusalem artichokes
- Leeks
- Nectarines
- Noodles
- Onions
- Pastries and biscuits, breads and cakes
- Pineapple
- Pizza
- Products that inulin has been added to, such as some cereals, chocolate and ice cream
- Raisins
- Semolina flour
- Shallots

## High amounts of galactans are found in:

- Beans
- Linseeds
- Lentils
- Oats
- Peas
- Soy products, including tofu
- Sprouts
- Wheat and other grains

# 2.4.3 The safe products list

| Fruit | Vegetables | Warm dishes |
|---|---|---|
| Blackberries | Avocado, green | Brandy vinegar |
| Currants | Basil | Caviar |
| Dates, fresh | Chard | Chinese oyster sauce |
| Figs, fresh | Chives | Fish, meat, shrimp and shellfish* |
| Goji berries | Coriander | |
| Lemon zest | Green peppers | Kraft® Italian Dressing |
| Loganberry | Horseradish | |
| Papaya | Kelp | Kraft® Mayonnaise |
| Passion fruit | Oregano | Oils |
| Rhubarb | Parsnips | Kraft® Thousand Island Dressing® |
| | Peppermint, fresh | |
| | Rice | Pepper and salt |
| | Rosemary | Rice bread |
| | Rutabaga | Rice noodles |
| | Squash: Butternut, calabash, giant and spaghetti | Soy oil |
| | Thyme | Spelt flour |
| | Yam | Tabasco® sauce |

*Non puréed and without breading and sauce.

| Beverages | Others | |
|---|---|---|
| Black coffee | Baking powder | Pecan nuts |
| Brandy | Brazil nuts | Pine nuts |
| Gin | Brown sugar | Pistachios |
| Jasmine tea | Cashews | Pumpkin seeds |
| Maté tea | Coconut | Rice bread |
| Peppermint tea | Gelatin | Spelt |
| Rum | Ginkgo | Walnuts |
| Tequila | Liquorice | White sugar |
| Tonic Water | Macadamia nuts | |
| Vodka | Maple syrup | |
| Water | Peanut butter | |
| Whisky | Peanuts | |

*This page has been intentionally left blank.*

# 2.5 For hosts

There will be someone in your circle of friends who has IBS or an intolerance towards one or more ingredients. Of course, as a host, you want to be considerate to your guests. In order to offer some suitable food options, ask whether anyone has an intolerance. This will give your guests a good impression, as you are demonstrating that their needs are important to you. Cut out the two leaflets from the preceding chapter. You can find therein the tolerable portions of a number of common foods. If one or more guests has a sorbitol intolerance, please ensure you cook sorbitol-containing ingredients separately.

Generally, you should be fine if you offer: black coffee, cheddar, corn flakes, eggs, fish and meat (non-breaded and without prepared sauce), French fries, kiwis, lettuce, lemons, margarine (not butter), nuts, oil with oregano, pepper and salt (as an alternative to sauce), oranges, peas, potatoes, rice, rice milk, salted popcorn, salted crisps, spinach, Stevia, sugar, tomatoes and water. Most herbs and spices, except for garlic and onions, are harmless. Adjusting to suit affected guests is actually quite straightforward. Just serve the tolerable foods separately from any sauces, garlic and onions, e.g., by using separate bowls for potatoes, butter, salad and dressing.

# 2.6 Stress management

Stress can affect your stomach and worsen irritable bowel symptoms. Hence, it is important to reduce it. Developing a solution-orientated way to manage your own worries can help you do so. How does that help? The more you stress over something, the more brain areas that are required for a reasonable decision are being set off. This happens, because in a certain way, our bodies are prepared for an earlier historical era. Dangerous situations like being attacked by a wolf pack left us with three options: fight, flight or playing dead. If we spent too much time thinking in such a situation, it was game over!

Now, completely different factors cause us to worry. In addition to such everyday concerns like air pollution, extreme temperatures and noise, many people worry about losing control over a situation. If you start to worry, fight and flight reactions are supported by the release of hormones that enable us to make quick, even if ill-conceived, decisions. Large parts of our brain are set aside for that purpose. You feel stress and tend to rather make impulsive then rational decisions. The third option your brain conceives in a dangerous situation, playing dead, somewhat corresponds to the extreme modern-day phenomena that is widely known as burnout.

You don't want to overreact or give up on your responsibilities and play dead like a hyena, so you need to maintain control of your body and mind. Appropriate actions in everyday life depend on rational thinking; this may require preventive measures. Once your body feels like it's in danger it is difficult to abruptly halt the rolling wheel of your body's emergency reactions. Yoga and progressive muscle relaxation before work are useful stress preventers. Using such techniques before going to work is sensible as it is seldom possible to take an hour off during the work day. Breaks and disruptions during your working hours are also **counterproductive** if you are dealing with complex tasks; they often lead to poor decisions, more stress and a short temper. Thus, try to avoid disruption when dealing with sophisticated tasks. However, interruptions of simple mental or physical labor lasting a few minutes, rather than seconds, are shown to offer slight positive effects. Taking breaks from hard physical labor, meanwhile, show even stronger benefits, lowering the risk of injuries and enhancing endurance.

Still, relaxation alone might not be the solution. Often, you can identify the source of your fears; when you are in the habit of regularly acknowledging the deeper causes of your stress, you will be able to deal with them and develop appropriate solutions that allow you to manage risks and arrive at your goals. By doing so, you can even use your fears—through the process of conquering them—to help you become more successful in your everyday life. Sit down at a quiet desk at the beginning or end of the day. Next, think about what you are worried about right now and which steps you need to take to prevent the feared outcomes.

It is helpful to create an Excel spreadsheet for doing so or to purchase the standardized and printer-optimized PaceAce-Version at a reasonable price at www.Laxiba.co.uk. If you want to create the table by yourself, call the first sheet "Worries" and the second one "Task List." Next, write down the following task headings in the first spreadsheet: "Current Worries," "Preventive measure A," "Preventive measure B" and "Preventive measure C." Then enter the following column titles in the second spreadsheet: "Task," "Priority," "Deadline," "Who does it?" and "Done."

You should write down your concerns in the first column of the first sheet. Then, think about what you'll need to do to prevent these worries from being realized. Think of three alternatives for each outcome. Enter these into the "Preventive measure A–C" fields next to each worry, A being the action you want to take first. Then, transfer "Preventive measure A" to the "Task List" sheet. Next, prioritize the tasks by employing an adapted version of the "Eisenhower method," an organization technique that takes importance and urgency into account, from A to E:

| Task is important | Action now | Better done soon |
|---|---|---|
| Task is unimportant | Chance for completion after everything important has been done. | Dull moment task |
| Efface (don't do) task | **Task is urgent** | **Task can be postponed** |

Carry out your daily tasks in order from A to D. The category E is for tasks that are ineffective and therefore, you leave it. Hence, you minimize stress over whether you are doing the right thing from moment to moment. After assessing the tasks from A to D, fill out the "Deadline" column, entering the date by which you want to accomplish the task. Additionally, either note "I" or the name of the person that you want to delegate the task to in the column "Who does it?". Finally, check off the cell in the column "Done" when you have finished the task.

Another important aspect is keeping your life balanced. This means that instead of delivering an over-the-top performance in one area but lousy results in all others, you want to do at least a satisfying job in all areas, in order to remain capable in the long run. Which of the family, spare time, relaxation and work quadrants are important is up to you, along with the results you're aiming for with them, such as spending time with those closest to you, taking daily walks, pursuing your hobbies and getting your work done properly. Furthermore, it is important to resist basing your success on external measures. You should nourish a healthy self-confidence and serenity in yourself. This also means knowing when the task you are doing has been done well enough. Some people get into time trouble because they over-deliver on some tasks and then have little time left to take care of other important tasks, which then causes stress.

| Family: | Relaxation: |
|---|---|
| Spend time with those closest to you | Go out for a walk on a daily basis |
| Spare time: | Work: |
| Pursue your hobbies regularly | Get your work done properly |

You can measure your progress with regard to the four quadrants on a monthly basis on a scale of 1 (very good) to 7 (very poor). Always assign 7 points to the area that you're happiest with and other numbers to the remaining quadrants in relation to that one. Afterward, consider whether you want to make any changes to how you're approaching these areas of your life and how you can make those changes. You can also use the spreadsheet you created to manage your worries.

One final point on the topic of stress: be mindful of your mood, and try to stay positive! What you need to do that depends on you. Sometimes simply deciding to be in a good mood can do more than most people realize. Everyone has a load of problems to carry, and it's easier to carry it if you commit yourself to a positive outlook.

Do things that excite you as often as possible. Plan your activities around what is most important to you in your life. What that means is obviously personal to you! It is your treasure, per se, so you have to dig it out yourself. Abraham Lincoln had this to say, to send you on your way: "That some achieve great success is proof to all that others can achieve it as well."

## 2.7 General summary

### 1. What you are dealing with

Do you have an intolerance and/or symptoms? Then your bowel is easily irritated by certain substances in food called "bricks." Problems develop when your body doesn't intercept such bricks before they can cause symptoms. With a brick in your belly, you are carrying a burden. It is often a chronic condition, but it does not cause cancer. In most cases, the symptoms can be reduced to an acceptable level if you follow an appropriate diet.

### 2. Are you a special case?

According to the World Gastroenterology Organisation (WGO), up to one billion people worldwide are affected by a dietary intolerance. In a way, you are lucky, as you can use this book to help you to reduce your symptoms.

### 3. Good reasons to follow this diet

An intolerance accompanies you for a long time, maybe even for the rest of your life. If the diet works, it is far cheaper than medical treatment and can sometimes be even more effective. Many medicines also have side effects. By examining different bricks one by one, you can find the one(s) that your body cannot tolerate. The level test will help you learn how to eat as freely as possible while continuing to gain nutritional benefits. You learn, as well, how to balance your diet despite reducing the consumption of certain foods. If the diet works for you, it will also lead to a general improvement in your well-being. You should find that you are ill less often, better able to concentrate, better at fulfilling social obligations, stronger at sports—your new diet can even positively affect your sex drive! Start today with the first LAXIBA® step: get the ball rolling by tracking your symptoms for four days using the symptom test sheet (page 51).

## 4. This is why you want to take the level test

Tolerance thresholds are different for everyone. The more bricks you are able to eat, the fewer restrictions you will face in your everyday diet. You might save yourself effort and be able to enjoy a more varied selection of food.

## 5. What you should pay attention to for the diet

Two things: First, keep your TLs by restricting your portion sizes accordingly. This means that you only eat as much of the bricks as your stomach can handle. If you do not consume any bricks, you will lose your ability to handle your interception shield well (see Chapter 1.5), and you will be back at square one. Second, eat in a balanced way by consuming fats, fibre and proteins each day (see Chapter 2.1.4).

## 6. The last trump of the vexed brick dragon

It is important that you really want the changes this book can help you achieve. Your first step is thus to understand that applying a working solution is going to help you lead a better life. If you recognize how the improvements in your diet relate to attaining your heartfelt ambitions, you will be more motivated to keep going, even if you face setbacks. This is a strategic plan, not an overnight miracle cure!

It may help you to set a time each Sunday to fill out the symptom test sheet—independent of the other tests. This will remind you of your goal and let you break down the necessary steps towards it on a weekly basis. What is also important is that you become aware of the hurdles you will face. It will be hard to restrict yourself with regard to the consumption of some foods that you have come to love. Especially at the beginning, it will be unnerving to ask for dietary considerations as a dinner guest. Your nutrition plan will be new to others; you may feel criticized for your insistence on maintaining your new eating habits. Explain that you need to do it for the sake of your health. At the same time, express your appreciation for others' support. Moreover, try not give dietary advice unless you are asked for it—respect the eating habits of others. This makes them more likely to accept yours.

The brick-eating dragons are betting on one last card: the influence of your old habits. They usually creep in after you have kept your new diet for a few days. It happens when you have started to feel better and become less alert to the dangers! Use your suggested weekly check as a countermeasure. It reminds you of your plan. Keep to it and it will help ensure your brick dragon cannot further agonize you. Take it easy. If you keep realigning your nutritional habits with your goals, you will get closer and closer to achieving them in the long run.

## 7. Are there hints for general nutrition?

Drink at least 1.5L of water every day. Eat a variety of foods. Even if you are lactose intolerant, you can try to eat dry cheese (for example) in order to cover your need for short-chain fatty acids. If you are a vegan, you should plan your protein intake, and consider your fiber consumption, if you are restricting your fructan and galactan intake. In addition to following your TL portion sizes and taking in linseeds or rice bran and a handful of nuts, you might also like to eat beans, lentils, peas and so forth: it is ok to eat foods that contain bricks; they can even be good for you, as long as you keep within your TL restrictions. To do even more for your health, work out regularly.

**What can you do if a fruit juice contains too many bricks to drink a regular glass full?** By diluting it with water you can multiply your tolerable portion.

**How can you save on cooking time?** Cook larger portion sizes. This only takes a little longer than smaller portions, and warming the food up is quick. Rice and potatoes, for instance, can be kept in the fridge for days. Purchase lockable glass containers to store your food keeping it fresh longer.

**If** you are suffering **acute symptoms**, take a walk and drink up to three liters of drinking water per day.

# 8. The LAXIBA® quickie

**Fructans & Galactans:** Eat fewer beans, lentils, peas and grain products, such as pastries and noodles.

**Fructose (& Sorbitol):** Avoid apple and peach juices and drink orange juice instead, for example. Be careful with soft drinks.

**Lactose:** Reduce your consumption of milk or use replacement products such as rice milk. Dry cheese like cheddar contains only a little lactose.

**Sorbitol:** Be wary of diabetic, diet and light products, as well as dried fruit.

# 3

# FOOD TABLES

## 3.1 Introduction to the tables

In the following section, you will learn about the tolerable portion sizes according to your TL for lactose, fructose, and the sum of nine sugar alcohols, fructans and galactans. The statements all relate to **one meal**, assuming **three meals** per day, consumed at roughly 7am, 1pm and 7pm, i.e., each with a **gap** of about **six hours**. (However, this is mainly just a reference point to align your consumption amounts with. You do not have to change your meal times!)

First, you find the lists are ordered by category. Juices are found under fast beverages, for example. Alternatively, you can use the alphabetical keyword index, e.g., if you are solely interested in finding the tolerable portion size of an orange juice. The sizes are shown next to the foods in the tables. In the **category tables,** the portions are based on the following TLs, which have been chosen according to the brick amounts for each level: **lactose: TL 1; fructose (with or without sorbitol adjustment): TL 0 (BTL); sorbitol: TL 0 and 1; fructans and galactans: TL 0 and TL1.** In the **alphabetical keyword index**, which begins after the **category tables**, only the sorbitol-adjusted fructose is shown at TL 0 and TL 1. In the first row of each table, you will find the multipliers to determine the portion size for the other three levels.

## 3.1.1 Your personal tolerance levels

Cross out all bricks that you are able to stomach without restrictions in the table below. The first column lists the bricks. The following columns list the TLs (the higher your TL, the less sensitive you are despite your intolerance towardss products that contain the respective brick) and the respective threshold amounts per meal. In the last two columns you should enter, in pencil, the TL that applies to you—before having done the level test this is the BTL, i.e., TL 0. The table is pretty much self-explanatory. In the field "combined TL" you should enter the TL you are able to stomach in combination with other bricks. In the field "single TL" you should enter the highest TL for the brick as you keep the BTLs of the remaining bricks.

| Brick | TL | g | Combined TL | Single TL |
|---|---|---|---|---|
| Free fructose g/meal | 0 | 0.5 | | |
| | 1 | 1 | | |
| | 2 | 2 | | |
| | 3 | 3 | | |
| Free sorbitol adjusted fructose g/meal | 0 | 0.5 | | |
| | 1 | 1 | | |
| | 2 | 2 | | |
| | 3 | 3 | | |
| Lactose g/meal | 0 | 1.5 | | |
| | 1 | 3 | | |
| | 2 | 6 | | |
| | 3 | 9 | | |
| Sorbitol and other sugar alcohols g/meal | 0 | 0 | | |
| | 1 | 0.1 | | |
| | 2 | 0.4 | | |
| | 3 | 0.7 | | |
| Fructans and galactans g/meal | 0 | 0.5 | | |
| | 1 | 1 | | |
| | 2 | 2 | | |
| | 3 | 3 | | |

# 3.1.2 Explanation of the abbreviations

## Overview

Here you can see an excerpt of a category table. The pattern for it is: "How many bananas/burgers/etc. can I eat per meal if I have an intolerance toward fructose/lactose/sorbitol (i.e. sugar alcohols) and/or fructans and galactans?"

| Food category name[a] | Unit[b] | Lactose[c] ↳ + Unit/⊂▶[c] | Fructose*[d] ↳ Fructose[d] ↳ | Sorbitol[e] ↳ Sorbitol[e] ↳ | Fruc/Galacta.[f] ↳📖 Fruc/Galacta.[f] ↳ |
|---|---|---|---|---|---|
| Baguette, wheat | slice(s) 1.49oz/42g | ☺ | ☺ ☺ | ☺ ☺ | ×1¾ [A] ×3½ |
| Grasshopper (drink) | glass(es) 8.4oz.fl/240mL | ×1¼[g] + ×1 unit[g] | ☺+ ×1¼ unit[h] ☺+ ×1½ unit[h] | ☹[i] ×¾ | ×7 ×14 |
| Red wine vinegar | tablespoon(s) 0.5oz.fl/14.8mL | ☺ | ☺[j] ☺[j] | ☹ ×20 | ☺ ☺ |

↳ Level 0[k]: lactose measure ×½
↳ Level 1[k]: fructose measure ×2
↳ Level 2[k]: fructose-/sorbitol measure ×4. the rest ×2
↳ Level 3[k]: sorbitol measure ×7. the rest ×3
📖: source of fruc/galactans data

+ Unit/⊂▶: added tolerated amount of unit per strong lactase capsule
Fructose*: fructose, sorbitol adjusted
☺+ ×[Amount] unit: Per unit consumed you can additionally tolerate up to [amount] × fructose(*)-unit of another product.

☹: avoid;  ☹¹: ¼ at TL 1;  ☹²: ¼ at TL 2;  ☹³: ¼ at TL 3;  ☺: only contains traces;  ☺: is free from it

## Explanation

| | |
|---|---|
| a | Category of the foods that are listed below. |
| b | The measurement unit that the measures in the ingredient columns relate to. Below you find the gram amount of that measurement unit. The measure is the number with which you have to multiply the measurement unit in order to determine the respective portion size that applies to you. |
| c | Lactose ↳ = Here you can find the tolerable lactose measures at TL (tolerance level) 1. Your TL for lactose refers to your sensitivity toward lactose if you are lactose intolerant. Apart from the basic tolerance level (BTL), TL 0, the TLs 1 to 3 may apply. The higher your TL, the less sensitive you are towardss products containing lactose, despite your intolerance, and the higher portion sizes you can tolerate of such products.<br>+ unit/⊂▶: Additionally tolerated measure per strong lactase capsule you |

| | |
|---|---|
| | take (only applicable to the restrictionts from the lactose content). |
| d | Fructose*↯ = Measure for free fructose with adjustment for the effect of sorbitol on the fructose absorption at TL 0.<br>Fructose↯ = Free fructose without adjustment for sorbitol at TL 0. |
| e | Sorbitol = Amounts if you have a sugar alcohol (sorbitol) intolerance above (↯) at TL 0 and below (↯) at TL 1. |
| f | Fruc/Galacta. = Tolerable amounts in case of a fructan and galactan malabsorbtion. Above (↯) at TL 0 and below (↯) at TL 1. If there is a letter in the column to the right, then it identifies the source for the shown amount. Otherwise, the amount is estimated based on the amount of lactose contained in the food and therefore refers to the minimum quantity of fructans and galactans contained in the food. |
| g | 1¼ = 250mL of the drink is tolerated even for a lactose intolerance at TL 0, as the statement is related to a 200mL glass (1.25 × 200mL = 250mL).<br>+ 1 unit/⌾ = For each lactase capsule taken, one further 200mL glass can be stomached, as this is the measurement unit here. |
| h | ☺+ ×[number] unit = More glucose than fructose is contained in the food. Hence, you can tolerate the product in case of fructose intolerance. What is more, due to the "neutralizing" effect of glucose on fructose (see Chapter 1.5.2), per consumed unit you will tolerate up to [number] times the TL 0 fructose amount of another food. For example, for a "grasshopper," 1¼× the fructose measure of another food can be additionally tolerated if the other food is consumed simultaneously. For safety you should halve the amount. |
| i | ☹ = Avoid the food when keeping TL 0 for sugar alcohols. |
| j | ☺ = You can stomach over 90 times the stated measurement unit.<br>☺ = The food is free of the respective brick. |
| k | Multipliers to calculate the portions, if a tolerance level other than the one named in the column header applies to you. If you want to determine the measure of lactose for a "grasshopper" for tolerance level (TL) 0, multiply the 1¼ with ½, which is about ½. Hence, you can tolerate half a glass, i.e., 100mL. |

**Note:** Please always consider the ingredients stated on packages, as well, as the composition may vary, especially for non-brand name products. You can find a guide to portion sizes and lactose content in fish and meat products at the end of Chapter 3.5.3 under the heading "Lactose hideouts."

# Table columns

| | |
|---|---|
| Unit | Measurement unit for foods. |
| Lactose +unit/⊙ | In the upper section you will find the amount of a **unit** that you can stomach if you have a lactose intolerance at TL 1.<br>In the lower section you will find the amount you will be able to additionally consume per strong (~12.000 FCC[13]) lactase capsule you take: +[number] unit, i.e., additional portion per capsule (this refers only to a lactose restriction). |
| Fructose* | Amount per **unit** that is tolerated in a fructose intolerance at TL 0, where the amount of sorbitol in the food is considered. In the keyword table, you will also find the **fructose*** amounts that apply for **fructose*** at TL 1.<br>Here you partially find the special labeling "☺+ ×[amount] unit," which means that the food contains more glucose than fructose. Thus, in the case of **simultaneous consumption** of one **unit** of the "☺+ ×[amount] unit" food, up to the stated [number] times the respective measure of a food that is restricted due to fructose can be additionally tolerated at TL 0. If for ice cream the **fructose*** cell states "☺+ ×3 unit," for example, then that means that you are now able to tolerate ¼ plus 3 × ¼, thus, up to a whole portion of **unit** of grapes, whose normally tolerable **fructose*** portion is limited to ¼ of **unit**, if you eat them simultaneously with the ice cream (simultaneously means that you chew both foods at the same time in your mouth). For safety, halve the stated "☺+ ×[number] unit" amount.<br>If a higher TL applies to you, you have to **divide** the ☺+ ×[number] unit" amount by the respective multiplier indicated in Chapter 3.1.3, as at a higher TL the **portions** are commensurably **larger**. For example, assume that your TL for **fructose*** is TL 2 and you read in the TL 1 row for **fructose*** in the Keyword Index that "+☺ +3¾ unit" applies to one apricot. The TL 2 multiplier of **fructose*** is 2. When you divide 3¾ by the multiplier 2, this is roughly 1¾. At TL 2 you can stomach one portion of grapes. If you eat an apricot at the same time, you can then stomach 1 portion plus 1¾ × 1, hence, 2¾ portions of grapes. |

---

[13] Food Chemical Codex, measurement unit for enzymes.

| | |
|---|---|
| Fructose | Amount per **unit in case of** fructose intolerance without consideration of the contained sorbitol for TL 0. Here you will also find the special labeling "☺+ ×[number] unit" explained above. Important: **Fructose** is only shown in the category tables and there at the bottom. |
| Sorbit | Amount per **unit** for a sorbitol (i.e., sugar alcohol) intolerance, above at TL 0 and below at TL 1. |
| Fruc/Gala ctans | Amount per **unit** for a fructans and galactans malabsorption, above at TL 0 and below at TL 1. |
| 📖 | Source upon which **fructans and galactans** calculations were based. If the field is **empty**, the indications are estimates based on the amount of lactose and thus are **less reliable**. |

# More elaborate explanation

In the **unit** column, beside the food name, you will find the portion measurement unit that applies to that food. The list of measurement units can be found at the top of this page. Below each measurement unit, you will also find the rough weight of a **unit.** In the columns to the right of **unit** you can find out how many **unit**s you can tolerate per meal dependent on which intolerance applies to you:

In the **Lactose** column you can find the tolerated amount of **unit** for tolerance level (TL) 1 and, below, the additionally consumable amount **unit** for each strong lactase capsule you take.

The **Fructose\*/Fructose** column shows you the tolerable amount in case you are fructose intolerant. At the top you will find the maximum portion size when the amount of sorbitol contained in the food is taken into consideration (**Fructose\*** shows the tolerable amount of **unit** due to the contained fructose and sorbitol in the product). Here, the amount of sorbitol is added to the amount of free fructose, and the portion is determined with regard to the TL of free fructose (see Chapter 1.5.2). In the category tables, the stated **Fructose\*** amounts refer to TL 0. In the keyword lists you will also find the **Fructose\*** TL 1 amounts below. In the category tables, however, below the **Fructose\*** TL 0 amounts you will find the TL 0 amounts for free fructose (**Fructose**) without taking sorbitol into account.

The **Sorbitol** column contains the amount of **unit** that holds if you have an intolerance toward sorbitol. The statement is based on the sum of nine sugar alcohols contained in the food, including sorbitol.

The **Fruc/Galactans** column shows the tolerable amount of **unit** that results from the sum of fructans and galactans. At the top, you will see the amount that applies to TL 0 and at the bottom the one for TL 1. The column "📖" refers to the source on which the calculation of the amount of **unit** for **fructan and galactan malabsorption** is based on, if any.[14] If **no source** is **listed**, the estimate is based on the amount of **lactose**[15] a food contains. In that case, concrete study results regarding the amount of fructans and galactans are not available for the respective food; the listed amount is less certain.

---

[14] A stands for Biesiekierski et al., 2011; B for Muir et al., 2009; C for Muir et al., 2007, D for Shepherd and Gibson, 2006, E for van Loo et al., 1995 and F for Muir et al., 2007, Van Loo et al., 1995, and G for Monash University, 2014.

[15] Balasubramanya, Sarwar, & Narayanan, 1993; Jensen, Blanc, & Patton, 1995.

## Amount symbols used:

| | |
|---|---|
| ☺ | Free consumption: the smiley shows you foods that are completely free of the given brick, such as fructose or sorbitol. |
| ☺ | Over 90 times **unit** can be tolerated. |
| ¼, ½, ¾, 1, 1¼, 1½, 1¾, 2, etc. | The tolerated amount of **unit**, e.g., "cookie/piece/½" means half a cookie of the respective type can be tolerated per meal, and "soup/portion/1¾" means one and three fourths of a **unit** of the soup. |
| ☹ | The tolerated amount is below ¼ of **unit** for TL 3, so it's best to avoid it. |
| ☹¹ | You can stomach ¼ of **unit** if TL 1 applies to you; otherwise ☹ applies. If TL 2 (or 3) applies to you, you can tolerate ½ (or ¾) of **unit**. ☹¹ is only shown in the category tables and is there only for **Fructose** and **Fructose***. |
| ☹² | You can tolerate ¼ of **unit** if TL 2 applies to you; otherwise ☹ applies. If TL 3 applies to you, the tolerable amount of **unit** increases to ½ for sugar alcohols only. |
| ☹³ | You can stomach ¼ of **unit** if TL 3 applies to you; otherwise ☹ applies. |
| + [number] unit | By taking a high-dosed lactase capsule, you can additionally tolerate the amount of **unit** with regard to lactose independent of your TL. If for example you consider drinking milk, and **unit** is one cup, +¼ unit in the bottom of the lactose row means that per lactase capsule you tolerate one fourth of a cup of milk more. |
| ☺+ × [number] unit | The product contains more glucose than free fructose. The **simultaneous** intake of a portion measurement unit (**unit**) of the respective food can enable you to eat up to [number] times the TL 0 amount that is shown for other fructose(*) containing foods. To be on the safe side, divide the [number] by two, as glucose is already partially absorbed by the mouth, and sometimes the food is not chewed completely. For example, for a Kellogg's® Corn Flakes 30g portion, "☺+ ×1½ unit" is shown. If you divide the statement by two, it means that instead of the |

normal amount of 1½ tbsp. of apple sauce you are now able to stomach the 1½ tbsp. + 1½ tbsp. × (1½ unit ÷2 [in case you halve the amount for safety]), and thus about 2½ tbsp. in total. If a higher TL applies to you, **divide** the [amount] by the respective level multiplier (Chapter 3.1.3), as for higher levels the portions are higher as well. In the keyword list you will also find the TL 1 amounts for **Fructose***.

If you are keeping the BTL (TL 0) for sorbitol, avoid all products without a ☺-smiley in the upper part of the **Sorbitol** column. Please consider the gram numbers indicated when using the tables. Common portion sizes may be smaller than you think, e.g., 30g for corn flakes.

# 3.1.3 Level multipliers

The multipliers are there to help you determine the tolerable amounts of each unit scale if your TL deviates from the underlying TL, i.e. the TL that the amounts in the table hold for. In the category tables the multipliers are based on TL 0 for fructose and on TL 1 for all other bricks. In the keyword tables, all multipliers are based on TL 1. The increments have been chosen primarily for their tolerability. For fructose you will also find the deviating multipliers for the keyword table in the right column.

**Lactose (Lactose)**, underlying TL: 1

| TL 0 = Amounts ÷ 2 |
|---|
| TL 2 = Amounts × 2 |
| TL 3 = Amounts × 3 |

**Sorbitol-adjusted free fructose (Fructose*)** as well as **free fructose without considering sorbitol (Fructose)**, underlying TL: 0

| TL 1 = Amounts × 2 |
|---|
| TL 2 = Amounts × 4 |
| TL 3 = Amounts × 6 |

**Sorbitol-adjusted fructose (Fructose*)**, underlying TL: 1

| TL 2 = Amounts × 2 |
|---|
| TL 3 = Amounts × 3 |

**Sugar alcohols (Sorbitol)**, underlying TL: 1

| TL 2 = Amounts × 4 |
|---|
| TL 3 = Amounts × 7 |

**Fructans and galactans (Fruc/Galactans)**, underlying TL: 1

| TL 2 = Amounts × 2 |
|---|
| TL 3 = Amounts × 3 |

# TABLES BY CATEGORY

| | | |
|---|---|---|
| 3.2 | Athletes | 114 |
| 3.3 | Beverages | 116 |
| 3.3.1 | Alcoholic | 116 |
| 3.3.2 | Hot beverages | 121 |
| 3.3.3 | Juices | 124 |
| 3.3.4 | Other beverages | 126 |
| 3.4 | Cold dishes | 129 |
| 3.4.1 | Bread | 129 |
| 3.4.2 | Cereals | 131 |
| 3.4.3 | Cold cut | 134 |
| 3.4.4 | Dairy products | 137 |
| 3.4.5 | Nuts and snacks | 141 |
| 3.4.6 | Sweet pastries | 144 |
| 3.4.7 | Sweets | 149 |
| 3.5 | Warm dishes | 154 |
| 3.5.1 | Meals | 154 |
| 3.5.2 | Meat and fish | 159 |
| 3.5.3 | Lactose hideouts | 161 |
| 3.5.4 | Sauces and spices | 162 |
| 3.5.5 | Side dishes | 167 |
| 3.6 | Fast food chains | 169 |
| 3.6.1 | Burger King® | 169 |
| 3.6.2 | KFC® | 171 |
| 3.6.3 | McDonald's® | 172 |
| 3.6.4 | Subway® | 174 |
| 3.7 | Fruit and vegetables | 176 |
| 3.7.1 | Fruit | 176 |
| 3.7.2 | Vegetables | 180 |
| 3.8 | Ice cream | 186 |
| 3.9 | Ingredients | 189 |

## 3.2 Athletes

| Athletes | Unit | Lactose + unit/💊 | Fructose* / Fructose | Sorbitol / Sorbitol | FrucGalactans / FrucGalactans |
|---|---|---|---|---|---|
| Clif Bar®, Chocolate Chip | piece<br>2.4oz/68g | 9<br>+7½ unit | ☺+ ×10 unit<br>☺+ ×10 unit | ☹<br>2¼ | ¾<br>1½ |
| Clif Bar®, Crunchy Peanut Butter | piece<br>2.4oz/68g | ☺ | ☺+ ×10¼ unit<br>☺+ ×10¼ unit | ☹<br>2½ | ☺<br>☺ |
| Clif Bar®, Oatmeal Raisin Walnut | piece<br>2.4oz/68g | ☺ | ☺+ ×10¼ unit<br>☺+ ×10½ unit | ☹<br>1¾ | 1¾ AG<br>3½ |
| Electrolyte replacement drink | glass<br>8.4oz/240g | ☺ | ☺+ ×9¾ unit<br>☺+ ×9¾ unit | ☺<br>☺ | ☺<br>☺ |
| Gatorade®, all flavors | glass<br>8.4oz/240g | 7½<br>+6¼ unit | ☺+ ×1¼ unit<br>☺+ ×1¼ unit | ☺<br>☺ | 41½<br>83¼ |
| Gatorade®, from dry mix, all flavors | glass<br>8.4oz/240g | ☺ | ☺+ ×10½ unit<br>☺+ ×10½ unit | ☺<br>☺ | ☺<br>☺ |
| Glaceau® Vitaminwater 10 | glass<br>8.4oz/240g | ☺ | ☹¹<br>☹¹ | ☹<br>☹² | ☺<br>☺ |
| Glaceau® Vitaminwater Energy | glass<br>8.4oz/240g | ☺ | ☹²<br>☹² | ☺<br>☺ | ☺<br>☺ |
| Glaceau® Vitaminwater Essential | glass<br>8.4oz/240g | ☺ | ☹²<br>☹² | ☺<br>☺ | ☺<br>☺ |
| Glaceau® Vitaminwater Focus | glass<br>8.4oz/240g | ☺ | ☹²<br>☹² | ☺<br>☺ | ☺<br>☺ |
| Glaceau® Vitaminwater Power-C | glass<br>8.4oz/240g | ☺ | ☹²<br>☹² | ☺<br>☺ | ☺<br>☺ |
| Glaceau® Vitaminwater Revive | glass<br>8.4oz/240g | ☺ | ☹²<br>☹² | ☺<br>☺ | ☺<br>☺ |
| High-protein bar, generic | piece<br>2.3oz/65g | 39¼<br>+32¾ unit | ¾<br>¾ | ☹<br>76¾ | ☺<br>☺ |
| Power Bar® 20g Protein Plus, Chocolate Crisp | piece<br>2.16oz/61g | 3<br>+2½ unit | ☹¹<br>☹¹ | ☹<br>☹ | 17<br>34¼ |
| Power Bar® 20g Protein Plus, Chocolate Peanut Butter | piece<br>2.16oz/61g | 3<br>+2½ unit | ☹²<br>☹² | ☹<br>☹ | 17<br>34¼ |
| Power Bar® 30g Protein Plus, Chocolate Brownie | piece<br>2.47oz/70g | 2<br>+1½ unit | ☺+ ×1½ unit<br>☺+ ×1½ unit | ☹<br>☺ | 11<br>22¼ |
| Power Bar® Harvest Energy®, Double Chocolate Crisp | piece<br>2.3oz/65g | 2¾<br>+2¼ unit | ☺+ ×5¾ unit<br>☺+ ×5¾ unit | ☹<br>10¾ | ¼ A<br>½ |
| Power Bar® Performance Energy®, Banana | piece<br>2.3oz/65g | ☺ | ¼<br>¼ | ☹<br>☺ | ☺<br>☺ |

| Athletes | Unit | Lactose 1 + unit/capsule | Fructose* 0 Fructose 0 | Sorbitol 0 Sorbitol 1 | FrucGalactans 0 FrucGalactans 1 📖 |
|---|---|---|---|---|---|
| Power Bar® Performance | piece | 😃 | ¼ | ☹ | 😃 |
| Energy®, Chocolate | 2.3oz/65g | | ¼ | 76¾ | 😃 |
| Power Bar® Performance | piece | 😃 | ¼ | ☹ | 😃 |
| Energy®, Cookie Dough | 2.3oz/65g | | ¼ | ☺ | 😃 |
| Power Bar® Performance | piece | 😃 | ¼ | ☹ | 😃 |
| Energy®, Mixed Berry Blast | 2.3oz/65g | | ¼ | 19 | 😃 |
| Power Bar® Performance | piece | 😃 | ¼ | ☹ | 😃 |
| Energy®, Vanilla Crisp | 2.3oz/65g | | ¼ | ☺ | 😃 |
| Powerade®, all flavors | glass | 7½ | 😃+ ×1¼ unit | 😃 | 41½ |
| | 8.4oz/240g | +6¼ unit | 😃+ ×1¼ unit | 😃 | 83¼ |

0 *Level 0:* lactose measure ×½
1 *Level 1:* fructose measure ×2

+ Unit/capsule: added tolerated amount of unit per strong lactase capsule
Fructose*: fructose, sorbitol adjusted

2 *Level 2:* fructose-/sorbitol measure ×4. the rest ×2
3 *Level 3:* sorbitol measure ×7. the rest ×3
📖: source of fruc/galactans data

😃+ ×[Amount] unit: Per unit consumed you can additionally tolerate up to [amount] × fructose(*)-unit of another product.

☹: avoid; ☹[1]: ¼ at TL 1; ☹[2]: ¼ at TL 2; ☹[3]: ¼ at TL 3; ☺: only contains traces; 😃: is free from it

# 3.3 Beverages

## 3.3.1 Alcoholic

| Alcoholic | Unit | Lactose<br>+ unit/ | Fructose*<br>Fructose | Sorbitol<br>Sorbitol | FrucGalactans<br>FrucGalactans |
|---|---|---|---|---|---|
| Advocaat, regular | glass | ¼ | ☺+ ×4¾ unit | ☺ | 1½ |
| | 8.4oz.fl/240ml | +0.24 unit | ☺+ ×4¾ unit | ☺ | 3¼ |
| Ale | glass | ☺ | 50 | ☹ | ☺ |
| | 8.4oz.fl/240ml | | ☺ | 10 | ☺ |
| Amaretto | glass | ☺ | ☺+ ×4½ unit | ☹ | ☺ |
| | 8.4oz.fl/240ml | | ☺+ ×5 unit | ¼ | ☺ |
| Applejack liquor | glass | ☺ | ☺ | ☺ | ☺ |
| | 8.4oz.fl/240ml | | ☺ | ☺ | ☺ |
| Aquavit | glass | ☺ | ☺ | ☺ | ☺ |
| | 8.4oz.fl/240ml | | ☺ | ☺ | ☺ |
| Beer | glass | ☺ | 50 | ☹ | ☺ |
| | 8.4oz.fl/240ml | | ☺ | 10 | ☺ |
| Beer, low alcohol | glass | ☺ | ☺+ ×2¼ unit | ☺ | ☺ |
| | 8.4oz.fl/240ml | | ☺+ ×2¼ unit | ☺ | ☺ |
| Black Russian | glass | ☺ | ☺ | ☹ | ☺ |
| | 8.4oz.fl/240ml | | ☺ | 8¼ | ☺ |
| Bloody Mary | glass | ☺ | 1¾ | ☹ | ☺ |
| | 8.4oz.fl/240ml | | 1¾ | ½ | ☺ |
| Bourbon | glass | ☺ | ☺ | ☺ | ☺ |
| | 8.4oz.fl/240ml | | ☺ | ☺ | ☺ |
| Brandy | glass | ☺ | ☺ | ☺ | ☺ |
| | 8.4oz.fl/240ml | | ☺ | ☺ | ☺ |
| Brandy, flavored | glass | ☺ | ☺+ ×4½ unit | ☹ | ☺ |
| | 8.4oz.fl/240ml | | ☺+ ×5 unit | ¼ | ☺ |
| Burgundy wine, red | glass | ☺ | 17¾ | ☹ | ☺ |
| | 8.4oz.fl/240ml | | ☺ | ½ | ☺ |
| Burgundy wine, white | glass | ☺ | 31¼ | ☹ | ☺ |
| | 8.4oz.fl/240ml | | ☺ | ¾ | ☺ |
| Campari® | glass | ☺ | ☺+ ×4½ unit | ☹ | ☺ |
| | 8.4oz.fl/240ml | | ☺+ ×5 unit | ¼ | ☺ |
| Cape Cod | glass | ☺ | ☺+ ×5 unit | ☹ | ☺ |
| | 8.4oz.fl/240ml | | ☺+ ×5 unit | 25 | ☺ |
| Champagne punch | glass | ☺ | ¾ | ☹ | ☺ |
| | 8.4oz.fl/240ml | | ¾ | 1 | ☺ |

| Alcoholic | Unit | Lactose ☹ + unit/💊 | Fructose* ☹ Fructose ☹ | Sorbitol ☹ Sorbitol ☹ | FrucGalactans ☹ FrucGalactans ☹ 📖 |
|---|---|---|---|---|---|
| Champagne, white | glass 8.4oz.fl/240ml | 🙂 | 3¼ 🙂 | ☹ ¾ | 🙂 🙂 |
| Chardonnay | glass 8.4oz.fl/240ml | 🙂 | 3¼ 🙂 | ☹ ¾ | 🙂 🙂 |
| Club soda | glass 8.4oz.fl/240ml | 🙂 | 🙂 🙂 | 🙂 🙂 | 🙂 🙂 |
| Cognac | glass 8.4oz.fl/240ml | 🙂 | 🙂 🙂 | 🙂 🙂 | 🙂 🙂 |
| Cointreau® | glass 8.4oz.fl/240ml | 🙂 | 🙂+ ×4½ unit 🙂+ ×5 unit | ☹ ¼ | 🙂 🙂 |
| Creme de Cocoa | glass 8.4oz.fl/240ml | 🙂 | 🙂 🙂 | ☹ 2½ | 🙂 🙂 |
| Creme de menthe | glass 8.4oz.fl/240ml | 🙂 | 🙂+ ×4½ unit 🙂+ ×5 unit | ☹ ¼ | 🙂 🙂 |
| Curacao | glass 8.4oz.fl/240ml | 🙂 | 🙂+ ×4½ unit 🙂+ ×5 unit | ☹ ¼ | 🙂 🙂 |
| Daiquiri | glass 8.4oz.fl/240ml | 🙂 | 🙂 🙂 | 🙂 🙂 | 🙂 🙂 |
| Fruit punch, alcoholic | glass 8.4oz.fl/240ml | 🙂 | ¾ ¾ | ☹ 1 | 🙂 🙂 |
| Gibson | glass 8.4oz.fl/240ml | 🙂 | 🙂 🙂 | ☹ 3¼ | 🙂 🙂 |
| Gin | glass 8.4oz.fl/240ml | 🙂 | 🙂 🙂 | 🙂 🙂 | 🙂 🙂 |
| Grand Marnier® | glass 8.4oz.fl/240ml | 🙂 | 🙂+ ×4½ unit 🙂+ ×5 unit | ☹ ¼ | 🙂 🙂 |
| Grasshopper | glass 8.4oz.fl/240ml | 1¼ +1 unit | 🙂+ ×1¼ unit 🙂+ ×1½ unit | ☹ ¾ | 7 14 |
| Harvey Wallbanger | glass 8.4oz.fl/240ml | 🙂 | 16½ 🙂 | ☹ ¼ | 🙂 🙂 |
| Kamikaze | glass 8.4oz.fl/240ml | 🙂 | 🙂+ ×1½ unit 🙂+ ×1¾ unit | ☹ 1 | 🙂 🙂 |
| Kirsch | glass 8.4oz.fl/240ml | 🙂 | 🙂+ ×4½ unit 🙂+ ×5 unit | ☹ ¼ | 🙂 🙂 |

☹ *Level 0*: lactose measure ×½  
☹ *Level 1*: fructose measure ×2  
☹ *Level 2*: fructose-/sorbitol measure ×4. the rest ×2  
☹ *Level 3*: sorbitol measure ×7. the rest ×3  
📖: source of fruc/galactans data  

+ Unit/💊: added tolerated amount of unit per strong lactase capsule  
Fructose*: fructose, sorbitol adjusted  
🙂+ ×[Amount] unit: Per unit consumed you can additionally tolerate up to [amount] × fructose(*)-unit of another product.  

☹: avoid;   ☹[1]: ¼ at TL 1;   ☹[2]: ¼ at TL 2;   ☹[3]: ¼ at TL 3;   🙂: only contains traces;   🙂: is free from it

| Alcoholic | Unit | Lactose ↯ + unit/🥛 | Fructose* ↯ Fructose ↯ | Sorbitol ↯ Sorbitol ↯ | FrucGalactans ↯ FrucGalactans ↯📖 |
|---|---|---|---|---|---|
| Liqueur, coffee flavored | glass 8.4oz.fl/240ml | ☺ | ☺ ☺ | ☹ 2½ | ☺ ☺ |
| Long Island iced tea | glass 8.4oz.fl/240ml | ☺ | ¾ ¾ | ☹ 16½ | ☺ ☺ |
| Mai Tai | glass 8.4oz.fl/240ml | ☺ | ☺+ ×½ unit ☺+ ×½ unit | ☹ 1¾ | ☺ ☺ |
| Malt liquor | glass 8.4oz.fl/240ml | ☺ | 50 ☺ | ☹ 10 | ☺ ☺ |
| Manhattan | glass 8.4oz.fl/240ml | ☺ | ½ ½ | ☹ 2 | ☺ ☺ |
| Margarita, frozen | glass 8.4oz.fl/240ml | ☺ | ☺+ ×¼ unit ☺+ ×¼ unit | ☹ 7 | ☺ ☺ |
| Martini® | glass 8.4oz.fl/240ml | ☺ | 83¼ ☺ | ☹ 3¼ | ☺ ☺ |
| Merlot, red | glass 8.4oz.fl/240ml | ☺ | 17¾ ☺ | ☹ ½ | ☺ ☺ |
| Merlot, white | glass 8.4oz.fl/240ml | ☺ | ¾ ¾ | ☺ ☺ | ☺ ☺ |
| Mint Julep | glass 8.4oz.fl/240ml | ☺ | ☺ ☺ | ☺ ☺ | ☺ ☺ |
| Mojito | glass 8.4oz.fl/240ml | ☺ | ☺ ☺ | ☺ ☺ | ☺ ☺ |
| Muscatel | glass 8.4oz.fl/240ml | ☺ | ☹² ☹² | ☹ ½ | ☺ ☺ |
| Non-alcoholic wine | glass 8.4oz.fl/240ml | ☺ | 2¼ 2¼ | ☹ 50 | ☺ ☺ |
| Ouzo | glass 8.4oz.fl/240ml | ☺ | ☺+ ×4½ unit ☺+ ×5 unit | ☹ ¼ | ☺ ☺ |
| Pina colada | glass 8.4oz.fl/240ml | ☺ | ☺+ ×1¼ unit ☺+ ×1¼ unit | ☹ 4 | ☺ ☺ |
| Port wine | glass 8.4oz.fl/240ml | ☺ | ☹² ☹² | ☹ ½ | ☺ ☺ |
| Riesling | glass 8.4oz.fl/240ml | ☺ | 31¼ ☺ | ☹ ¾ | ☺ ☺ |
| Rob Roy | glass 8.4oz.fl/240ml | ☺ | ¼ ¼ | ☹ 2½ | ☺ ☺ |
| Rompope (eggnog with alcohol) | glass 8.4oz.fl/240ml | ¼ +¼ unit | ☺ ☺ | ☺ ☺ | 2¾ 5½ |
| Root beer | glass 8.4oz.fl/240ml | ☺ | ½ ½ | ☺ ☺ | ☺ ☺ |

| Alcoholic | Unit | Lactose + unit/ 🍼 | Fructose* Fructose | Sorbitol Sorbitol | FrucGalactans FrucGalactans |
|---|---|---|---|---|---|
| Rose wine, other types | glass | ☺ | ¾ | ☺ | ☺ |
|  | 8.4oz.fl/240ml |  | ¾ | ☺ | ☺ |
| Rum | glass | ☺ | ☺ | ☺ | ☺ |
|  | 8.4oz.fl/240ml |  | ☺ | ☺ | ☺ |
| Rum and cola | glass | ☺ | 1 | ☺ | ☺ |
|  | 8.4oz.fl/240ml |  | 1 | ☺ | ☺ |
| Rusty nail | glass | ☺ | ☺+ ×1¾ unit | ☹ | ☺ |
|  | 8.4oz.fl/240ml |  | ☺+ ×2 unit | ¾ | ☺ |
| Sake | glass | ☺ | ☹² | ☹ | ☺ |
|  | 8.4oz.fl/240ml |  | ☹² | ½ | ☺ |
| Sambuca | glass | ☺ | ☺+ ×4½ unit | ☹ | ☺ |
|  | 8.4oz.fl/240ml |  | ☺+ ×5 unit | ¼ | ☺ |
| Sangria | glass | ☺ | 7¾ | ☹ | ☺ |
|  | 8.4oz.fl/240ml |  | 11¼ | ¾ | ☺ |
| Schnapps, all flavors | glass | ☺ | ☺+ ×2¼ unit | ☹ | ☺ |
|  | 8.4oz.fl/240ml |  | ☺+ ×2½ unit | ½ | ☺ |
| Scotch and soda | glass | ☺ | ☺ | ☺ | ☺ |
|  | 8.4oz.fl/240ml |  | ☺ | ☺ | ☺ |
| Screwdriver | glass | ☺ | 2 | ☹ | ☺ |
|  | 8.4oz.fl/240ml |  | 2 | ¼ | ☺ |
| Seabreeze | glass | ☺ | ☺+ ×5¼ unit | ☹ | ☺ |
|  | 8.4oz.fl/240ml |  | ☺+ ×5¼ unit | 2½ | ☺ |
| Singapore sling | glass | ☺ | ☺+ ×¼ unit | ☹ | ☺ |
|  | 8.4oz.fl/240ml |  | ☺+ ×¼ unit | 4½ | ☺ |
| Sloe gin | glass | ☺ | ☺+ ×4½ unit | ☹ | ☺ |
|  | 8.4oz.fl/240ml |  | ☺+ ×5 unit | ¼ | ☺ |
| Sloe gin fizz | glass | ☺ | ☺+ ×¾ unit | ☹ | ☺ |
|  | 8.4oz.fl/240ml |  | ☺+ ×¾ unit | 1½ | ☺ |
| Southern Comfort® | glass | ☺ | ☺ | ☺ | ☺ |
|  | 8.4oz.fl/240ml |  | ☺ | ☺ | ☺ |
| Sylvaner | glass | ☺ | 31¼ | ☹ | ☺ |
|  | 8.4oz.fl/240ml |  | ☺ | ¾ | ☺ |
| Tequila | glass | ☺ | ☺ | ☺ | ☺ |
|  | 8.4oz.fl/240ml |  | ☺ | ☺ | ☺ |

↻ *Level 0*: lactose measure ×½    + Unit/🍼: added tolerated amount of unit per strong lactase capsule
↡ *Level 1*: fructose measure ×2    Fructose*: fructose, sorbitol adjusted
↡ *Level 2*: fructose-/sorbitol measure ×4. the rest ×2    ☺+ ×[Amount] unit: Per unit consumed you can
↡ *Level 3*: sorbitol measure ×7. the rest ×3    additionally tolerate up to [amount] ×
📖: source of fruc/galactans data    fructose(*)-unit of another product.
☹: avoid;   ☹¹: ¼ at TL 1;   ☹²: ¼ at TL 2;   ☹³: ¼ at TL 3;   ☺: only contains traces;   ☺: is free from it

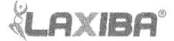 The Nutrition Navigator

| Alcoholic | Unit | Lactose ↓<br>+ unit/🥛 | Fructose* ☹<br>Fructose ☹ | Sorbitol ☹<br>Sorbitol ↓ | FrucGalactans ☹<br>FrucGalactans ↓ 📖 |
|---|---|---|---|---|---|
| Tokaji Wine | glass<br>8.4oz.fl/240ml | ☺ | ☹²<br>☹² | ☹<br>½ | ☺<br>☺ |
| Tom Collins | glass<br>8.4oz.fl/240ml | ☺ | 31¼<br>31¼ | ☹<br>16½ | ☺<br>☺ |
| Triple Sec | glass<br>8.4oz.fl/240ml | ☺ | ☺+ ×4½ unit<br>☺+ ×5 unit | ☹<br>¼ | ☺<br>☺ |
| Vodka | glass<br>8.4oz.fl/240ml | ☺ | ☺<br>☺ | ☺<br>☺ | ☺<br>☺ |
| Whiskey | glass<br>8.4oz.fl/240ml | ☺ | ☺<br>☺ | ☺<br>☺ | ☺<br>☺ |
| Whiskey sour | glass<br>8.4oz.fl/240ml | ☺ | 9½<br>9½ | ☹<br>6¼ | ☺<br>☺ |
| White Russian | glass<br>8.4oz.fl/240ml | 1½<br>+1¼ unit | ☺<br>☺ | ☹<br>8¼ | 9<br>18¼ |
| Wine spritzer | glass<br>8.4oz.fl/240ml | ☺ | 27¾<br>☺ | ☹<br>1 | ☺<br>☺ |

# 3.3.2 Hot beverages

| Hot beverages | Unit | Lactose ↯ + unit/💊 | Fructose* ☯ Fructose ↯ | Sorbitol ☯ Sorbitol ↯ | FrucGalactans ☯ FrucGalactans ↯ 📖 |
|---|---|---|---|---|---|
| Americano, decaf, without flavored syrup | cup 5.2oz.fl/150ml | ☺ | ☺ ☺ | ☺ ☺ | ☺ ☺ |
| Americano, with flavored syrup | cup 5.2oz.fl/150ml | ☺ | ☺ ☺ | ☺ ☺ | ☺ ☺ |
| Americano, without flavored syrup | cup 5.2oz.fl/150ml | ☺ | ☺ ☺ | ☺ ☺ | ☺ ☺ |
| Brown sugar | tbsp. 0.5oz/14.21ml | ☺ | ☺ ☺ | ☺ ☺ | ☺ ☺ |
| Cafe au lait, without flavored syrup | cup 5.2oz.fl/150ml | 1 +¾ unit | ☺ ☺ | ☺ ☺ | 6½ 13 |
| Cafe latte, with flavored syrup | cup 5.2oz.fl/150ml | ½ +¼ unit | ☺ ☺ | ☺ ☺ | 3 6 |
| Cafe latte, without flavored syrup | cup 5.2oz.fl/150ml | ¼ +¼ unit | ☺ ☺ | ☺ ☺ | 2¾ 5½ |
| Camomile tea | glass 8.5oz.fl/242ml | ☺ | ☺ ☺ | ☺ ☺ | ☺ G ☺ |
| Cappuccino, bottled or canned | cup 5.2oz.fl/150ml | ½ +½ unit | ☺ ☺ | ☺ ☺ | 4 8 |
| Cappuccino, decaf, with flavored syrup | cup 5.2oz.fl/150ml | ½ +¼ unit | ☺ ☺ | ☺ ☺ | 3 6¼ |
| Cappuccino, decaf, without flavored syrup | cup 5.2oz.fl/150ml | ½ +¼ unit | ☺ ☺ | ☺ ☺ | 2¾ 5¾ |
| Chicory coffee | cup 5.2oz.fl/150ml | ☺ | ☺ ☺ | ☹ 11 | ☹ E ☹ |
| Coffee substitute, prepared | cup 5.2oz.fl/150ml | ☺ | ☺ ☺ | ☺ ☺ | ☺ ☺ |
| Coffee, prepared from flavored mix, sugar free | cup 5.2oz.fl/150ml | ☺ | ☺ ☺ | ☹ 66½ | ☺ ☺ |
| Demitasse | cup 5.2oz.fl/150ml | ☺ | ☺ ☺ | ☺ ☺ | ☺ ☺ |

☯ *Level 0*: lactose measure ×½   + Unit/💊: added tolerated amount of unit per strong lactase capsule
↯ *Level 1*: fructose measure ×2   Fructose*: fructose, sorbitol adjusted
↯ *Level 2*: fructose-/sorbitol measure ×4. the rest ×2   ☺+ ×[Amount] unit: Per unit consumed you can
↯ *Level 3*: sorbitol measure ×7. the rest ×3   additionally tolerate up to [amount] ×
📖: source of fruc/galactans data   fructose(*)-unit of another product.

☹: avoid;   ☹¹: ¼ at TL 1;   ☹²: ¼ at TL 2;   ☹³: ¼ at TL 3;   ☺: only contains traces;   ☺: is free from it

| Hot beverages | Unit | Lactose ↧ + unit/🥛 | Fructose* ↧ Fructose ↧ | Sorbitol ↧ Sorbitol ↧ | FrucGalactans ↧ FrucGalactans ↧ |
|---|---|---|---|---|---|
| Dove® Promises, Milk Chocolate | cup 5.2oz.fl/150ml | ¼ +0.21 unit | ☺ ☺ | ☹ ☺ | 1¾ 3¾ |
| Earl Grey, strong | glass 8.4oz.fl/240ml | ☺ | ½ ½ | ☺ ☺ | ☺G ☺ |
| Espresso, without flavored syrup | cup 5.2oz.fl/150ml | ☺ | ☺ ☺ | ☺ ☺ | ☺ ☺ |
| Evaporated milk, diluted, skim (fat free) | cup 5.2oz.fl/150ml | ¼ +¼ unit | ☺ ☺ | ☺ ☺ | 1¾ 3¾ |
| Fennel tea | glass 8.6oz.fl/247ml | ☺ | ☺ ☺ | ☺ ☺ | ☺G ☺ |
| Frappuccino® | cup 5.2oz.fl/150ml | ½ +½ unit | ☺ ☺ | ☺ ☺ | 3¾ 7½ |
| Frappuccino®, bottled or canned | cup 5.2oz.fl/150ml | ½ +½ unit | ☺ ☺ | ☺ ☺ | 3½ 7 |
| Frappuccino®, bottled or canned, light | cup 5.2oz.fl/150ml | ½ +½ unit | ☺ ☺ | ☺ ☺ | 4 8 |
| Green tea, strong | glass 8.7oz.fl/248ml | ☺ | ☺ ☺ | ☺ ☺ | ☺ ☺ |
| Herbal tea | glass 8.6oz.fl/246ml | ☺ | ☺ ☺ | ☺ ☺ | ☺G ☺ |
| Hershey's® Bliss Hot Drink White Chocolate, prepared | cup 5.2oz.fl/150ml | ¼ +¼ unit | ☺+ ×½ unit ☺+ ×½ unit | ☺ ☺ | 1¾ 3¾ |
| Hot chocolate, homemade | cup 5.2oz.fl/150ml | ¼ +¼ unit | 27¾ 27¾ | ☹ 66½ | 1¾ 3¾ |
| Instant coffee mix, unprepared | cup 5.2oz.fl/150ml | ☺ | 8¼ 8¼ | ☹ ☹[2] | ☺ ☺ |
| Irish coffee with alcohol and whipped cream | cup 5.2oz.fl/150ml | 3¾ +3 unit | ☺ ☺ | ☺ ☺ | 21 42 |
| Jasmine tea | glass 8.4oz.fl/241ml | ☺ | ☺ ☺ | ☺ ☺ | ☺G ☺ |
| Light cream | portion 0.53oz.fl/15ml | 5¼ +4½ unit | ☺ ☺ | ☺ ☺ | 30¼ 60½ |
| Milk, lactose reduced (Lactaid®), skim (fat free) | cup 5.2oz.fl/150ml | ☺ | ☺+ ×7½ unit ☺+ ×7½ unit | ☺ ☺ | ☺ ☺ |
| Milk, lactose reduced (Lactaid®), whole | cup 5.2oz.fl/150ml | ☺ | ☺+ ×7½ unit ☺+ ×7½ unit | ☺ ☺ | ☺ ☺ |
| Milk, unprepared dry powder, nonfat, instant | portion 0.78oz.fl/22ml | ¼ +0.21 unit | ☺ ☺ | ☺ ☺ | 1¼ 2¾ |
| Mocha, without flavored syrup | cup 5.2oz.fl/150ml | ½ +¼ unit | ☺+ ×1¾ unit ☺+ ×1¾ unit | ☺ ☺ | 3 6 |

| Hot beverages | Unit | Lactose 1<br>+ unit/capsule | Fructose* 0<br>Fructose 0 | Sorbitol 0<br>Sorbitol 1 | FrucGalactans 0<br>FrucGalactans 1 📖 |
|---|---|---|---|---|---|
| Nestle® Hot Cocoa Dark Chocolate, prepared | cup<br>5.2oz.fl/150ml | ¼<br>+¼ unit | ☺+ ×½ unit<br>☺+ ×½ unit | ☹<br>☺ | 1¾<br>3¾ |
| Nestle® Hot Cocoa Rich Milk Chocolate, prepared | cup<br>5.2oz.fl/150ml | ¼<br>+¼ unit | ☺<br>☺ | ☺<br>☺ | 1¾<br>3¾ |
| Nestle® Nesquik®, chocolate flavors, unprepared dry | glass<br>8.4oz/240g | ☺ | 1½<br>1½ | ☹<br>5½ | ☺<br>☺ |
| Soy milk, chocolate, sweetened with sugar, not fortified, ready-to-drink | cup<br>5.2oz.fl/150ml | ☺ | ☺<br>☺ | ☹<br>4¼ | ¼ A<br>½ |
| Splenda® | portion<br>0oz.fl/0ml | ☺ | ☺<br>☺ | ☺<br>☺ | ☺<br>☺ |
| Starbucks® Hot Cocoa Double Chocolate, prepared | cup<br>5.2oz.fl/150ml | ¼<br>+¼ unit | 37<br>37 | ☹<br>66½ | 1¾<br>3¾ |
| Starbucks® Hot Cocoa Salted Caramel, prepared | cup<br>5.2oz.fl/150ml | ¼<br>+¼ unit | 33¼<br>33¼ | ☹<br>66½ | 1¾<br>3¾ |
| Sugar, white granulated | tbsp.<br>0.5oz/14.21ml | ☺ | ☺<br>☺ | ☺<br>☺ | ☺<br>☺ |
| Sweetened condensed milk | portion<br>1.35oz.fl/38ml | ½<br>+½ unit | ☺<br>☺ | ☺<br>☺ | 3¾<br>7½ |
| Sweetened condensed milk, reduced fat | portion<br>1.38oz.fl/39ml | ½<br>+½ unit | ☺<br>☺ | ☺<br>☺ | 3½<br>7¼ |
| Whipped cream, aerosol | portion<br>0.25oz.fl/7ml | ☺ | ☺<br>☺ | ☺<br>☺ | ☺<br>☺ |
| Whipped cream, aerosol, fat free | portion<br>0.18oz.fl/5ml | 18¾<br>+15¾ unit | ☺+ ×¼ unit<br>☺+ ×¼ unit | ☺<br>☺ | ☺<br>☺ |
| Zsweet® | portion<br>0.18oz.fl/5ml | ☺ | ☺<br>☺ | ☹<br>☹ | ☺<br>☺ |

0 *Level 0:* lactose measure ×½
1 *Level 1:* fructose measure ×2
2 *Level 2:* fructose-/sorbitol measure ×4. the rest ×2
3 *Level 3:* sorbitol measure ×7. the rest ×3
📖: source of fruc/galactans data

+ Unit/capsule: added tolerated amount of unit per strong lactase capsule
Fructose*: fructose, sorbitol adjusted
☺+ ×[Amount] unit: Per unit consumed you can additionally tolerate up to [amount] × fructose(*)-unit of another product.

☹: avoid; ☹[1]: ¼ at TL 1; ☹[2]: ¼ at TL 2; ☹[3]: ¼ at TL 3; ☺: only contains traces; ☺: is free from it

# 3.3.3 Juices

| Juices | Unit | Lactose ︎ + unit/ | Fructose* ︎ Fructose ︎ | Sorbitol ︎ Sorbitol ︎ | FrucGalactans ︎ FrucGalactans ︎ |
|---|---|---|---|---|---|
| Apple banana strawberry juice | glass 8.4oz.fl/240ml | ☺ | ☹¹ ☹¹ | ☹ ☹² | ¾ FB 1¾ |
| Apple grape juice | glass 8.4oz.fl/240ml | ☺ | ☹² ☹² | ☹ ☹² | 1½ CB 3 |
| Apricot nectar | glass 8.4oz.fl/240ml | ☺ | ☺+ ×4¾ unit ☺+ ×5 unit | ☹ ¼ | ☺ ☺ |
| Arby's® orange juice | glass 8.4oz.fl/240ml | ☺ | 1½ 1½ | ☹ ¼ | ☺ B ☺ |
| Black cherry juice | glass 8.4oz.fl/240ml | ☺ | ¼ ¼ | ☹ 2½ | ☺ ☺ |
| Black currant juice | glass 8.4oz.fl/240ml | ☺ | ☺+ ×1½ unit ☺+ ×1½ unit | ☹ 1½ | ☺ ☺ |
| Blackberry juice | glass 8.4oz.fl/240ml | ☺ | ¼ ¼ | ☺ ☺ | ☺ ☺ |
| Capri Sun®, all flavors | glass 8.4oz.fl/240ml | ☺ | ☺+ ×1 unit ☺+ ×1 unit | ☹ 2 | ☺ ☺ |
| Carrot juice | glass 8.4oz.fl/240ml | ☺ | ☺+ ×1 unit ☺+ ×1 unit | ☹ 4 | ☺ B ☺ |
| Cranberry juice cocktail, with apple juice | glass 8.4oz.fl/240ml | ☺ | ☹¹ ☹¹ | ☹ ☹² | 1½ CB 3 |
| Cranberry juice cocktail, with blueberry juice | glass 8.4oz.fl/240ml | ☺ | ☹¹ ☹¹ | ☹ ☹² | ☺ ☺ |
| Fruit drink or punch, ready to drink | glass 8.4oz.fl/240ml | ☺ | ☺+ ×1 unit ☺+ ×1 unit | ☹ 2 | 1½ C 3 |
| Grapefruit juice, unsweetened, white | glass 8.4oz.fl/240ml | ☺ | ☺+ ×5 unit ☺+ ×5 unit | ☹ ¼ | 1 CB 2 |
| Kern's® Mango-Orange Nectar | glass 8.4oz.fl/240ml | ☺ | ☹¹ ☹¹ | ☹ 2 | 3 B 6¼ |
| Kern's® Strawberry Nectar | glass 8.4oz.fl/240ml | ☺ | ☹¹ ☹¹ | ☹ ¾ | ☺ C ☺ |
| Lemon juice, fresh | glass 8.4oz.fl/240ml | ☺ | 2¼ 2¼ | ☹ 1½ | 2¼ B 4½ |
| Libby's® Apricot Nectar | glass 8.4oz.fl/240ml | ☺ | ☹¹ ☹¹ | ☹ ¼ | ☺ ☺ |
| Libby's® Banana Nectar | glass 8.4oz.fl/240ml | ☺ | ☹¹ ☹¹ | ☹ 25 | ½ FB 1 |

| Juices | Unit | Lactose ↯ + unit/💊 | Fructose* ☹ Fructose ☹ | Sorbitol ☹ Sorbitol ↯ | FrucGalactans ☹ FrucGalactans ↯ 📖 |
|---|---|---|---|---|---|
| Libby's® Juicy Juice®, Apple Grape | glass 8.4oz.fl/240ml | ☺ | ☹¹ ☹¹ | ☹ ¼ | 1½ CB 3 |
| Libby's® Juicy Juice®, Grape | glass 8.4oz.fl/240ml | ☺ | ☹¹ ☹¹ | ☹ ¼ | 1½ CB 3 |
| Libby's® Pear Nectar | glass 8.4oz.fl/240ml | ☺ | ☹² ☹² | ☹ ☹² | ☺ B ☺ |
| Lime juice, fresh | glass 8.4oz.fl/240ml | ☺ | ☺+ ×¾ unit ☺+ ×¾ unit | ☺ ☺ | 2¼ B 4½ |
| Mango nectar | glass 8.4oz.fl/240ml | ☺ | 1 1 | ☹ 1¼ | ☺ B ☺ |
| Northland® Cranberry Juice, all flavors | glass 8.4oz.fl/240ml | ☺ | ☺+ ×7¼ unit ☺+ ×7¼ unit | ☹ 25 | ☺ ☺ |
| Orange kiwi passion juice | glass 8.4oz.fl/240ml | ☺ | ☹ ☹ | ☹ ¾ | ☺ B ☺ |
| Passion fruit juice | glass 8.4oz.fl/240ml | ☺ | ☺+ ×3¾ unit ☺+ ×3¾ unit | ☹ ☹ | ☺ ☺ |
| Peach juice | glass 8.4oz.fl/240ml | ☺ | ¾ ¾ | ☹ ¾ | ½ B 1¼ |
| Pear juice | glass 8.4oz.fl/240ml | ☺ | ☹² ☹² | ☹ ☹³ | 1½ C 3 |
| Pineapple juice | glass 8.4oz.fl/240ml | ☺ | ☺+ ×3¼ unit ☺+ ×3¼ unit | ☹ 1¾ | 1½ CB 3 |
| Pineapple orange drink | glass 8.4oz.fl/240ml | ☺ | ¾ ¾ | ☺ ☺ | 1½ CB 3 |
| Pomegranate juice | glass 8.4oz.fl/240ml | ☺ | ¾ 2¾ | ☹ ☹² | ☺ ☺ |
| Raspberry juice | glass 8.4oz.fl/240ml | ☺ | ☹² ☹² | ☹ ☹² | ¾ B 1½ |
| Tomato juice | glass 8.4oz.fl/240ml | ☺ | 1¼ 1¼ | ☹ ¼ | 2¾ B 5½ |
| V-8® 100% A-C-E Vitamin Rich Vegetable Juice | glass 8.4oz.fl/240ml | ☺ | ¼ ¼ | ☹ 3 | 2¾ B 5½ |
| Veryfine Cranberry Raspberry | glass 8.4oz.fl/240ml | ☺ | ☹¹ ☹¹ | ☹ ☹² | ¾ B 1½ |

↯ Level 0: lactose measure ×½  + Unit/💊: added tolerated amount of unit per strong lactase capsule
↯ Level 1: fructose measure ×2  Fructose*: fructose, sorbitol adjusted
↯ Level 2: fructose-/sorbitol measure ×4. the rest ×2   ☺+ ×[Amount] unit: Per unit consumed you can additionally tolerate up to [amount] × fructose(*)-unit of another product.
↯ Level 3: sorbitol measure ×7. the rest ×3
📖: source of fruc/galactans data

☹: avoid;   ☹¹: ¼ at TL 1;   ☹²: ¼ at TL 2;   ☹³: ¼ at TL 3;   ☺: only contains traces;   ☺: is free from it

# 3.3.4 Other beverages

| Other beverages | Unit | Lactose ☺ + unit/🥛 | Fructose* ☺ Fructose ☺ | Sorbitol ☺ Sorbitol ☺ | FrucGalactans ☺ FrucGalactans ☺ |
|---|---|---|---|---|---|
| 7 UP® | glass 8.4oz.fl/240ml | ☺ | ☹² ☹² | ☺ ☺ | ☺ ☺ |
| Cherry Coke® | glass 8.4oz.fl/240ml | ☺ | ½ ½ | ☺ ☺ | ☺ ☺ |
| Coke Zero® | glass 8.4oz.fl/240ml | ☺ | ☺ ☺ | ☺ ☺ | ☺ ☺ |
| Coke® | glass 8.4oz.fl/240ml | ☺ | ½ ½ | ☺ ☺ | ☺ ☺ |
| Coke® with Lime | glass 8.4oz.fl/240ml | ☺ | ½ ½ | ☺ ☺ | ☺ ☺ |
| Diet 7 UP® | glass 8.4oz.fl/240ml | ☺ | ☺ ☺ | ☺ ☺ | ☺ ☺ |
| Diet Coke® | glass 8.4oz.fl/240ml | ☺ | ☺ ☺ | ☺ ☺ | ☺ ☺ |
| Diet Dr. Pepper® | glass 8.4oz.fl/240ml | ☺ | ☺ ☺ | ☺ ☺ | ☺ ☺ |
| Diet Pepsi®, fountain | glass 8.4oz.fl/240ml | ☺ | ☺ ☺ | ☺ ☺ | ☺ ☺ |
| Fanta Zero®, fruit flavors | glass 8.4oz.fl/240ml | ☺ | ☺ ☺ | ☺ ☺ | ☺ ☺ |
| Fanta® Red | glass 8.4oz.fl/240ml | ☺ | ☹¹ ☹¹ | ☺ ☺ | ☺ ☺ |
| Fanta®, fruit flavors | glass 8.4oz.fl/240ml | ☺ | 8¼ 8¼ | ☺ ☺ | ☺ ☺ |
| Ginger ale | glass 8.4oz.fl/240ml | ☺ | ☹² ☹² | ☺ ☺ | ☺ ☺ |
| Lipton® Iced Tea Mix, sweetened with sugar, prepared | glass 8.4oz.fl/240ml | ☺ | ☺ ☺ | ☺ ☺ | ☺ ☺ |
| Lipton® Instant 100% Tea, unsweetened, prepared | glass 8.4oz.fl/240ml | ☺ | ☺ ☺ | ☺ ☺ | ☺ ☺ |
| Mineral Water | glass 8.4oz.fl/240ml | ☺ | ☺ ☺ | ☺ ☺ | ☺ ☺ |
| Monster® Energy® | glass 8.4oz.fl/240ml | ☺ | ☺+ ×17½ unit ☺+ ×17½ unit | ☺ ☺ | ☺ ☺ |
| Monster® Khaos | portion 8.47oz.fl/240ml | ☺ | ☺+ ×9 unit ☺+ ×9½ unit | ☹ ¼ | ☺ ☺ |

| Other beverages | Unit | Lactose ☝ + unit/💊 | Fructose* ☝☝ Fructose ☝ | Sorbitol ☝☝ Sorbitol ☝ | FrucGalactans ☝☝ FrucGalactans ☝ 📖 |
|---|---|---|---|---|---|
| Mountain Dew® | glass 8.4oz.fl/240ml | ☺ | ☹[1] ☹[1] | ☺ ☺ | ☺ ☺ |
| Mountain Dew® Code Red | glass 8.4oz.fl/240ml | ☺ | ☹[1] ☹[1] | ☺ ☺ | ☺ ☺ |
| Nestea® 100% Tea, unsweetened, dry | glass 8.4oz.fl/240ml | ☺ | ☺+ ×22 unit ☺+ ×22 unit | ☺ ☺ | ☺ ☺ |
| Nestea® Iced Tea, Sugar Free, dry | glass 8.4oz.fl/240ml | ☺ | ☺+ ×11½ unit ☺+ ×11½ unit | ☺ ☺ | ☺ ☺ |
| Nestea® Iced Tea, Sugar Free, prepared | glass 8.4oz.fl/240ml | ☺ | ☺ ☺ | ☺ ☺ | ☺ ☺ |
| Nestea® Iced Tea, sweetened with sugar, dry | glass 8.4oz.fl/240ml | ☺ | ☺ ☺ | ☺ ☺ | ☺ ☺ |
| No Fear® | glass 8.4oz.fl/240ml | ☺ | ☺+ ×6¼ unit ☺+ ×6¼ unit | ☹ 50 | ☺ ☺ |
| No Fear® Sugar Free | glass 8.4oz.fl/240ml | ☺ | ☺ ☺ | ☺ ☺ | ☺ ☺ |
| Pepsi® | glass 8.4oz.fl/240ml | ☺ | ½ ½ | ☺ ☺ | ☺ ☺ |
| Pepsi® Max | glass 8.4oz.fl/240ml | ☺ | ☺ ☺ | ☺ ☺ | ☺ ☺ |
| Pepsi® Twist | glass 8.4oz.fl/240ml | ☺ | ½ ½ | ☺ ☺ | ☺ ☺ |
| Red Bull® Energy Drink | glass 8.4oz.fl/240ml | ☺ | ☺+ ×7¾ unit ☺+ ×7¾ unit | ☺ ☺ | ☺ ☺ |
| Red Bull® Energy Drink Sugar Free | glass 8.4oz.fl/240ml | ☺ | ☺ ☺ | ☺ ☺ | ☺ ☺ |
| Rockstar Original® | glass 8.4oz.fl/240ml | ☺ | ☺+ ×23¾ unit ☺+ ×23¾ unit | ☹ 5 | ☺ ☺ |
| Rockstar Original® Sugar Free | glass 8.4oz.fl/240ml | ☺ | ☺ ☺ | ☹ 5 | ☺ ☺ |
| Schweppes® Bitter Lemon | glass 8.4oz.fl/240ml | ☺ | ☹[2] ☹[2] | ☺ ☺ | ☺ ☺ |
| Spearmint tea | glass 8.4oz.fl/240ml | ☺ | ☺ ☺ | ☺ ☺ | ☺ ☺ |

☝ *Level 0*: lactose measure ×½
☝ *Level 1*: fructose measure ×2
☝☝ *Level 2*: fructose-/sorbitol measure ×4. the rest ×2
☝☝ *Level 3*: sorbitol measure ×7. the rest ×3
📖: source of fruc/galactans data

+ Unit/💊: added tolerated amount of unit per strong lactase capsule
Fructose*: fructose, sorbitol adjusted
☺+ ×[Amount] unit: Per unit consumed you can additionally tolerate up to [amount] × fructose(*)-unit of another product.

☹: avoid;  ☹[1]: ¼ at TL 1;  ☹[2]: ¼ at TL 2;  ☹[3]: ¼ at TL 3;  ☺: only contains traces;  ☺: is free from it

| Other beverages | Unit + unit/ | Lactose | Fructose* / Fructose | Sorbitol / Sorbitol | FrucGalactans / FrucGalactans |
|---|---|---|---|---|---|
| Sprite® | glass 8.4oz.fl/240ml | ☺ | ☹² ☹² | ☺ ☺ | ☺ ☺ |
| Sprite® Zero | glass 8.4oz.fl/240ml | ☺ | ☺ ☺ | ☺ ☺ | ☺ ☺ |
| Tap water | glass 8.4oz.fl/240ml | ☺ | ☺ ☺ | ☺ ☺ | ☺ ☺ |
| Tonic water | glass 8.4oz.fl/240ml | ☺ | ☹² ☹² | ☺ ☺ | ☺ ☺ |
| Tonic water, diet | glass 8.4oz.fl/240ml | ☺ | ☺ ☺ | ☺ ☺ | ☺ ☺ |
| Vanilla Coke® | glass 8.4oz.fl/240ml | ☺ | ½ ½ | ☺ ☺ | ☺ ☺ |
| Yerba® Mate tea | glass 8.4oz.fl/240ml | ☺ | ☺ ☺ | ☺ ☺ | ☺ ☺ |

# 3.4 Cold dishes

## 3.4.1 Bread

| Bread | Unit | Lactose ☾<br>+ unit/ 💊 | Fructose* ☾<br>Fructose ☾ | Sorbitol ☾<br>Sorbitol ☾ | FrucGalactans ☾<br>FrucGalactans ☾📖 |
|---|---|---|---|---|---|
| Baguette | slice<br>1.49oz/42g | ☺ | ☺<br>☺ | ☺<br>☺ | 1¾ ᴬ<br>3½ |
| Cracked wheat bread, with raisins | slice<br>1.49oz/42g | ☺ | 1¼<br>1½ | ☹<br>4¼ | 1¾ ᴬ<br>3½ |
| English muffin bread | slice<br>1.49oz/42g | ☺ | 38¼<br>38¼ | ☺<br>☺ | 1¾ ᴬ<br>3½ |
| Focaccia bread | slice<br>1.49oz/42g | ☺ | ☺<br>☺ | ☺<br>☺ | 1¼ ᴬ<br>2½ |
| French or Vienna roll | slice<br>1.49oz/42g | ☺ | ☺<br>☺ | ☺<br>☺ | 1¼ ᴬ<br>2½ |
| GG® Scandinavian Bran Crispbread (Health Valley®) | slice<br>1.49oz/42g | ☺ | ☺<br>☺ | ☺<br>☺ | ¼ ᴬ<br>½ |
| Gluten free bread | slice<br>1.49oz/42g | ☺ | ☺<br>☺ | ☺<br>☺ | 3½ ᴬ<br>7 |
| Newman's Own® Organic Pretzels, Spelt | slice<br>1.49oz/42g | ☺ | ☺+ ×½ unit<br>☺+ ×½ unit | ☺<br>☺ | ¾ ᴬ<br>1½ |
| Potato bread | slice<br>1.2oz/34g | 6¼<br>+5¼ unit | ☺<br>☺ | ☹<br>☺ | 1½ ᴬ<br>3 |
| Pumpernickel roll | slice<br>1.49oz/42g | ☺ | ☺<br>☺ | ☺<br>☺ | ½ ᴬ<br>1¼ |
| Rice bread | slice<br>1.49oz/42g | ☺ | ☺<br>☺ | ☺<br>☺ | ☺ ᴬ<br>☺ |
| Rye bread | slice<br>1.49oz/42g | ☺ | ☺<br>☺ | ☺<br>☺ | ¾ ᴬ<br>1¾ |
| Rye roll | slice<br>1.49oz/42g | ☺ | ☺<br>☺ | ☺<br>☺ | ¾ ᴬ<br>1¾ |
| Sourdough bread | slice<br>1.49oz/42g | ☺ | ☺<br>☺ | ☺<br>☺ | ¾ ᴬ<br>1½ |

☾ *Level 0:* lactose measure ×½
☾ *Level 1:* fructose measure ×2
☾ *Level 2:* fructose-/sorbitol measure ×4. the rest ×2
☾ *Level 3:* sorbitol measure ×7. the rest ×3
📖: source of fruc/galactans data

+ Unit/ 💊: added tolerated amount of unit per strong lactase capsule
Fructose*: fructose, sorbitol adjusted
☺+ ×[Amount] unit: Per unit consumed you can additionally tolerate up to [amount] × fructose(*)-unit of another product.

☹: avoid;   ☹¹: ¼ at TL 1;   ☹²: ¼ at TL 2;   ☹³: ¼ at TL 3;   ☺: only contains traces;   ☺: is free from it

| Bread | Unit | Lactose ⚠ + unit/💊 | Fructose* 😕 Fructose 😕 | Sorbitol 😕 Sorbitol ⚠ | FrucGalactans 😕 FrucGalactans ⚠📖 |
|---|---|---|---|---|---|
| Soy bread | slice | 3½ | 11 | ☹ | 1 [A] |
|  | 1.49oz/42g | +3 unit | 11 | 2 | 2 |
| Toast, cinnamon and sugar, whole wheat bread | slice | 49½ | 1½ | ☺ | ¾ [A] |
|  | 1.49oz/42g | +41¼ unit | 1½ | ☺ | 1¾ |
| Toast, wheat bread, with butter | slice | 62½ | 1¾ | ☺ | 1¼ [A] |
|  | 1.49oz/42g | +52 unit | 1¾ | ☺ | 2½ |
| Triticale bread | slice | ☺ | 2½ | ☺ | 1 [A] |
|  | 1.49oz/42g |  | 2½ | ☺ | 2 |
| White bread, store bought | slice | ☺ | 1¼ | ☺ | 1¼ [A] |
|  | 1.49oz/42g |  | 1¼ | ☺ | 2½ |
| White whole grain wheat bread | slice | ☺ | ¾ | ☹ | ¾ [A] |
|  | 1.49oz/42g |  | ¾ | 26¼ | 1¾ |
| Whole wheat bread, store bought | slice | ☺ | 1¼ | ☺ | 1 [A] |
|  | 1.49oz/42g |  | 1¼ | ☺ | 2¼ |

# 3.4.2 Cereals

| Cereals | Unit | Lactose ↴ + unit/💊 | Fructose* ↴ Fructose ↴ | Sorbitol ↴ Sorbitol ↴ | FrucGalactans ↴ FrucGalactans ↴ 📖 |
|---|---|---|---|---|---|
| All-Bran® Original (Kellogg's®) | portion 1.06oz/30g | ☺ | ☺+ ×¼ unit ☺+ ×¼ unit | ☺ ☺ | ¼ ᴬ ¾ |
| Amaranth Flakes (Arrowhead Mills) | portion 1.06oz/30g | ☺ | 3 3¾ | ☹ 2½ | ¾ ᴳ 1½ |
| Cascadian Farm® Organic Chewy Granola Bar, Trail Mix Dark Chocolate Cranberry | piece 1.24oz/35g | ☺ | ☺+ ×4¼ unit ☺+ ×4¼ unit | ☹ 71¼ | ½ ᴬ 1 |
| Chocolate Chex® (General Mills®) | tbsp. 0.5ozfl/14.21ml | ☺ | ¼ ¼ | ☹ ☺ | 1¼ ᴬ 2¾ |
| Cinnamon toast crunch® (General Mills®) | portion 1.06oz/30g | ☺ | ¼ ¼ | ☺ ☺ | 1½ ᴬ 3 |
| Cinnamon Toasters® (Malt-O-Meal®) | portion 1.06oz/30g | ☺ | 2 2 | ☺ ☺ | 1½ ᴬ 3 |
| Cocoa Krispies® (Kellogg's®) | portion 1.06oz/30g | ☺ | ☺ ☺ | ☹ ☺ | 1½ ᴬ 3 |
| Cocoa Puffs® (General Mills®) | portion 1.06oz/30g | ☺ | ☺+ ×2 unit ☺+ ×2 unit | ☹ ☺ | ½ ᴬ 1¼ |
| Corn Chex® (General Mills®) | portion 1.06oz/30g | ☺ | ☺ ☺ | ☹ ☺ | ½ ᴬ 1¼ |
| Corn Flakes (Kellogg's®) | portion 1.06oz/30g | ☺ | ☺+ ×1½ unit ☺+ ×1½ unit | ☹ ☺ | 1½ ᴬ 3 |
| Crunchy Nut Roasted Nut & Honey (Kellogg's®) | portion 1.06oz/30g | ☺ | 23¾ 24 | ☹ 15 | 1½ ᴬ 3 |
| Essentials Oat Bran cereal (Quaker®) | portion 1.95oz/55g | ☺ | ☺ ☺ | ☺ ☺ | 1¼ ᴬ 2¾ |
| Evaporated milk, diluted, skim (fat free) | glass 8.4oz/240g | ¼ +0.21 unit | ☺ ☺ | ☺ ☺ | 1¼ 2¾ |
| Familia Swiss Muesli®, Original Recipe | portion 1.95oz/55g | ☺ | 1 1 | ☹ 1 | ¼ ᴬ ¾ |
| Fiber One Original® (General Mills®) | portion 1.06oz/30g | ☺ | 41½ 41½ | ☺ ☺ | ½ ᴬ 1¼ |

↴ Level 0: lactose measure ×½
↴ Level 1: fructose measure ×2
↴ Level 2: fructose-/sorbitol measure ×4. the rest ×2
↴ Level 3: sorbitol measure ×7. the rest ×3
📖: source of fruc/galactans data

+ Unit/💊: added tolerated amount of unit per strong lactase capsule
Fructose*: fructose, sorbitol adjusted
☺+ ×[Amount] unit: Per unit consumed you can additionally tolerate up to [amount] × fructose(*)-unit of another product.

☹: avoid; ☹¹: ¼ at TL 1; ☹²: ¼ at TL 2; ☹³: ¼ at TL 3; ☺: only contains traces; ☺: is free from it

| Cereals | Unit + unit/🍽 | Lactose | Fructose* / Fructose | Sorbitol / Sorbitol | FrucGalactans / FrucGalactans 📖 |
|---|---|---|---|---|---|
| Fiber One® Nutty Clusters & Almonds (General Mills®) | portion 1.95oz/55g | ☺ | ☺ ☺ | ☺ ☺ | ¼ A ¾ |
| Froot Loops® (Kellogg's®) | portion 1.06oz/30g | ☺ | ☺ ☺ | ☺ ☺ | ½ A 1¼ |
| Frosted Flakes® (Kellogg's®) | portion 1.06oz/30g | ☺ | ☺ ☺ | ☹ ☺ | 1½ A 3 |
| Frosted Flakes® Reduced Sugar (Kellogg's®) | portion 1.06oz/30g | ☺ | ☺+ ×¼ unit ☺+ ×¼ unit | ☹ ☺ | 1½ A 3 |
| Frosted Mini-Wheats Big Bite® (Kellogg's®) | portion 1.95oz/55g | ☺ | ☺+ ×¼ unit ☺+ ×¼ unit | ☺ ☺ | ¼ A ¾ |
| GoLEAN® Crisp! Cereal, Cinnamon Crumble (Kashi®) | portion 1.95oz/55g | ☺ | ☺+ ×1¼ unit ☺+ ×1¼ unit | ☹ 25¾ | ¼ A ¾ |
| GoLEAN® Crunch! Cereal, Honey Almond Flax (Kashi®) | portion 1.95oz/55g | ☺ | ☺+ ×1 unit ☺+ ×1 unit | ☹ 18 | ¼ A ¾ |
| Health Valley® Multigrain Chewy Granola Bar, Chocolate Chip | piece 1.03oz/29g | 29½ +24¾ unit | ☺+ ×1 unit ☺+ ×1 unit | ☹ ☺ | ½ A 1¼ |
| Honey | tbsp. 0.5oz/14.21ml | ☺ | ½ ½ | ☹ 1¾ | ☺ ☺ |
| Honey Nut Chex® (General Mills®) | portion 1.06oz/30g | ☺ | ☺ ☺ | ☹ 37 | ½ A 1¼ |
| Honey Smacks® (Kellogg's®) | portion 1.06oz/30g | ☺ | ☺+ ×12 unit ☺+ ×12 unit | ☹ 83¼ | ½ A 1¼ |
| Kashi® Chewy Granola Bar, Cherry Dark Chocolate | piece 1.24oz/35g | ☺ | ☺+ ×1 unit ☺+ ×1 unit | ☹ 1 | ½ A 1 |
| Maple syrup, pure | tbsp. 0.5oz/14.21ml | ☺ | ☺+ ×¼ unit ☺+ ×¼ unit | ☺ ☺ | ☺ ☺ |
| Milk, lactose reduced (Lactaid®), skim (fat free) | glass 8.4oz/240g | ☺ | ☺+ ×10 unit ☺+ ×10 unit | ☺ ☺ | ☺ ☺ |
| Milk, lactose reduced, skim (fat free), fortified with calcium (Lactaid®) | glass 8.4oz/240g | ☺ | ☺+ ×10 unit ☺+ ×10 unit | ☺ ☺ | ☺ ☺ |
| Mueslix® (Kellogg's®) | portion 1.95oz/55g | ☺ | ☺+ ×¾ unit ☺+ ×¾ unit | ☹ 2¾ | ¼ A ¾ |
| Rice Krispies® (Kellogg's®) | portion 1.06oz/30g | ☺ | ☺ ☺ | ☺ ☺ | 1½ A 3 |
| Sorghum | portion 1.06oz/30g | ☺ | ☺ ☺ | ☺ ☺ | ☺ ☺ |
| Special K® Blueberry cereal (Kellogg's®) | portion 1.06oz/30g | ☺ | ☺+ ×½ unit ☺+ ×½ unit | ☹ 15 | ½ A 1¼ |

| Cereals | Unit | Lactose + unit/🔵 | Fructose* Fructose | Sorbitol Sorbitol | FrucGalactans FrucGalactans 📖 |
|---|---|---|---|---|---|
| Special K® Cinnamon Pecan cereal (Kellogg's®) | portion 1.06oz/30g | ☺ | ☺ ☺ | ☺ ☺ | ½ A 1¼ |
| Special K® Original cereal (Kellogg's®) | portion 1.06oz/30g | 13 +10¾ unit | ☺ ☺ | ☺ ☺ | ½ A 1¼ |
| Special K® Red Berries cereal (Kellogg's®) | portion 1.06oz/30g | ☺ | ☺ ☺ | ☹ 41½ | ½ A 1¼ |
| Sprinkles Cookie Crisp® (General Mills®) | portion 1.06oz/30g | ☺ | ☺+ ×¼ unit ☺+ ×¼ unit | ☹ ☺ | ¾ A 1¾ |
| Sunbelt Bakery® Chewy Granola Bar, Banana Harvest | piece 0.89oz/25g | 49 +40¾ unit | ☺+ ×½ unit ☺+ ×¾ unit | ☹ ¾ | ¾ A 1½ |
| Sunbelt Bakery® Chewy Granola Bar, Blueberry Harvest | piece 0.89oz/25g | 49 +40¾ unit | ☺+ ×½ unit ☺+ ×¾ unit | ☹ ¾ | ¾ A 1½ |
| Sunbelt Bakery® Chewy Granola Bar, Golden Almond | piece 0.99oz/28g | 4 +3¼ unit | 1½ ☺+ ×¾ unit | ☹ ☹² | ½ A 1¼ |
| Sunbelt Bakery® Chewy Granola Bar, Low Fat Oatmeal Raisin | piece 1.06oz/30g | 11¾ +9¾ unit | ½ ☺ | ☹ ☹² | ½ A 1¼ |
| Sunbelt Bakery® Chewy Granola Bar, Oats & Honey | piece 0.96oz/27g | 17½ +14¾ unit | 5¾ ☺+ ×¾ unit | ☹ ☹² | ½ A 1¼ |
| Sunbelt Bakery® Fudge Dipped Chewy Granola Bar, Coconut | piece 1.03oz/29g | 17¼ +14½ unit | ¾ ☺+ ×1¾ unit | ☹ ☹² | ½ A 1¼ |
| Weetabix® Organic Crispy Flakes & Fiber (Barbara's Bakery®) | portion 1.95oz/55g | ☺ | ☺+ ×¾ unit ☺+ ×¾ unit | ☺ ☺ | ¼ A ¾ |
| Wheaties® (General Mills®) | portion 1.06oz/30g | c | 83¼ 83¼ | ☺ ☺ | ½ A 1¼ |

🔵 *Level 0*: lactose measure ×½     + Unit/🔵: added tolerated amount of unit per strong lactase capsule
🔵 *Level 1*: fructose measure ×2    Fructose*: fructose, sorbitol adjusted
🔵 *Level 2*: fructose-/sorbitol measure ×4. the rest ×2    ☺+ ×[Amount] unit: Per unit consumed you can
🔵 *Level 3*: sorbitol measure ×7. the rest ×3    additionally tolerate up to [amount] ×
📖: source of fruc/galactans data    fructose(*)-unit of another product.

☹: avoid;    ☹¹: ¼ at TL 1;    ☹²: ¼ at TL 2;    ☹³: ¼ at TL 3;    ☺: only contains traces;    ☺: is free from it

# 3.4.3 Cold cut

| Cold cut | Unit | Lactose ☝︎ + unit/ 📖 | Fructose* ☝︎ Fructose ☝︎ | Sorbitol ☝︎ Sorbitol ☝︎ | FrucGalactans ☝︎ FrucGalactans ☝︎ 📖 |
|---|---|---|---|---|---|
| Alpine Lace 25% Reduced Fat, Mozzarella | portion 1.06oz/30g | 37¼ +31 unit | ☺ ☺ | ☺ ☺ | ☺ ☺ |
| American cheese, processed | portion 1.06oz/30g | 4½ +3¾ unit | ☺ ☺ | ☺ ☺ | 25¾ 51½ |
| Blue cheese | portion 1.06oz/30g | 20 +16½ unit | ☺ ☺ | ☺ ☺ | ☺ ☺ |
| Bologna, beef ring | portion 1.95oz/55g | ☺ | ☺+ ×5¾ unit ☺+ ×5¾ unit | ☺ ☺ | ☺ ☺ |
| Bologna, combination of meats, light (reduced fat) | portion 1.95oz/55g | ☺ | ☺+ ×½ unit ☺+ ×½ unit | ☺ ☺ | ☺ ☺ |
| Brie cheese | portion 1.06oz/30g | 22 +18½ unit | ☺ ☺ | ☺ ☺ | ☺ ☺ |
| Butter, light, salted | portion 0.5oz/14g | ☺ | ☺ ☺ | ☺ ☺ | ☺ ☺ |
| Butter, unsalted | portion 0.5oz/14g | ☺ | ☺ ☺ | ☺ ☺ | ☺ ☺ |
| Camembert cheese | portion 1.06oz/30g | 21½ +18 unit | ☺ ☺ | ☺ ☺ | ☺ ☺ |
| Cheddar cheese, natural | portion 1.06oz/30g | 43¼ +36 unit | ☺ ☺ | ☺ ☺ | ☺ ☺ |
| Cheese sauce, store bought | portion 2.33oz/66g | ¼ +¼ unit | ☺ ☺ | ☺ ☺ | 1¾ 3¾ |
| Colby Jack cheese | portion 1.06oz/30g | 27¼ +22¾ unit | ☺ ☺ | ☺ ☺ | ☺ ☺ |
| Cottage cheese, 1% fat, lactose reduced | portion 3.89oz/110g | 3¼ +2¾ unit | ☺+ ×1¾ unit ☺+ ×1¾ unit | ☺ ☺ | 18¾ 37¾ |
| Cottage cheese, uncreamed dry curd | portion 1.95oz/55g | 3½ +2¾ unit | ☺ ☺ | ☺ ☺ | 19¾ 39½ |
| Cream cheese spread | portion 1.06oz/30g | 2¾ +2¼ unit | ☺ ☺ | ☺ ☺ | 15¾ 31½ |
| Cream cheese, whipped, flavored | portion 1.06oz/30g | 2½ +2 unit | ☺ ☺ | ☺ ☺ | 14 28 |
| Cream cheese, whipped, plain | portion 1.06oz/30g | 3 +2½ unit | ☺ ☺ | ☺ ☺ | 17¼ 34½ |
| Edam cheese | portion 1.06oz/30g | 6¾ +5¾ unit | ☺ ☺ | ☺ ☺ | 38¾ 77½ |

| Cold cut | Unit | Lactose ↳ + unit/💊 | Fructose* ↳ Fructose ↳ | Sorbitol ↳ Sorbitol ↳ | FrucGalactans ↳ FrucGalactans ↳ 📖 |
|---|---|---|---|---|---|
| Fleischmann's® Move Over Butter Margarine, tub, whipped | portion 0.32oz/9g | 21¾ +18 unit | ☺ ☺ | ☺ ☺ | ☺ ☺ |
| Goats cheese, hard | portion 1.06oz/30g | 4½ +3¾ unit | ☺ ☺ | ☺ ☺ | 25½ 51 |
| Gorgonzola cheese | portion 1.06oz/30g | 20 +16½ unit | ☺ ☺ | ☺ ☺ | ☺ ☺ |
| Gouda cheese | portion 1.06oz/30g | 4½ +3¾ unit | ☺ ☺ | ☺ ☺ | 25 50 |
| Honey | portion 0.75oz/21g | ☺ | ¼ ¼ | ☹ 1¼ | ☺ ☺ |
| Hot dog, combination of meats, plain | portion 1.95oz/55g | ☺ | ☺+ ×3 unit ☺+ ×3 unit | ☺ ☺ | ☺ ☺ |
| Jam or preserves | portion 0.71oz/20g | ☺ | ☺+ ×2¾ unit ☺+ ×2¾ unit | ☹ 1¾ | ☺ ☺ |
| Jam or preserves, reduced sugar | portion 0.71oz/20g | ☺ | 7 7 | ☹ 41½ | ☺ ☺ |
| Jam or preserves, sugar free with aspartame | portion 0.6oz/17g | ☺ | 15¾ 17½ | ☹ 5¼ | ☺ ☺ |
| Jam or preserves, sugar free with saccharin | portion 0.5oz/14g | ☺ | 2¼ 2¼ | ☹ 19¼ | ☺ ☺ |
| Jam or preserves, sugar free with sucralose | portion 0.6oz/17g | ☺ | ☺ ☺ | ☹ 65¼ | ☺ ☺ |
| Jam or preserves, without sugar or artificial sweetener | tbsp. 0.5ozfl/14.21ml | ☺ | ¼ ¼ | ☹ ☹² | ☺ ☺ |
| Kraft® Cheese Spread, Roka Blue | portion 1.06oz/30g | 1¾ +1¼ unit | ☺ ☺ | ☺ ☺ | 9¾ 19½ |
| Limburger cheese | portion 1.06oz/30g | 20¼ +17 unit | ☺ ☺ | ☺ ☺ | ☺ ☺ |
| Maple syrup, pure | tbsp. 0.5oz/14.21ml | ☺ | ☺+ ×¼ unit ☺+ ×¼ unit | ☺ ☺ | ☺ ☺ |
| Margarine, diet, fat free | portion 0.5oz/14g | 15½ +13 unit | ☺ ☺ | ☺ ☺ | 86¾ ☺ |

↳ *Level 0*: lactose measure ×½  
↳ *Level 1*: fructose measure ×2  
↳ *Level 2*: fructose-/sorbitol measure ×4. the rest ×2  
↳ *Level 3*: sorbitol measure ×7. the rest ×3  
📖: source of fruc/galactans data

+ Unit/💊: added tolerated amount of unit per strong lactase capsule  
Fructose*: fructose, sorbitol adjusted  
☺+ ×[Amount] unit: Per unit consumed you can additionally tolerate up to [amount] × fructose(*)-unit of another product.

☹: avoid;   ☹¹: ¼ at TL 1;   ☹²: ¼ at TL 2;   ☹³: ¼ at TL 3;   ☺: only contains traces;   ☺: is free from it

| Cold cut | Unit | Lactose ↓ + unit/⊙ | Fructose* ☺ Fructose ☺ | Sorbitol ☺ Sorbitol ↓ | FrucGalactans ☺ FrucGalactans ↓ |
|---|---|---|---|---|---|
| Margarine, tub, salted, sunflower oil | portion 0.5oz/14g | 30 +25 unit | ☺ ☺ | ☺ ☺ | ☺ ☺ |
| Marmalade, sugar free with aspartame | portion 0.6oz/17g | ☺ | 15¾ 17½ | ☹ 5¼ | ☺ ☺ |
| Marmalade, sugar free with saccharin | portion 0.57oz/16g | ☺ | 2 2 | ☹ 16¾ | ☺ ☺ |
| Marmalade, sugar free with sucralose | portion 0.6oz/17g | ☺ | ☺ ☺ | ☹ 65¼ | ☺ ☺ |
| Mascarpone | portion 1.06oz/30g | 2½ +2 unit | ☺ ☺ | ☺ ☺ | 13¾ 27¾ |
| Mortadella | portion 1.95oz/55g | ☺ | ☺+ ×¼ unit ☺+ ×¼ unit | ☺ ☺ | ☺ ☺ |
| Muenster cheese, natural | portion 1.06oz/30g | 8¾ +7¼ unit | ☺ ☺ | ☺ ☺ | 49½ ☺ |
| Nutella® (filbert spread) | portion 1.31oz/37g | 32¼ +27 unit | 67½ 67½ | ☹ 20¾ | ☺ ☺ |
| Roquefort cheese | portion 1.06oz/30g | 5 +4 unit | ☺ ☺ | ☺ ☺ | 27¾ 55½ |
| Smart Balance® Light with Flax Oil Margarine, tub | portion 0.5oz/14g | 32¼ +27 unit | ☺ ☺ | ☺ ☺ | ☺ ☺ |
| Smart Balance® Margarine | portion 0.5oz/14g | 31 +25¾ unit | ☺ ☺ | ☺ ☺ | ☺ ☺ |
| Soy Kaas Fat Free, all flavors | portion 1.06oz/30g | 9 +7½ unit | 55½ 55½ | ☹ 18½ | 1¼ A 2¾ |
| Swiss cheese, natural | portion 1.06oz/30g | ☺ | ☺+ ×¼ unit ☺+ ×¼ unit | ☺ ☺ | ☺ ☺ |
| Swiss cheese, natural, low sodium | portion 1.06oz/30g | ☺ | ☺+ ×¼ unit ☺+ ×¼ unit | ☺ ☺ | ☺ ☺ |
| Tilsit cheese | portion 1.06oz/30g | 5¼ +4¼ unit | ☺ ☺ | ☺ ☺ | 29½ 59 |

# 3.4.4 Dairy products

| Dairy products | Unit | Lactose ☹<br>+ unit/💊 | Fructose* ☹<br>Fructose ☹ | Sorbitol ☹<br>Sorbitol ☹ | FrucGalactans ☹<br>FrucGalactans ☹📖 |
|---|---|---|---|---|---|
| Almond milk, vanilla or other flavors, unsweetened | glass<br>8.4oz/240g | ☺ | ☺<br>☺ | ☺<br>☺ | ☹ᴬ<br>☹² |
| Breyers® Light! Boosts Immunity Yogurt, all flavors | piece<br>4oz/114g | ½<br>+¼ unit | 28¾<br>31 | ☹<br>14¼ | 3<br>6 |
| Breyers® No Sugar Added Ice Cream, Vanilla | tbsp.<br>0.5ozfl/14.21ml | 3¼<br>+2½ unit | ¾<br>☺ | ☹<br>☹² | 18¼<br>36½ |
| Breyers® YoCrunch Light Nonfat Yogurt, with granola | piece<br>6.5oz/185g | ¼<br>+0.24 unit | ☺<br>☺ | ☹<br>6½ | 1½<br>3 |
| Cabot® Non Fat Yogurt, plain | piece<br>8.01oz/227g | ¼<br>+0.22 unit | ☺<br>☺ | ☺<br>☺ | 1¼<br>2¾ |
| Cabot® Non Fat Yogurt, vanilla | piece<br>8.01oz/227g | ¼<br>+¼ unit | 30¼<br>33¼ | ☹<br>13¼ | 2¼<br>4½ |
| Chobani® Nonfat Greek Yogurt, Black Cherry | tbsp.<br>0.5ozfl/14.21ml | 5¼<br>+4½ unit | ☺<br>☺ | ☹<br>3¾ | 30¼<br>60¾ |
| Chobani® Nonfat Greek Yogurt, Lemon | piece<br>6.04oz/171g | ½<br>+¼ unit | ☺+ ×½ unit<br>☺+ ×½ unit | ☺<br>☺ | 3<br>6 |
| Chobani® Nonfat Greek Yogurt, Peach | piece<br>6.04oz/171g | ¼<br>+¼ unit | ☺+ ×1 unit<br>☺+ ×1 unit | ☹<br>4¼ | 1¾<br>3½ |
| Chobani® Nonfat Greek Yogurt, Raspberry | piece<br>6.04oz/171g | ¼<br>+¼ unit | ☺+ ×¾ unit<br>☺+ ×¾ unit | ☹<br>20 | 1¾<br>3½ |
| Chobani® Nonfat Greek Yogurt, Strawberry | piece<br>6.04oz/171g | ¼<br>+¼ unit | ☺+ ×¾ unit<br>☺+ ×¾ unit | ☹<br>3½ | 1¾<br>3½ |
| Chocolate pudding, store bought | piece<br>3.5oz/98g | ¾<br>+½ unit | ☺<br>☺ | ☹<br>25 | 4¾<br>9¾ |
| Chocolate pudding, store bought, sugar free | tbsp.<br>0.5ozfl/14.21ml | 89¼<br>+74¼ unit | ¾<br>☺ | ☹<br>☹² | ☺<br>☺ |
| Cottage cheese, uncreamed dry curd | portion<br>1.95oz/55g | 3½<br>+2¾ unit | ☺<br>☺ | ☺<br>☺ | 19¾<br>39½ |
| Danone® Activia® Light Yogurt, vanilla | piece<br>4oz/115g | ¼<br>+¼ unit | ¼<br>¼ | ☺<br>☺ | 2<br>4 |

☹ *Level 0:* lactose measure ×½
☹ *Level 1:* fructose measure ×2
☹ *Level 2:* fructose-/sorbitol measure ×4. the rest ×2
☹ *Level 3:* sorbitol measure ×7. the rest ×3
📖: source of fruc/galactans data

+ Unit/💊: added tolerated amount of unit per strong lactase capsule
Fructose*: fructose, sorbitol adjusted

☺+ ×[Amount] unit: Per unit consumed you can additionally tolerate up to [amount] × fructose(*)-unit of another product.

☹: avoid;   ☹¹: ¼ at TL 1;   ☹²: ¼ at TL 2;   ☹³: ¼ at TL 3;   ☺: only contains traces;   ☺: is free from it

| Dairy products | Unit | Lactose ↯ + unit/ | Fructose* ↯ Fructose ↯ | Sorbitol ↯ Sorbitol ↯ | FrucGalactans ↯ FrucGalactans ↯ |
|---|---|---|---|---|---|
| Danone® Activia® Yogurt, plain | piece 4oz/115g | ½ +¼ unit | ☺ ☺ | ☺ ☺ | 2¾ 5½ |
| Danone® Greek Yogurt, Honey | piece 5.3oz/150g | ½ +¼ unit | ¼ ¼ | ☹ 3¼ | 2¾ 5¾ |
| Danone® Greek Yogurt, Plain | piece 5.3oz/150g | ½ +¼ unit | ☺ ☺ | ☺ ☺ | 1¼ 2½ |
| Danone® la Crème Yogurt, fruit flavors | piece 4oz/115g | ¼ +¼ unit | ¼ ¼ | ☹ 10¾ | 2 4 |
| Evaporated milk, diluted, 2% fat (reduced fat) | glass 8.4oz/240g | ¼ +0.22 unit | ☺ ☺ | ☺ ☺ | 1½ 3 |
| Evaporated milk, diluted, skim (fat free) | glass 8.4oz/240g | ¼ +0.21 unit | ☺ ☺ | ☺ ☺ | 1¼ 2¾ |
| Evaporated milk, diluted, whole | glass 8.4oz/240g | ¼ +0.24 unit | ☺ ☺ | ☺ ☺ | 1½ 3 |
| Feta cheese | portion 1.06oz/30g | 2¼ +2 unit | ☺ ☺ | ☺ ☺ | 13½ 27 |
| Feta cheese, fat free | portion 1.06oz/30g | ¾ +¾ unit | ☺ ☺ | ☺ ☺ | 5 10¼ |
| Fondue sauce | portion 1.87oz/53g | ☺ | ☺+ ×¼ unit ☺+ ×¼ unit | ☹ 5 | ☺ ☺ |
| GO Veggie!™ Rice Slices, all flavors | portion 1.06oz/30g | 12 +10 unit | ☺ ☺ | ☺ ☺ | 67¼ A ☺ |
| Greek yogurt, plain, nonfat, | piece 5.3oz/150g | ¼ +¼ unit | ☺ ☺ | ☺ ☺ | 2½ 5 |
| Half and half | portion 1.06oz/30g | 2¼ +1¾ unit | ☺ ☺ | ☺ ☺ | 12¾ 25¾ |
| Kefir | portion 8.65oz/245g | ¼ +¼ unit | ☺ ☺ | ☺ ☺ | 1¾ 3¾ |
| Laughing Cow® Mini Babybel®, Cheddar | piece 0.75oz/21g | ☺ | ☺ ☺ | ☺ ☺ | ☺ ☺ |
| Laughing Cow® Mini Babybel®, Original | piece 0.75oz/21g | 12¾ +10½ unit | ☺ ☺ | ☺ ☺ | 70¾ ☺ |
| Licuado, mango | glass 8.4oz/240g | ¼ +¼ unit | ¼ ¼ | ☹ 1 | 2½ 5 |
| Light cream | portion 0.53oz/15g | 5¼ +4½ unit | ☺ ☺ | ☺ ☺ | 30¼ 60½ |
| Milk, lactose reduced (Lactaid®), skim (fat free) | glass 8.4oz/240g | ☺ | ☺+ ×10 unit ☺+ ×10 unit | ☺ ☺ | ☺ ☺ |
| Milk, lactose reduced (Lactaid®), whole | glass 8.4oz/240g | ☺ | ☺+ ×10 unit ☺+ ×10 unit | ☺ ☺ | ☺ ☺ |

| Dairy products | Unit | Lactose ↳ + unit/💊 | Fructose* ↳ Fructose ↳ | Sorbitol ↳ Sorbitol ↳ | FrucGalactans ↳ FrucGalactans ↳ 📖 |
|---|---|---|---|---|---|
| Milk, lactose reduced, skim (fat free), fortified with calcium (Lactaid®) | glass 8.4oz/240g | ☺ | ☺+ ×10 unit ☺+ ×10 unit | ☺ ☺ | ☺ ☺ |
| Mozzarella cheese, fat free | portion 1.06oz/30g | ½ +½ unit | ☺ ☺ | ☺ ☺ | 3½ 7¼ |
| Mozzarella cheese, whole milk | portion 1.06oz/30g | 9¾ +8¼ unit | ☺ ☺ | ☺ ☺ | 55 ☺ |
| Oat milk | glass 8.4oz/240g | ☺ | ☺ ☺ | ☺ ☺ | ¼ A ¾ |
| Parmesan cheese, dry (grated) | portion 0.18oz/5g | ☺ | ☺ ☺ | ☺ ☺ | ☺ ☺ |
| Parmesan cheese, dry (grated), nonfat | portion 0.18oz/5g | ☺ +75¾ unit | ☺ ☺ | ☺ ☺ | ☺ ☺ |
| Pudding mix, other flavors, cooked type | portion 0.88oz/24.75g | ☺ | ☺ ☺ | ☺ ☺ | ☺ ☺ |
| Rice milk, plain or original, unsweetened, enriched, ready-to-drink | glass 8.4oz/240g | ☺ | ☺+ ×¼ unit ☺+ ×¼ unit | ☺ ☺ | ☺ A ☺ |
| Rice pudding (arroz con leche), coconut, raisins | piece 7.06oz/200g | ½ +¼ unit | 27¾ ☺ | ☹ 1¼ | 3¼ 6½ |
| Rice pudding (arroz con leche), plain | piece 7.06oz/200g | ½ +¼ unit | ☺+ ×½ unit ☺+ ×½ unit | ☺ ☺ | 2¾ 5¾ |
| Rice pudding (arroz con leche), raisins | piece 7.06oz/200g | ½ +¼ unit | 3¾ 8 | ☹ 1¼ | 3 6 |
| Ricotta cheese, part skim milk | portion 1.95oz/55g | 17½ +14½ unit | ☺ ☺ | ☺ ☺ | ☺ ☺ |
| Slim-Fast® Easy to Digest, Vanilla, ready-to-drink can | glass 8.4oz/240g | 2½ +2 unit | ☺ ☺ | ☺ ☺ | 14¼ 28¾ |
| Sour cream | portion 1.06oz/30g | 3¼ +2¾ unit | ☺ ☺ | ☺ ☺ | 19¼ 38½ |
| Soy milk, plain or original, sweetened with artificial sweetener, ready-to-drink | glass 8.4oz/240g | ☺ | 4¾ 4¾ | ☹ 1½ | ☹ A ¼ |

↳ *Level 0*: lactose measure ×½   + Unit/💊: added tolerated amount of unit per strong lactase capsule
↳ *Level 1*: fructose measure ×2   Fructose*: fructose, sorbitol adjusted
↳ *Level 2*: fructose-/sorbitol measure ×4. the rest ×2   ☺+ ×[Amount] unit: Per unit consumed you can
↳ *Level 3*: sorbitol measure ×7. the rest ×3   additionally tolerate up to [amount] ×
📖: source of fruc/galactans data   fructose(*)-unit of another product.
☹: avoid;   ☹[1]: ¼ at TL 1;   ☹[2]: ¼ at TL 2;   ☹[3]: ¼ at TL 3;   ☺: only contains traces;   ☺: is free from it

| Dairy products | Unit | Lactose ↓<br>+ unit/ 🥛 | Fructose* ⚊<br>Fructose ↓ | Sorbitol ⚊<br>Sorbitol ↓ | FrucGalactans ⚊<br>FrucGalactans ↓ 📖 |
|---|---|---|---|---|---|
| Soy milk, vanilla or other flavors, sweetened with sugar, fat free, ready-to-drink | glass<br>8.4oz/240g | ☺ | ☺+ ×¾ unit<br>☺+ ×¾ unit | ☹<br>7 | ☹ A<br>¼ |
| Stonyfield® Oikos Greek Yogurt, Blueberry | piece<br>5.3oz/150g | ¼<br>+¼ unit | ☺+ ×1 unit<br>☺+ ×1 unit | ☺<br>☺ | 1¾<br>3½ |
| Stonyfield® Oikos Greek Yogurt, Caramel | piece<br>4.03oz/114g | ½<br>+½ unit | ☺+ ×½ unit<br>☺+ ×½ unit | ☺<br>☺ | 4<br>8 |
| Stonyfield® Oikos Greek Yogurt, Chocolate | piece<br>4.03oz/114g | ½<br>+¼ unit | 66½<br>66½ | ☺<br>☺ | 3<br>6¼ |
| Stonyfield® Oikos Greek Yogurt, Strawberry | piece<br>5.3oz/150g | ¼<br>+¼ unit | 4<br>4¼ | ☹<br>2 | 1¾<br>3½ |
| Strawberry milk, plain, prepared | glass<br>8.4oz/240g | ¼<br>+¼ unit | ☺<br>☺ | ☺<br>☺ | 1¾<br>3½ |
| Sweetened condensed milk | portion<br>1.35oz/38g | ½<br>+½ unit | ☺<br>☺ | ☺<br>☺ | 3¾<br>7½ |
| Sweetened condensed milk, reduced fat | portion<br>1.38oz/39g | ½<br>+½ unit | ☺<br>☺ | ☺<br>☺ | 3½<br>7¼ |
| Tofu, raw (not silken), cooked, low fat | portion<br>3oz/85g | ☺ | 2¼<br>2¼ | ☹<br>¾ | ½ A<br>1 |
| Whipped cream, aerosol | portion<br>0.25oz/7g | ☺ | ☺<br>☺ | ☺<br>☺ | ☺<br>☺ |
| Whipped cream, aerosol, chocolate | portion<br>0.18oz/5g | 9¾<br>+8 unit | ☺<br>☺ | ☹<br>☺ | 54½<br>☺ |
| Whipped cream, aerosol, fat free | portion<br>0.18oz/5g | 18¾<br>+15¾ unit | ☺+ ×¼ unit<br>☺+ ×¼ unit | ☺<br>☺ | ☺<br>☺ |
| Yogurt, chocolate or coffee flavors, nonfat, sweetened with aspartame | tbsp.<br>0.5ozfl/14.21ml | 4<br>+3¼ unit | ☺<br>☺ | ☺<br>☺ | 22½<br>45 |
| Yogurt, chocolate or coffee flavors, whole milk, sweetened with sucralose | piece<br>6.04oz/171g | ¼<br>+¼ unit | 40<br>40 | ☺<br>☺ | 1½<br>3¼ |
| Yogurt, fruited, whole milk | tbsp.<br>0.5ozfl/14.21ml | 2¾<br>+2¼ unit | ¾<br>¾ | ☹<br>60½ | 16<br>32¼ |

# 3.4.5 Nuts and snacks

| Nuts and snacks | Unit | Lactose ↓ + unit/💊 | Fructose* ☺ Fructose ☺ | Sorbitol ☺ Sorbitol ↓ | FrucGalactans ☺ FrucGalactans ↓ 📖 |
|---|---|---|---|---|---|
| Almonds, raw | hand<br>1.06oz/30g | ☺ | ☺<br>☺ | ☺<br>☺ | ½ G<br>1¼ |
| Baby food, double baked (zwieback) | portion<br>0.25oz/7g | ☺ | ☺<br>☺ | ☺<br>☺ | 1½ A<br>3 |
| Brazil nuts, unsalted | hand<br>1.06oz/30g | ☺ | ☺<br>☺ | ☺<br>☺ | ☺<br>☺ |
| Caramel or sugar coated popcorn, store bought | hand<br>0.75oz/21g | ☺ | ☺+ ×1 unit<br>☺+ ×1 unit | ☺<br>☺ | ☺ C<br>☺ |
| Cashews, raw | hand<br>1.06oz/30g | ☺ | ☺<br>☺ | ☺<br>☺ | ¼ G<br>¾ |
| Cheese cracker | piece<br>0.11oz/3g | ☺ | ☺<br>☺ | ☺<br>☺ | 3½ A<br>7 |
| Chestnuts, roasted | portion<br>1.06oz/30g | ☺ | ☺<br>☺ | ☹<br>3 | ☺<br>☺ |
| Chia seeds | hand<br>1.06oz/30g | ☺ | ☺<br>☺ | ☺<br>☺ | 1¼ G<br>2¾ |
| Coconut cream (liquid from grated meat) | hand<br>1.06oz/30g | ☺ | 20¾<br>20¾ | ☺<br>☺ | ☺<br>☺ |
| Coconut milk, fresh (liquid from grated meat, water added) | glass<br>8.4oz/240g | ☺ | ☺+ ×1 unit<br>☺+ ×1 unit | ☺<br>☺ | 1¾ G<br>3½ |
| Coconut, dried, shredded or flaked, unsweetened | hand<br>1.06oz/30g | ☺ | ☺+ ×¾ unit<br>☺+ ×¾ unit | ☺<br>☺ | 12¼<br>24½ |
| Coconut, fresh | portion<br>0.53oz/15g | ☺ | ☺+ ×¼ unit<br>☺+ ×¼ unit | ☺<br>☺ | 24½ G<br>49 |
| Doritos® Tortilla Chips, Nacho Cheese | hand<br>0.75oz/21g | ☺ | ☺<br>☺ | ☹<br>☺ | 10¾ A<br>21½ |
| Filberts, raw | hand<br>1.06oz/30g | ☺ | ☺<br>☺ | ☹<br>8¼ | 2¾ G<br>5¾ |
| Flax seeds, not fortifed | tbsp.<br>0.5oz/14.21ml | ☺ | ☺<br>☺ | ☺<br>☺ | 2 G<br>4¼ |

☺ *Level 0*: lactose measure ×½　　+ Unit/💊: added tolerated amount of unit per strong lactase capsule
↓ *Level 1*: fructose measure ×2　　Fructose*: fructose, sorbitol adjusted
↓ *Level 2*: fructose-/sorbitol measure ×4. the rest ×2　　☺+ ×[Amount] unit: Per unit consumed you can additionally tolerate up to [amount] × fructose(*)-unit of another product.
↓ *Level 3*: sorbitol measure ×7. the rest ×3
📖: source of fruc/galactans data

☹: avoid;　　☹1: ¼ at TL 1;　　☹2: ¼ at TL 2;　　☹3: ¼ at TL 3;　　☺: only contains traces;　　☺: is free from it

| Nuts and snacks | Unit | Lactose ↓ + unit/ | Fructose* ↓ Fructose ↓ | Sorbitol ↓ Sorbitol ↓ | FrucGalactans ↓ FrucGalactans ↓ |
|---|---|---|---|---|---|
| Ginko nuts, dried | hand 1.06oz/30g | ☺ | ☺ ☺ | ☺ ☺ | ☺ ☺ |
| Hickorynuts | hand 1.06oz/30g | ☺ | ☺ ☺ | ☺ ☺ | 2¾ G 5¾ |
| Lay's® Potato Chips, Classic | hand 0.75oz/21g | ☺ | 41¾ 41¾ | ☹ 79¼ | 10¾ A 21½ |
| Lay's® Potato Chips, Salt & Vinegar | hand 0.75oz/21g | ☺ | 41¾ 41¾ | ☹ 79¼ | 10¾ A 21½ |
| Lay's® Potato Chips, Sour Cream & Onion | hand 0.75oz/21g | ☺ | 41¾ 41¾ | ☹ 79¼ | 10¾ A 21½ |
| Lay's® Stax Potato Crisps, Cheddar | hand 0.75oz/21g | ☺ | 41¾ 41¾ | ☹ 79¼ | 10¾ A 21½ |
| Lay's® Stax Potato Crisps, Hot 'n Spicy Barbecue | hand 0.75oz/21g | ☺ | 54 54 | ☹ ☺ | 10¾ A 21½ |
| Macadamia nuts, raw | hand 1.06oz/30g | ☺ | ☺ ☺ | ☺ ☺ | ☺ ☺ |
| Melba Toast®, Classic (Old London®) | portion 0.53oz/15g | ☺ | ☺+ ×¼ unit ☺+ ×¼ unit | ☹ ☺ | ½ A 1¼ |
| Old Dutch® Crunch Curls | hand 0.75oz/21g | 4 +3¼ unit | ☺ ☺ | ☹ ☺ | 7¼ A 14½ |
| Peanut butter, unsalted | portion 1.13oz/32g | ☺ | ☺+ ×¼ unit ☺+ ×¼ unit | ☺ ☺ | ☺ G ☺ |
| Peanuts, dry roasted, salted | hand 1.06oz/30g | ☺ | ☺ ☺ | ☺ ☺ | ☺ G ☺ |
| Pine nuts, pignolias | hand 1.06oz/30g | ☺ | ☺ ☺ | ☺ ☺ | ☺ ☺ |
| Pistachio nuts, raw | hand 0.75oz/21g | ☺ | ☺ ☺ | ☺ ☺ | ☺ ☺ |
| Poore Brothers® Potato Chips, Salt & Cracked Pepper | hand 0.75oz/21g | ☺ | 54 54 | ☹ ☺ | 10¾ A 21½ |
| Potato chips, salted | hand 0.75oz/21g | ☺ | 41¾ 41¾ | ☹ 79¼ | 10¾ A 21½ |
| Potato sticks | hand 0.75oz/21g | ☺ | ☺ ☺ | ☹ 79¼ | 10¾ A 21½ |
| Pretzels, hard, unsalted, sticks | hand 0.75oz/21g | ☺ | ☺ ☺ | ☺ ☺ | 1½ A 3¼ |
| Pringles® Light Fat Free Potato Crisps, Barbecue | hand 0.75oz/21g | ☺ | 37 37 | ☹ 79¼ | 10¾ A 21½ |
| Pringles® Potato Crisps Loaded Baked Potato | hand 0.75oz/21g | ☺ | 41¾ 41¾ | ☹ 79¼ | 10¾ A 21½ |

| Nuts and snacks | Unit | Lactose ↓ + unit/💊 | Fructose* ↺ Fructose ↓ | Sorbitol ↺ Sorbitol ↓ | FrucGalactans ↺ FrucGalactans ↓ 📖 |
|---|---|---|---|---|---|
| Pringles® Potato Crisps, Original | hand 0.75oz/21g | ☺ | 76¾ 76¾ | ☹ ☺ | 10¾ A 21½ |
| Pringles® Potato Crisps, Salt & Vinegar | hand 0.75oz/21g | ☺ | 41¾ 41¾ | ☹ 79¼ | 10¾ A 21½ |
| Pumpkin or squash seeds, shelled, unsalted | hand 1.06oz/30g | ☺ | ☺ ☺ | ☺ ☺ | 2¾ G 5¾ |
| Rice cake | piece 0.32oz/9g | ☺ | ☺ ☺ | ☺ ☺ | 7½ A 15 |
| Ritz Cracker (Nabisco®) | portion 1.06oz/30g | ☺ | ☺ ☺ | ☺ ☺ | ¼ A ½ |
| Sesame sticks | hand 0.75oz/21g | ☺ | ☺ ☺ | ☹ ☺ | 1½ A 3¼ |
| Soy chips | hand 0.75oz/21g | 5¼ +4¼ unit | 15 15 | ☹ 1 | 2 A 4 |
| Sunflower seeds, raw | hand 1.06oz/30g | ☺ | ☺ ☺ | ☺ ☺ | 1 A 2¼ |
| Taco John's® nachos | hand 0.75oz/21g | 28 +23¼ unit | ☺ ☺ | ☹ ☺ | 10 A 20 |
| Tortilla, white, store bought, fried | piece 2.05oz/58g | ☺ | ☺ ☺ | ☺ ☺ | ¾ A 1¾ |
| Walnuts | hand 1.06oz/30g | ☺ | ☺ ☺ | ☺ ☺ | ☺ ☺ |
| Wise Onion Flavored Rings | Portion 30 g | ☺ | ☺ ☺ | ☹ ☺ | 10¼ AC 20¾ |

↺ *Level 0*: lactose measure ×½
↓ *Level 1*: fructose measure ×2
↯ *Level 2*: fructose-/sorbitol measure ×4. the rest ×2
↳ *Level 3*: sorbitol measure ×7. the rest ×3
📖: source of fruc/galactans data

+ Unit/💊: added tolerated amount of unit per strong lactase capsule
Fructose*: fructose, sorbitol adjusted
☺+ ×[Amount] unit: Per unit consumed you can additionally tolerate up to [amount] × fructose(*)-unit of another product.

☹: avoid;   ☹¹: ¼ at TL 1;   ☹²: ¼ at TL 2;   ☹³: ¼ at TL 3;   ☺: only contains traces;   ☺: is free from it

# 3.4.6 Sweet pastries

| Sweet pastries | Unit | Lactose<br>+ unit/ | Fructose*<br>Fructose | Sorbitol<br>Sorbitol | FrucGalactans<br>FrucGalactans |
|---|---|---|---|---|---|
| Almond cookies | piece<br>0.44oz/12.4g | ☺ | ☺<br>☺ | ☺<br>☺ | 3 A<br>6 |
| Apple cake, glazed | piece<br>1.59oz/45g | ☺ | ¾<br>1 | ☹<br>½ | 1¼ A<br>2½ |
| Apple strudel | piece<br>2.26oz/64g | ☺ | ¼<br>¼ | ☹<br>¼ | ¾ A<br>1¾ |
| Archway® Oatmeal Raisin Cookies | piece<br>0.92oz/26g | 23¾<br>+19¾ unit | ☺<br>☺ | ☹<br>10¼ | 2¼ A<br>4¾ |
| Archway® Peanut Butter Cookies | piece<br>1.2oz/34g | 23¾<br>+19¾ unit | 2<br>2 | ☹<br>10¾ | 1½ A<br>3 |
| Biscotti, chocolate, nuts | piece<br>0.73oz/20.5g | ☺ | ☺<br>☺ | ☹<br>☺ | 2½ A<br>5 |
| Brownie, chocolate, fat free | piece<br>1.56oz/44g | 3<br>+2½ unit | 71<br>71 | ☹<br>☺ | 1 A<br>2¼ |
| Butter cracker | piece<br>0.15oz/4g | ☺ | ☺<br>☺ | ☺<br>☺ | 10 A<br>20 |
| Carrot cake, glazed, homemade | piece<br>0.98oz/27.72g | ☺ | ☺+ ×¼ unit<br>☺+ ×¼ unit | ☹<br>8 | 2 A<br>4 |
| Cheesecake, plain or flavored, graham cracker crust, homemade | piece<br>7.77oz/220g | ½<br>+½ unit | ☺+ ×½ unit<br>☺+ ×½ unit | ☺<br>☺ | ☹ A<br>¼ |
| Cherry pie, bottom crust only | piece<br>4.31oz/122g | ☺ | 1<br>☺+ ×1½ unit | ☹<br>☹2 | ¼ A<br>¾ |
| Chips Ahoy!® Chewy Gooey Caramel Cookies (Nabisco®) | piece<br>0.55oz/15.5g | 12¼<br>+10¼ unit | ½<br>½ | ☹<br>☺ | 3 A<br>6¼ |
| Chocolate cake, glazed, store bought | piece<br>1.03oz/29g | ☺ | ☺+ ×½ unit<br>☺+ ×½ unit | ☹<br>☺ | 1¾ A<br>3¾ |
| Chocolate chip cookies, store bought | piece<br>0.36oz/10g | ☺ | ☺<br>☺ | ☹<br>☺ | 2½ A<br>5¼ |
| Chocolate cookies, iced, store bought | piece<br>0.36oz/10g | ☺ | ☺<br>☺ | ☹<br>☺ | 5 A<br>10¼ |
| Chocolate sandwich cookies, double filling | piece<br>0.52oz/14.5g | ☺ | ☺<br>☺ | ☹<br>☺ | 3½ A<br>7 |
| Chocolate sandwich cookies, sugar free | piece<br>0.43oz/12g | ☺ | 13¾<br>☺ | ☹<br>☹ | 4¼ A<br>8½ |
| Cinnamon Roll with Icing, all flavours | piece<br>1.56oz/44g | 9<br>+7½ unit | ☺+ ×8¼ unit<br>☺+ ×8¼ unit | ☺<br>☺ | 1 A<br>2¼ |

| Sweet pastries | Unit | Lactose ↳ + unit/🗩 | Fructose* ↯ Fructose ↳ | Sorbitol ↯ Sorbitol ↳ | FrucGalactans ↯ FrucGalactans ↳ 📖 |
|---|---|---|---|---|---|
| Crepe, plain | piece 1.95oz/55g | 1¼ +1 unit | ☺ ☺ | ☺ ☺ | ¾ ᴬ 1¾ |
| Croissant, chocolate | piece 2.44oz/69g | 3½ +3 unit | ☺+ ×1 unit ☺+ ×1 unit | ☹ ☺ | ¾ ᴬ 1½ |
| Croissant, fruit | piece 2.62oz/74g | 3½ +3 unit | ☺+ ×2½ unit ☺+ ×2½ unit | ☹ 2 | ½ ᴬ 1¼ |
| Danish pastry, frosted or glazed, with cheese filling | piece 4.41oz/125g | 3 +2½ unit | ☺ ☺ | ☺ ☺ | ¼ ᴰ ½ |
| Dare Breaktime Ginger Cookies | piece 0.27oz/7.5g | ☺ | ☺ ☺ | ☺ ☺ | 8½ ᴬ 17¼ |
| Dare® Lemon Crème Cookies | piece 0.69oz/19.5g | 32½ +27 unit | ☺ ☺ | ☺ ☺ | 2½ ᴬ 5¼ |
| Doughnut, raised, glazed, coconut topping | piece 2.79oz/79g | 4¾ +4 unit | ☺ ☺ | ☺ ☺ | ½ ᴬ 1¼ |
| Doughnut, raised, glazed, plain | piece 2.72oz/77g | 4¾ +4 unit | ☺ ☺ | ☺ ☺ | ½ ᴬ 1¼ |
| Doughnut, raised, sugared | piece 2.56oz/72.5g | 4¾ +4 unit | ☺ ☺ | ☺ ☺ | ¾ ᴬ 1½ |
| EGG® bread roll | piece 1.24oz/35g | 5¼ +4¼ unit | ☺ ☺ | ☺ ☺ | 1½ ᴬ 3 |
| Elephant ear (crispy) | piece 2.09oz/59g | 4¼ +3½ unit | ☺ ☺ | ☺ ☺ | 1 ᴬ 2 |
| English muffin, whole wheat, with raisins | piece 2.33oz/66g | 1¼ +1 unit | 2 2½ | ☹ 2¼ | ¾ ᴬ 1½ |
| French toast, homemade, French bread | piece 4.63oz/131g | 1¼ +1 unit | ☺+ ×½ unit ☺+ ×½ unit | ☺ ☺ | ¼ ᴬ ¾ |
| Frozen custard, chocolate or coffee flavors | portion 3.09oz/87.5g | ½ +¼ unit | ☺+ ×2¼ unit ☺+ ×2¼ unit | ☹ ☺ | ½ ᴬ 1 |
| German chocolate cake, glazed, homemade | piece 1.03oz/29g | ☺ | ☺+ ×½ unit ☺+ ×½ unit | ☹ ☺ | 1¾ ᴬ 3¾ |
| Girl Scout® Lemonades | piece 0.55oz/15.5g | ☺ | ☺ ☺ | ☺ ☺ | 4 ᴬ 8¼ |
| Girl Scout® Peanut Butter Patties | piece 0.45oz/12.5g | ☺ | ☺ ☺ | ☹ ☺ | 4 ᴬ 8¼ |

↯ *Level 0*: lactose measure ×½
↳ *Level 1*: fructose measure ×2
↯ *Level 2*: fructose-/sorbitol measure ×4. the rest ×2
↳ *Level 3*: sorbitol measure ×7. the rest ×3
📖: source of fruc/galactans data

\+ Unit/🗩: added tolerated amount of unit per strong lactase capsule
Fructose*: fructose, sorbitol adjusted

☺+ ×[Amount] unit: Per unit consumed you can additionally tolerate up to [amount] × fructose(*)-unit of another product.

☹: avoid;   ☹¹: ¼ at TL 1;   ☹²: ¼ at TL 2;   ☹³: ¼ at TL 3;   ☺: only contains traces;   ☺: is free from it

| Sweet pastries | Unit + unit/ | Lactose | Fructose* / Fructose | Sorbitol / Sorbitol | FrucGalactans / FrucGalactans |
|---|---|---|---|---|---|
| Girl Scout® Samoas® | piece | 52¼ | 10¼ | ☹ | 3½ A |
|  | 0.52oz/14.5g +43½ unit |  | ☺ | ¾ | 7 |
| Girl Scout® Shortbread® | piece | 18½ | ☺ | ☺ | 3¼ A |
|  | 0.4oz/11.34g +15½ unit |  | ☺ | ☺ | 6¾ |
| Girl Scout® Thin Mints | piece | 32½ | ☺ | ☹ | 6¼ A |
|  | 0.29oz/8g +27 unit |  | ☺ | ☺ | 12½ |
| Halvah | portion | ☺ | ☺+ ×1½ unit | ☺ | 1¼ A |
|  | 1.42oz/40g |  | ☺+ ×1½ unit | ☺ | 2¾ |
| Lebkuchen | piece | ☺ | 6¼ | ☹ | 2 A |
|  | 1.15oz/32.4g |  | 6¼ | 6½ | 4 |
| Little Debbie® Coffee Cake, Apple Streusel | piece | ☺ | ☺+ ×5¼ unit | ☺ | 1 A |
|  | 1.84oz/52g |  | ☺+ ×5¼ unit | ☺ | 2 |
| Little Debbie® Fudge Brownies with English Walnuts | piece | ☺ | ☺+ ×4¼ unit | ☹ | 1¾ A |
|  | 1.08oz/30.5g |  | ☺+ ×4¼ unit | ☺ | 3½ |
| Long John or bismarck, glazed, cream or custard filled, with nuts | piece | 2¼ | ☺ | ☺ | ½ A |
|  | 3.71oz/105g +2 unit |  | ☺ | ☺ | 1 |
| Molasses cookies, store bought | piece | ☺ | ☺ | ☺ | 3¼ A |
|  | 0.53oz/15g |  | ☺ | ☺ | 6¾ |
| Muffins, banana | piece | 2½ | ☺+ ×¼ unit | ☹ | ¼ A |
|  | 3.99oz/113g +2 unit |  | ☺+ ×¼ unit | 29¼ | ¾ |
| Muffins, blueberry, store bought | piece | 1½ | ☺ | ☺ | ¼ A |
|  | 3.99oz/113g +1¼ unit |  | ☺ | ☺ | ¾ |
| Muffins, carrot, homemade, with nuts | piece | 1½ | ☺ | ☹ | ¼ A |
|  | 3.99oz/113g +1¼ unit |  | ☺ | 3¼ | ¾ |
| Muffins, oat bran or oatmeal, store bought | piece | 1¼ | ☺+ ×¼ unit | ☺ | ½ A |
|  | 3.99oz/113g +1 unit |  | ☺+ ×¼ unit | ☺ | 1 |
| Muffins, pumpkin, store bought | piece | 1¾ | ☺+ ×¼ unit | ☹ | ¼ A |
|  | 3.99oz/113g +1¼ unit |  | ☺+ ×¼ unit | 14½ | ¾ |
| Murray® Sugar Free Oatmeal Cookies | piece | ☺ | ½ | ☹ | 4½ A |
|  | 0.39oz/11g |  | ☺ | ☹2 | 9 |
| Murray® Sugar Free Shortbread | piece | ☺ | 1½ | ☹ | 10½ A |
|  | 0.14oz/3.75g |  | ☺ | ☹2 | 21¼ |
| Nabisco® 100 Calorie Packs, Honey Maid Cinnamon Roll Thin Crisps | piece | ☺ | ☺ | ☹ | 4¾ A |
|  | 0.46oz/13g |  | ☺ | 42½ | 9¾ |
| Nilla Wafers® (Nabisco®) | piece | 32½ | ☺ | ☺ | 12¼ A |
|  | 0.14oz/3.75g +27 unit |  | ☺ | ☺ | 24¾ |
| Nutter Butter® Cookies (Nabisco®) | portion | ☺ | ☺ | ☺ | 3½ A |
|  | 0.5oz/14g |  | ☺ | ☺ | 7¼ |

| Sweet pastries | Unit | Lactose ↙ + unit/💊 | Fructose* ↙↗ Fructose ↙ | Sorbitol ↙↗ Sorbitol ↙ | FrucGalactans ↙↗ FrucGalactans ↙ 📖 |
|---|---|---|---|---|---|
| Oatmeal cookies, store bought | piece 0.46oz/13g | 45¾ +38 unit | ☺ ☺ | ☺ ☺ | 3¾ ᴬ 7½ |
| Oreo® Brownie Cookies (Nabisco®) | piece 1.5oz/42.5g | ☺ | ¼ ¼ | ☹ ☺ | 1 ᴬ 2¼ |
| Oreo® Cookies (Nabisco®) | piece 0.43oz/12g | ☺ | ☺ ☺ | ☹ ☺ | 4¼ ᴬ 8½ |
| Oreo® Cookies, Sugar Free (Nabisco®) | piece 0.43oz/12g | ☺ | 13¾ ☺ | ☹ ☹ | 4¼ ᴬ 8½ |
| Pancake, buckwheat, from mix, add water only | piece 1.56oz/44g | ☺ | ☺ ☺ | ☹ 3¾ | 1¼ ᴬ 2½ |
| Pancake, whole wheat, homemade | piece 1.56oz/44g | 2½ +2 unit | ☺ ☺ | ☺ ☺ | 1 ᴬ 2¼ |
| Peach pie, bottom crust only | piece 4.31oz/122g | ☺ | 2¾ 5¾ | ☹ 1 | ¼ ᴬ ¾ |
| Pepperidge Farm® Sweet & Simple, Soft Baked Sugar Cookies | piece 0.48oz/13.5g | ☺ | ☹¹ ☹¹ | ☺ ☺ | 4¾ ᴬ 9½ |
| Pepperidge Farm® Turnover, Apple | piece 3.14oz/89g | 9 +7½ unit | ½ ½ | ☹ ¼ | ½ ᴬ 1¼ |
| Pillsbury® Big Deluxe White Chunk Macadamia Nut Cookies | piece 1.35oz/38g | 6¾ +5½ unit | ☺ ☺ | ☺ ☺ | ½ ᴬ 1¼ |
| Popcorn, store bought (prepopped), "buttered" | portion 1.06oz/30g | 36¾ +30¾ unit | ☺ ☺ | ☺ ☺ | ☺ ᶜᴮ ☺ |
| Rhubarb pie, bottom crust only | piece 4.31oz/122g | ☺ | ☺ ☺ | ☺ ☺ | ¼ ᴬ ¾ |
| Sandwich cookies, vanilla | piece 0.53oz/15g | 9 +7½ unit | ☺ ☺ | ☺ ☺ | 3 ᴬ 6¼ |
| Sticky bun | piece 2.51oz/71g | 8¾ +7¼ unit | ☺+ ×¾ unit ☺+ ×¾ unit | ☺ ☺ | ½ ᴰ 1 |
| Strawberry pie, bottom crust only | piece 4.31oz/122g | ☺ | 1¾ 2 | ☹ ¾ | ¼ ᴬ ¾ |
| Sugar cookies, iced, store bought | piece 0.53oz/15g | ☺ | ☺ ☺ | ☺ ☺ | 3¼ ᴬ 6½ |

↗ *Level 0:* lactose measure ×½    + Unit/💊: added tolerated amount of unit per strong lactase capsule
↙ *Level 1:* fructose measure ×2    Fructose*: fructose, sorbitol adjusted
↗ *Level 2:* fructose-/sorbitol measure ×4. the rest ×2    ☺+ ×[Amount] unit: Per unit consumed you can
↙ *Level 3:* sorbitol measure ×7. the rest ×3    additionally tolerate up to [amount] ×
📖: source of fruc/galactans data    fructose(*)-unit of another product.

☹: avoid;    ☹¹: ¼ at TL 1;    ☹²: ¼ at TL 2;    ☹³: ¼ at TL 3;    ☺: only contains traces;    ☺: is free from it

| Sweet pastries | Unit | Lactose + unit/ | Fructose* Fructose | Sorbitol Sorbitol | FrucGalactans FrucGalactans |
|---|---|---|---|---|---|
| Sweet potato bread | slice | ☺ | ☺ ☺ | ☺ ☺ | 1½ A |
|  | 1.49oz/42g |  |  |  | 3¼ |
| Tiramisu | portion | 2½ | ☺ ☺ | ☺ ☺ | 13¾ A |
|  | 1.95oz/55g | +2 unit |  |  | 27¾ |
| Twix® | piece | 2 | ☺+ ×1½ unit | ☺ ☺ | 2 A |
|  | 1.8oz/51g | +1¾ unit | ☺+ ×1½ unit |  | 4 |
| Waffles, bran | piece | ¾ | ☺+ ×¼ unit | ☺ ☺ | ¼ A |
|  | 3.36oz/95g | +¾ unit | ☺+ ×¼ unit |  | ¾ |
| Waffles, whole wheat, from mix, add milk, fat and egg | piece | 1 | ☺+ ×¼ unit | ☺ ☺ | ½ A |
|  | 3.36oz/95g | +¾ unit | ☺+ ×¼ unit |  | 1 |
| Windmill cookies | piece(s) | c | ☺ ☺ | ☺ ☺ | 6¼ A |
|  | 0.75oz/21g |  |  |  | 12¾ |

# 3.4.7 Sweets

| Sweets | Unit | Lactose ↯ + unit/ 💊 | Fructose* ☹ Fructose ☹ | Sorbitol ☹ Sorbitol ↯ | FrucGalactans ☹ FrucGalactans ↯ 📖 |
|---|---|---|---|---|---|
| 3 Musketeers® | piece 2.14oz/60.4g | 1¾ +1½ unit | ☺+ ×3¾ unit ☺+ ×3¾ unit | ☺ ☺ | 6¼ 12½ |
| After Eight® Thin Chocolate Mints | piece 0.29oz/8g | 10¼ +8½ unit | ☺ ☺ | ☺ ☺ | 57¾ ☺ |
| Almond paste (Marzipan) | portion 0.99oz/28g | ☺ | ☺ ☺ | ☹ 20½ | ½ G 1¼ |
| Almonds, honey roasted | hand 1.06oz/30g | ☺ | 2 2 | ☹ 5½ | ½ G 1¼ |
| Breath mint, regular | portion 0.08oz/2g | ☺ | ☺+ ×¼ unit ☺+ ×¼ unit | ☺ ☺ | ☺ ☺ |
| Breath mint, sugar free | portion 0.08oz/2g | ☺ | ¼ ☺ | ☹ ☹³ | ☺ ☺ |
| Brown sugar | tbsp. 0.5oz/14.21ml | ☺ | ☺ ☺ | ☺ ☺ | ☺ ☺ |
| Buttermels® (Switzer's®) | piece 0.25oz/6.9g | 8 +6½ unit | ☺+ ×½ unit ☺+ ×½ unit | ☺ ☺ | 44¾ 89¾ |
| Candy necklace | piece 0.75oz/21g | ☺ | ☺+ ×3¼ unit ☺+ ×3¼ unit | ☺ ☺ | ☺ ☺ |
| Chewing gum | piece 0.11oz/3g | ☺ | ☺ ☺ | ☺ ☺ | ☺ ☺ |
| Chewing gum, sugar free | piece 0.08oz/2g | ☺ | ¼ ☺ | ☹ ☹² | ☺ ☺ |
| Chocolate truffles | piece 0.58oz/16.2g | 2½ +2 unit | ☺ ☺ | ☺ ☺ | 14¼ 28¾ |
| Classic Fruit Chocolates (Liberty Orchards®) | piece 0.53oz/15g | 56½ +47 unit | ☺+ ×¼ unit ☺+ ×¼ unit | ☹ 31½ | ☺ ☺ |
| Coconut bars, nuts | piece 1.49oz/42g | 45¼ +37¾ unit | ☺ ☺ | ☺ ☺ | ☺ ☺ |
| Dark chocolate bar 45%-59% cacoa | bar 4.77oz/135g | 1¼ +1 unit | ☺ ☺ | ☹ 8 | ¼ ¾ |

↯ *Level 0*: lactose measure ×½  
↯ *Level 1*: fructose measure ×2  
↯ *Level 2*: fructose-/sorbitol measure ×4. the rest ×2  
↯ *Level 3*: sorbitol measure ×7. the rest ×3  
📖: source of fruc/galactans data  

\+ Unit/ 💊: added tolerated amount of unit per strong lactase capsule  
Fructose*: fructose, sorbitol adjusted  
☺+ ×[Amount] unit: Per unit consumed you can additionally tolerate up to [amount] × fructose(*)-unit of another product.  

☹: avoid;   ☹¹: ¼ at TL 1;   ☹²: ¼ at TL 2;   ☹³: ¼ at TL 3;   ☺: only contains traces;   ☺: is free from it

| Sweets | Unit | Lactose ⌄ + unit/ | Fructose* ⌄ Fructose ⌄ | Sorbitol ⌄ Sorbitol ⌄ | FrucGalactans ⌄ FrucGalactans ⌄ |
|---|---|---|---|---|---|
| Dark chocolate bar 60%-69% cacao | bar 4.77oz/135g | 7½ +6¼ unit | ☺ ☺ | ☹ 6½ | ¼ ¾ |
| Dark chocolate bar 70%-85% cacao | bar 4.77oz/135g | ☺ | ☺ ☺ | ☹ 5 | ¼ ¾ |
| Dark chocolate bar, sugar free | piece 0.43oz.fl/12g | 26¾ +22¼ unit | 34 34 | ☹ ☹ | 4¼ 8¾ |
| Dark Fruit Chocolates (Liberty Orchards®) | piece 0.53oz/15g | 56½ +47 unit | ☺+ ×¼ unit ☺+ ×¼ unit | ☹ 31½ | ☺ ☺ |
| Dark Fruit Chocolates, Sugar Free (Liberty Orchards®) | piece 0.6oz/17g | 37¾ +31¼ unit | ☹² ☺ | ☹ ☹ | ☺ ☺ |
| Fifty 50® Sugar Free Low Glycemic Butterscotch Hard Candy | piece 0.14oz/3.75g | ☺ | ☺ ☺ | ☹ ☹ | ☺ ☺ |
| French Burnt Peanuts | hand 1.06oz/30g | ☺ | ☺+ ×1¾ unit ☺+ ×1¾ unit | ☺ ☺ | ☺ G ☺ |
| Gelatin (jello) powder, flavored, sugar free | piece 0.18oz/5g | ☺ | ☺ ☺ | ☺ ☺ | ☺ ☺ |
| Gelatin (jello) powder, plain | piece 0.07oz/1.75g | ☺ | ☺ ☺ | ☺ ☺ | ☺ ☺ |
| Gum drops | hand 1.06oz/30g | ☺ | ☺+ ×2¼ unit ☺+ ×2¼ unit | ☺ ☺ | ☺ ☺ |
| Gum drops, sugar free | tsp. 0.16ozfl/4.74ml | ☺ | ☺ ☺ | ☹ ☹ | ☺ ☺ |
| Gummi bears | hand 1.06oz/30g | ☺ | ☺+ ×3½ unit ☺+ ×3½ unit | ☹ ☺ | ☺ ☺ |
| Gummi bears, sugar free | tsp. 0.16ozfl/4.74ml | ☺ | 10 ☺ | ☹ ☹³ | ☺ ☺ |
| Gummi dinosaurs | hand 1.06oz/30g | ☺ | ☺+ ×3½ unit ☺+ ×3½ unit | ☹ ☺ | ☺ ☺ |
| Gummi dinosaurs, sugar free | tsp. 0.16ozfl/4.74ml | ☺ | 10 ☺ | ☹ ☹³ | ☺ ☺ |
| Gummi worms | hand 1.06oz/30g | ☺ | ☺+ ×3½ unit ☺+ ×3½ unit | ☹ ☺ | ☺ ☺ |
| Gummi worms, sugar free | tsp. 0.16ozfl/4.74ml | ☺ | 10 ☺ | ☹ ☹³ | ☺ ☺ |
| Hard candy | piece 0.22oz/6g | ☺ | ☺+ ×¾ unit ☺+ ×¾ unit | ☺ ☺ | ☺ ☺ |
| Hard candy, sugar free | piece 0.11oz/3g | ☺ | ☹¹ ☺ | ☹ ☹ | ☺ ☺ |

| Sweets | Unit | Lactose ꝯ + unit/ 📖 | Fructose* ꝯ Fructose ꝯ | Sorbitol ꝯ Sorbitol ꝯ | FrucGalactans ꝯ FrucGalactans ꝯ 📖 |
|---|---|---|---|---|---|
| Hershey's® Caramel Filled Chocolates Sugar Free | piece 0.31oz/8.6g | 74½ +62 unit | 21¾ ☺ | ☹ ☹ | ☺ ☺ |
| Hershey's® Milk Chocolate Bar | bar 4.77oz/135g | ¼ +¼ unit | ☺ ☺ | ☺ ☺ | ¼ G ¾ |
| Jelly beans® | hand 1.06oz/30g | ☺ | ☺+ ×9¾ unit ☺+ ×9¾ unit | ☺ ☺ | ☺ ☺ |
| Jelly beans®, sugar free | tsp. 0.16ozfl/4.74ml | ☺ | 12¼ ☺ | ☹ ☹ | ☺ ☺ |
| Jujyfruits® | hand 1.06oz/30g | ☺ | ☺+ ×12¼ unit ☺+ ×12¼ unit | ☺ ☺ | ☺ ☺ |
| Kit Kat® | piece 1.52oz/43g | 2 +1¾ unit | ☺ ☺ | ☹ ☺ | 2 A 4¼ |
| Kit Kat® White | piece 1.49oz/42g | ¾ +½ unit | ☺ ☺ | ☺ ☺ | 1½ A 3¼ |
| Licorice | piece 0.39oz/11g | ☺ | ☺+ ×1½ unit ☺+ ×1½ unit | ☺ ☺ | ☺ ☺ |
| Little Debbie® Nutty Bars | piece 1.01oz/28.5g | ☺ | ☺+ ×13¾ unit ☺+ ×13¾ unit | ☹ ☺ | 4¼ A 8½ |
| M & M's® Peanut | portion 1.42oz/40g | 2½ +2 unit | ☺ ☺ | ☺ ☺ | 8¾ 17¾ |
| Mamba® Fruit Chews | portion 1.42oz/40g | ☺ | ☺ ☺+ ×22¼ unit | ☹ ☹ | ☺ ☺ |
| Mamba® Sour Fruit Chews | portion 1.42oz/40g | ☺ | ☹² ☺+ ×17½ unit | ☹ ☹ | ☺ ☺ |
| Marshmallow | portion 1.06oz/30g | ☺ | ☺+ ×4½ unit ☺+ ×4½ unit | ☺ ☺ | ☺ ☺ |
| Mentos® | piece 0.11oz/3g | ☺ | ☺ ☺ | ☺ ☺ | ☺ ☺ |
| Milk chocolate bar, cereal | bar 4.77oz/135g | ½ +½ unit | ☺ ☺ | ☹ 40 | ¼ A ¾ |
| Milk chocolate bar, cereal, sugar free | piece 0.43oz.fl/12g | 26½ +22 unit | 80 80 | ☹ ☹ | 4½ A 9 |
| Milk chocolate bar, sugar free | piece 0.43oz.fl/12g | 32½ +27 unit | 80 80 | ☹ ☹ | 4½ 9 |

ꝯ *Level 0*: lactose measure ×½
ꝯ *Level 1*: fructose measure ×2
ꝯ *Level 2*: fructose-/sorbitol measure ×4. the rest ×2
ꝯ *Level 3*: sorbitol measure ×7. the rest ×3
📖: source of fruc/galactans data

+ Unit/ 📖: added tolerated amount of unit per strong lactase capsule
Fructose*: fructose, sorbitol adjusted
☺+ ×[Amount] unit: Per unit consumed you can additionally tolerate up to [amount] × fructose(*)-unit of another product.

☹: avoid;   ☹¹: ¼ at TL 1;   ☹²: ¼ at TL 2;   ☹³: ¼ at TL 3;   ☺: only contains traces;   ☺: is free from it

| Sweets | Unit | Lactose ↯ + unit/ 🥛 | Fructose* ⊙↯ Fructose ⊙↯ | Sorbitol ⊙↯ Sorbitol ↯ | FrucGalactans ⊙↯ FrucGalactans ↯📖 |
|---|---|---|---|---|---|
| Milk chocolate bar, sugar free | piece 0.43oz.fl/12g | 32½ +27 unit | 80 80 | ☹ ☹ | 4½ 9 |
| Milk Chocolate covered raisins | hand 1.06oz/30g | 2¾ +2¼ unit | ☺+ ×¼ unit ☺+ ×¼ unit | ☹ 3¼ | 16 32 |
| Molasses, dark | tbsp. 0.5oz/14.21ml | ☺ | 3¾ 3¾ | ☺ ☺ | ☺ ☺ |
| Nougat | bar 4.77oz/135g | ☺ | ☺+ ×18 unit ☺+ ×18 unit | ☺ ☺ | ☺ ☺ |
| Pecan praline | piece 1.95oz/55g | 3½ +2¾ unit | ☺+ ×1¼ unit ☺+ ×1¼ unit | ☺ ☺ | 19½ 39¼ |
| Riesen® | piece 0.32oz/9g | 12¾ +10½ unit | ½ ☺+ ×2¾ unit | ☹ ☹³ | 71 ☺ |
| Smarties® | hand 1.06oz/30g | ☺ | ☺+ ×55 unit ☺+ ×55 unit | ☺ ☺ | ☺ ☺ |
| Snickers® | piece 2.08oz/58.7g | 1½ +1¼ unit | ☺+ ×7 unit ☺+ ×7 unit | ☺ ☺ | 8¾ 17½ |
| Snickers®, Almond | piece 1.77oz/49.9g | 1¾ +1½ unit | ☺+ ×8¾ unit ☺+ ×8¾ unit | ☺ ☺ | 6½ ᴳ 13¼ |
| Splenda® | portion 0oz/0g | ☺ | ☺ ☺ | ☺ ☺ | ☺ ☺ |
| Starburst®, Original | piece 0.18oz/5g | ☺ | ☺+ ×½ unit ☺+ ×½ unit | ☹ 30¼ | ☺ ☺ |
| Suckers®, sugar free | piece 0.5oz/14g | ☺ | ☹ ☺ | ☹ ☹ | ☺ ☺ |
| Sugar, white granulated | tbsp. 0.5oz/14.21ml | ☺ | ☺ ☺ | ☺ ☺ | ☺ ☺ |
| Taffy | piece 0.31oz/8.6g | ☺ | ☺+ ×4¼ unit ☺+ ×4¼ unit | ☺ ☺ | ☺ ☺ |
| Tic Tacs® | 2 piece 0.05oz/1.15g | ☺ | ☺ ☺ | ☺ ☺ | ☺ ☺ |
| Toblerone® Swiss Dark Chocolate with Honey & Almond Nougat | piece 0.89oz/25g | 7¼ +6 unit | ☺ ☺ | ☹ 40 | 40¼ 80¾ |
| Toblerone® Swiss Milk Chocolate with Honey & Almond Nougat | piece 0.89oz/25g | 1½ +1¼ unit | ☺ ☺ | ☺ ☺ | 8¾ 17½ |
| Toblerone® Swiss White Confection with Honey & Almond Nougat | piece 0.89oz/25g | 1 +1 unit | ☺ ☺ | ☺ ☺ | 6¾ 13½ |

| Sweets | Unit | Lactose ꟼ + unit/💊 | Fructose* ꟼ Fructose ꟼ | Sorbitol ꟼ Sorbitol ꟼ | FrucGalactans ꟼ FrucGalactans ꟼ 📖 |
|---|---|---|---|---|---|
| Toffee | piece<br>0.25oz/7g | 40¾<br>+34 unit | ☺<br>☺ | ☺<br>☺ | ☺<br>☺ |
| Toffifay® | piece<br>0.29oz/8.2g | 7½<br>+6¼ unit | ½<br>☺+ ×¼ unit | ☹<br>☹² | 42¾<br>85½ |
| Tootsie Pops® | piece<br>0.6oz/17g | ☺ | ☺+ ×2½ unit<br>☺+ ×2½ unit | ☺<br>☺ | ☺<br>☺ |
| Werther's® Original Caramel Coffee Hard Candies | piece<br>0.15oz/4g | 17¾<br>+14¾ unit | ☺+ ×½ unit<br>☺+ ×½ unit | ☺<br>☺ | ☺<br>☺ |
| White chocolate bar | piece<br>0.43oz.fl/12g | 2½<br>+2 unit | ☺<br>☺ | ☺<br>☺ | 14<br>28¼ |
| Wild 'n Fruity Gummi Bears (Brach's®) | hand<br>1.06oz/30g | ☺ | ☺+ ×3½ unit<br>☺+ ×3½ unit | ☹<br>☺ | ☺<br>☺ |
| Zsweet® | portion<br>0.18oz/5g | ☺ | ☺<br>☺ | ☹<br>☹ | ☺<br>☺ |

ꟼ *Level 0:* lactose measure ×½  
ꟼ *Level 1:* fructose measure ×2  
ꟼ *Level 2:* fructose-/sorbitol measure ×4. the rest ×2  
ꟼ *Level 3:* sorbitol measure ×7. the rest ×3  
📖: source of fruc/galactans data  

+ Unit/💊: added tolerated amount of unit per strong lactase capsule  
Fructose*: fructose, sorbitol adjusted  
☺+ ×[Amount] unit: Per unit consumed you can additionally tolerate up to [amount] × fructose(*)-unit of another product.  

☹: avoid;   ☹¹: ¼ at TL 1;   ☹²: ¼ at TL 2;   ☹³: ¼ at TL 3;   ☺: only contains traces;   ☺: is free from it

## 3.5 Warm dishes

### 3.5.1 Meals

| Meals | Unit | Lactose ↓ + unit/💊 | Fructose* ↓ Fructose ↓ | Sorbitol ↓ Sorbitol ↓ | FrucGalactans ↓ FrucGalactans ↓📖 |
|---|---|---|---|---|---|
| Arby's® macaroni and cheese | portion 7.66oz/217g | 21½ +18 unit | ☺ ☺ | ☺ ☺ | ½ ᴬ 1¼ |
| Asian noodle bowl, vegetables only | portion 7.06oz/200g | ☺ | ☺+ ×1 unit ☺+ ×1 unit | ☹ 10 | 1½ ᴬ 3¼ |
| Baby food, Gerber Graduates® Organic Pasta Pick-Ups Three Cheese Ravioli | Portion 170 g | 88 | ☺ ☺ | ☺ ☺ | ¾ ᴬ 1½ |
| Beef with noodles soup, condensed | portion 4.45oz/126g | ☺ | ☺ ☺ | ☹ 4¼ | 4 ᴬ 8¼ |
| Butternut squash soup | portion 8.65oz/245g | 13½ +11¼ unit | ☺ ☺ | ☹ 2½ | ½ ᴳ 1 |
| Calzone, cheese | piece 5.93oz/168g | 12¼ +10¼ unit | ☺ ☺ | ☹ 2¾ | ¼ ᴬ ½ |
| Casserole, pasta with turkey, gravy base, vegetables other than dark green, with cheese | portion 8.05oz/228g | 3¾ +3 unit | ☺ ☺ | ☹ 1¼ | ½ ᴬ 1 |
| Casserole rice with beef, tomato base, vegetables other than dark green, with cheese | portion 8.61oz/244g | 9¾ +8¼ unit | ☺+ ×1 unit ☺+ ×1 unit | ☹ ¼ | ¼ ᴬ ¾ |
| Chicken and dumplings soup, condensed | portion 4.45oz/126g | 7¼ +6 unit | ☺ ☺ | ☹ 2¼ | 2¼ 4½ |
| Chicken noodle soup with vegetables, ready-to-serve can | portion 8.65oz/245g | ☺ | ☺ ☺ | ☹ 1 | 1¼ 2½ |
| Chicken wonton soup, prepared from condensed can | portion 8.65oz/245g | ☺ | ☺ ☺ | ☹ 40¾ | ☺ ☺ |
| Chili with beans, beef, canned | tbsp. 0.5oz.fl/14.8ml | ☺ | ☺ ☺ | ☹ 55½ | 3 ᴬᶜ 6 |
| Chop suey, chicken, no noodles | portion 5.86oz/166g | ☺ | ☺ ☺ | ☹ ¼ | ¼ ᴬᴮ ¾ |
| Chop suey, tofu, no noodles | portion 5.86oz/166g | ☺ | ☺ ☺ | ☹ ¼ | ☺ ☺ |
| Cream of asparagus soup, prepared from condensed can | tbsp. 0.5ozfl/14.21ml | 6½ +5½ unit | ☺ ☺ | ☹ ☺ | 1½ 3 |
| Cream of broccoli soup, condensed | portion 4.45oz/126g | 5 +4¼ unit | ☺ ☺ | ☹ 19¾ | 1 ᶜ 2¼ |

| Meals | Unit | Lactose ↓ + unit/ 💊 | Fructose* ○↓ Fructose ↓ | Sorbitol ○↓ Sorbitol ↓ | FrucGalactans ○↓ FrucGalactans ↓ 📖 |
|---|---|---|---|---|---|
| Cream of celery soup, homemade | portion 8.65oz/245g | ½ +½ unit | ☺ ☺ | ☹ ¼ | ¼ ½ |
| Cream of chicken soup, condensed | portion 4.45oz/126g | 6½ +5½ unit | ☺ ☺ | ☹ 26¼ | 37¼ CB 74¾ |
| Cream of mushroom soup, prepared from condensed can | portion 8.65oz/245g | 8½ +7 unit | ☺ ☺ | ☹ ¼ | ½ 1 |
| Cream of potato soup mix, dry | portion 0.82oz/23g | 3¼ +2¾ unit | ☺ ☺ | ☹ 3 | 5 10 |
| Cream of spinach soup mix, dry | portion 0.57oz/16g | ☻ | ☻+ ×¼ unit ☻+ ×¼ unit | ☹ 18¼ | ☻ ☻ |
| Dairy Queen® Foot Long Hot Dog | piece 7.02oz/199g | ☺ | ☻+ ×1¾ unit ☻+ ×1¾ unit | ☹ 8¼ | ¼ A ½ |
| Fettuccini Alfredo®, no meat, vegetables other than dark green | tbsp. 0.5oz.l/14.21ml | 66¾ +55½ unit | ☺ ☺ | ☹ 2¾ | 81½ A ☻ |
| Fettuccini Alfredo®, no meat, with carrots or dark green vegetables | portion 7.06oz/200g | 5 +4 unit | ☺ ☺ | ☻ ☻ | 27¾ 55½ |
| Fruit sauce, jelly-based | portion 1.42oz/40g | ☺ | ☻+ ×5¼ unit ☻+ ×5¼ unit | ☹ ¾ | ☻ ☻ |
| German style potato salad, with bacon and vinegar dressing | portion 4.94oz/140g | ☺ | ☻+ ×¼ unit ☻+ ×¼ unit | ☹ 4¾ | 1 CB 2 |
| Green pea soup, prepared from condensed can | tbsp. 0.5ozfl/14.21ml | ☺ | ☻ ☻ | ☹ 20 | 3¼ AC 6¾ |
| Hardee's® Loaded Omelet Biscuit | piece 5.58oz/158g | 12 +10 unit | ☻+ ×9¼ unit ☻+ ×9¼ unit | ☻ ☻ | ¼ A ½ |
| Lasagna, homemade, beef | portion 4.94oz/140g | 23¼ +19¼ unit | ☻+ ×¼ unit ☻+ ×¼ unit | ☹ 1 | ¾ A 1½ |
| Lasagna, homemade, cheese, no vegetables | portion 4.94oz/140g | 25¾ +21½ unit | 11 12¼ | ☹ ¾ | ¾ A 1½ |
| Lasagna, homemade, spinach, no meat | portion 4.94oz/140g | 8½ +7 unit | 9¾ 11 | ☹ ½ | ¾ A 1½ |

○↓ *Level 0*: lactose measure ×½  
↓ *Level 1*: fructose measure ×2  
↕ *Level 2*: fructose-/sorbitol measure ×4. the rest ×2  
↨ *Level 3*: sorbitol measure ×7. the rest ×3  
📖: source of fruc/galactans data  

+ Unit/ 💊: added tolerated amount of unit per strong lactase capsule  
Fructose*: fructose, sorbitol adjusted  
☻+ ×[Amount] unit: Per unit consumed you can additionally tolerate up to [amount] × fructose(*)-unit of another product.  

☹: avoid;  ☹¹: ¼ at TL 1;  ☹²: ¼ at TL 2;  ☹³: ¼ at TL 3;  ☺: only contains traces;  ☻: is free from it

| Meals | Unit + unit/🍽 | Lactose 💧 | Fructose* 💧 Fructose 💧 | Sorbitol 💧 Sorbitol 💧 | FrucGalactans 💧 FrucGalactans 💧📖 |
|---|---|---|---|---|---|
| Lentil soup, condensed | portion 4.45oz/126g | ☺ | ☺ ☺ | ☹ 1 | 5½ AC 11¼ |
| Lyonnaise (potatoes and onions) | portion 2.47oz/70g | ☺ | ☺ ☺ | ☹ 15¾ | ☺ ☺ |
| Macaroni or pasta salad, with meat, egg, mayo dressing | portion 4.94oz/140g | ☺ | ☺+ ×¼ unit ☺+ ×½ unit | ☹ 1¼ | ☺ A ☺ |
| Meat ravioli, with tomato sauce | portion 8.82oz/250g | ☺ | ☺+ ×½ unit ☺+ ×½ unit | ☹ ½ | ¼ A ¾ |
| Minestrone soup, condensed | portion 4.45oz/126g | ☺ | ☺ ☺ | ☹ ¾ | ½ 1 |
| Minestrone soup, homemade | portion 8.65oz/245g | ☺ | ☺ ☺ | ☹ 1 | ¼ ½ |
| Noodle soup mix, dry | portion 0.57oz/16g | ☺ | ☺+ ×¼ unit ☺+ ×¼ unit | ☺ ☺ | ☺ ☺ |
| Omelet, made with bacon | portion 3.89oz/110g | 34¾ +29 unit | ☺+ ×1¾ unit ☺+ ×1¾ unit | ☺ ☺ | ☺ ☺ |
| Omelet, made with sausage, potatoes, onions, cheese | portion 3.89oz/110g | 52¼ +43½ unit | ☺+ ×1 unit ☺+ ×1 unit | ☹ 6¾ | ¼ CB ½ |
| Pad thai, without meat | portion 4.94oz/140g | ☺ | ☺ ☺ | ☹ 3¾ | ☺ A ☺ |
| Paella | portion 8.47oz/240g | ☺ | 2¼ 2¼ | ☹ 2¼ | 1 2 |
| Pasta salad with vegetables, Italian dressing | portion 4.94oz/140g | ☺ | 3¾ 3¾ | ☹ 1½ | 1½ A 3¼ |
| Pho soup (Vietnamese noodle soup) | portion 8.65oz/245g | ☺ | ☺ ☺ | ☹ 6¾ | ¾ 1¾ |
| Pizza Hut® cheese bread stick | piece 1.98oz/56g | 61½ +51¼ unit | ☺+ ×¼ unit ☺+ ×¼ unit | ☺ ☺ | 1¼ A 2½ |
| Pizza Hut® Pepperoni Lover's pizza, stuffed crust | portion 4.94oz/140g | 30 +25 unit | ☺ ☺ | ☹ 1 | ¾ A 1½ |
| Pizza Hut® Personal Pan, supreme | piece 9.03oz/256g | 16¾ +14 unit | ☺ ☺ | ☹ ¼ | 4¾ A 9½ |
| Pizza, homemade or restaurant, cheese, thin crust | piece 7.38oz/209g | 12¼ +10¼ unit | ☺+ ×¾ unit ☺+ ×¾ unit | ☹ ¾ | ½ A 1 |
| Potato salad, with egg, mayo dressing | portion 4.94oz/140g | ☺ | ☺+ ×½ unit ☺+ ×½ unit | ☹ 2 | 1 CB 2 |
| Potato soup with broccoli and cheese | portion 8.65oz/245g | 29¾ +24¾ unit | ☺ ☺ | ☹ 13½ | ½ AC 1 |
| Ratatouille | portion 3.89oz/110g | ☺ | ☺ ☺ | ☹ 1¼ | 4 B 8 |

| Meals | Unit | Lactose ↳ + unit/ 💊 | Fructose* ☹ Fructose ☹ | Sorbitol ☹ Sorbitol ↳ | FrucGalactans ☹ FrucGalactans ↳ 📖 |
|---|---|---|---|---|---|
| Red beans and rice soup mix, dry | portion 1.8oz/51g | ☺ | ¼ ¼ | ☹ ¼ | 1¼ AC 2¾ |
| Scrambled egg with bacon | portion 3.89oz/110g | 2¼ +1¾ unit | ☺+ ×1¾ unit ☺+ ×1¾ unit | ☺ ☺ | 12½ 25¼ |
| Sesame chicken | portion 8.89oz/252g | ☺ | ☺ ☺ | ☹ 3¾ | ☺ ☺ |
| Soup base | tbsp. 0.5oz/14.21ml | ☺ | 64 64 | ☹ 74 | ☺ ☺ |
| Spaghetti, with carbonara sauce | portion 7.09oz/201g | 13½ +11¼ unit | ☺+ ×¾ unit ☺+ ×¾ unit | ☹ 6 | ½ A 1 |
| Spinach ravioli, with tomato sauce | portion 8.82oz/250g | 5½ +4½ unit | ☺+ ×¼ unit ☺+ ×¼ unit | ☹ ½ | ½ A 1 |
| Spring roll | portion 4.94oz/140g | ☺ | 21 21 | ☹ 2¾ | ¼ ½ |
| Squash or pumpkin ravioli, with cream sauce | portion 8.82oz/250g | ½ +½ unit | ☺+ ×¼ unit ☺+ ×¼ unit | ☹ 40 | ½ A 1 |
| Stewed green peas with sofrito | tbsp. 0.5oz.fl/14.8ml | ☺ +2¾ unit | ☺ ☺ | ☹ 5½ | 1¼ AB 2½ |
| Sushi, with fish | portion 4.94oz/140g | ☺ | 10½ 32¼ | ☹ 2½ | ☺ ☺ |
| Sushi, with fish and vegetables in seaweed | portion 4.94oz/140g | ☺ | ☺ ☺ | ☹ 2 | ☺ ☺ |
| Sushi, with vegetables in seaweed | portion 4.94oz/140g | ☺ | ☺ ☺ | ☹ 1½ | ☺ ☺ |
| Swedish Meatballs | portion 4.94oz/140g | 1½ +1¼ unit | ☺ ☺ | ☹ 71¼ | 9 18 |
| Sweet and sour chicken | tbsp. 0.5ozfl/14.21ml | ☺ | 2½ 2½ | ☹ ☺ | ☺ ☺ |
| Taco Bell® 7-Layer Burrito | portion 4.94oz/140g | 25½ +21¼ unit | ☺ ☺ | ☹ 5¾ | ¼ A ¾ |
| Taco Bell® Crunchwrap Supreme | piece 8.65oz/245g | 4¼ +3½ unit | ☺ ☺ | ☹ 5 | ☹ A ¼ |
| Taco Bell® Mexican Pizza | piece 7.52oz/213g | 13¾ +11½ unit | 23¼ 29¼ | ☹ 1 | ¼ A ¾ |

↳ Level 0: lactose measure ×½   + Unit/💊: added tolerated amount of unit per strong lactase capsule
↳ Level 1: fructose measure ×2   Fructose*: fructose, sorbitol adjusted
↳ Level 2: fructose-/sorbitol measure ×4. the rest ×2   ☺+ ×[Amount] unit: Per unit consumed you can
↳ Level 3: sorbitol measure ×7. the rest ×3   additionally tolerate up to [amount] ×
📖: source of fruc/galactans data   fructose(*)-unit of another product.

☹: avoid;   ☹¹: ¼ at TL 1;   ☹²: ¼ at TL 2;   ☹³: ¼ at TL 3;   ☺: only contains traces;   ☺: is free from it

| Meals | Unit + unit/🍽 | Lactose ↓ | Fructose* ↓ Fructose ↓ | Sorbitol ↓ Sorbitol ↓ | FrucGalactans ↓ FrucGalactans ↓ |
|---|---|---|---|---|---|
| Taco Bell® Nachos Supreme | portion<br>4.94 oz/140g | 6¼<br>+5¼ unit | ☺<br>☺ | ☹<br>7¾ | 35¾ B<br>71½ |
| Taco, soft corn shell, with beans, cheese | portion<br>4.94 oz/140g | ☺<br>+77 unit | 12¾<br>13 | ☺<br>4¼ | ¼ A<br>½ |
| Tomato relish | portion<br>0.53 oz/15g | ☺ | ☺<br>☺ | ☹<br>5¼ | 33<br>66¼ |
| Tomato soup mix, dry | portion<br>1.2 oz/34g | ¼<br>+0.24 unit | 13<br>13¾ | ☹<br>2 | 1¼ B<br>2¾ |
| Vegetable soup, condensed | portion<br>4.45 oz/126g | ☺ | ☺+ ×¼ unit<br>☺+ ×¼ unit | ☹<br>1 | 19¾<br>39½ |
| Vichyssoise soup | portion<br>8.65 oz/245g | ¾<br>+½ unit | ☺+ ×¼ unit<br>☺+ ×¼ unit | ☹<br>1¼ | 4¼ AB<br>8½ |
| Wendy's® Strawberry Shake | glass<br>8.4 oz/240g | ¼<br>+¼ unit | ☺+ ×4¼ unit<br>☺+ ×4¼ unit | ☹<br>3¼ | 1¾<br>3¾ |
| White bean stew with sofrito | tbsp.<br>0.5ozfl/14.21ml | ☺ | ☺<br>☺ | ☹<br>☺ | 3 AC<br>6 |

# 3.5.2 Meat and fish

| Meat and fish | Unit | Lactose ℓ +unit/💊 | Fructose* ℓ Fructose ℓ | Sorbitol ℓ Sorbitol ℓ | FrucGalactans ℓ FrucGalactans ℓ 📖 |
|---|---|---|---|---|---|
| Arby's® Chicken Cordon Bleu Sandwich, crispy | portion 4.94oz/140g | 32¼ +27 unit | 2 2 | ☺ ☺ | 1 A 2¼ |
| Beef bacon (kosher) | portion 0.53oz/15g | ☺ | ☺ ☺ | ☺ ☺ | ☺ ☺ |
| Beef steak, chuck, visible fat eaten | portion 3oz/85g | ☺ | ☺ ☺ | ☺ ☺ | ☺ ☺ |
| Boston Market® 1/4 white rotisserie chicken, with skin | portion 3oz/85g | ☺ | ☺ ☺ | ☺ ☺ | ☺ ☺ |
| Boston Market® roasted turkey breast | portion 3oz/85g | ☺ | ☺ ☺ | ☺ ☺ | ☺ ☺ |
| Bratwurst | portion 1.95oz/55g | ☺ | ☺+ ×¼ unit ☺+ ×¼ unit | ☺ ☺ | ☺ ☺ |
| Bratwurst, beef | portion 1.95oz/55g | ☺ | ☺+ ×1 unit ☺+ ×1 unit | ☺ ☺ | ☺ ☺ |
| Bratwurst, light (reduced fat) | portion 1.95oz/55g | ☺ | ☺+ ×2¾ unit ☺+ ×2¾ unit | ☺ ☺ | ☺ ☺ |
| Bratwurst, made with beer | portion 1.95oz/55g | ☺ | ☺+ ×¼ unit ☺+ ×¼ unit | ☹ ☺ | ☺ ☺ |
| Bratwurst, made with beer, cheese-filled | portion 1.95oz/55g | ☺ | ☺+ ×½ unit ☺+ ×½ unit | ☹ ☺ | ☺ ☺ |
| Bratwurst, turkey | portion 1.95oz/55g | ☺ | ☺+ ×1½ unit ☺+ ×1½ unit | ☺ ☺ | ☺ ☺ |
| Braunschweiger (liver sausage) | portion 1.95oz/55g | ☺ | ☺ ☺ | ☺ ☺ | ☺ ☺ |
| Caviar | tbsp. 0.5oz/14.21ml | ☺ | ☺ ☺ | ☺ ☺ | ☺ ☺ |
| Chicken fricassee with gravy, American style | portion 8.61oz/244g | ☺ | ☺ ☺ | ☺ ☺ | 5¾ C 11½ |
| Clams, stuffed with mushroom, onions, and bread | portion 4.94oz/140g | 24½ +20½ unit | ☺ ☺ | ☹ ½ | 3¼ CB 6¾ |

ℓ *Level 0:* lactose measure ×½  
ℓ *Level 1:* fructose measure ×2  
ℓ *Level 2:* fructose-/sorbitol measure ×4. the rest ×2  
ℓ *Level 3:* sorbitol measure ×7. the rest ×3  
📖: source of fruc/galactans data  

+ Unit/💊: added tolerated amount of unit per strong lactase capsule  
Fructose*: fructose, sorbitol adjusted  

☺+ ×[Amount] unit: Per unit consumed you can additionally tolerate up to [amount] × fructose(*)-unit of another product.  

☹: avoid;   ☹¹: ¼ at TL 1;   ☹²: ¼ at TL 2;   ☹³: ¼ at TL 3;   ☺: only contains traces;   ☺: is free from it

| Meat and fish | Unit + unit/ | Lactose ☺ | Fructose* ☺ Fructose ☺ | Sorbitol ☺ Sorbitol ☺ | FrucGalactans ☺ FrucGalactans ☺ |
|---|---|---|---|---|---|
| Fish croquette | portion 3oz/85g | 2¼ +1¾ unit | ☺ ☺ | ☹ ☺ | 1¾ A 3½ |
| Fish sticks, patties, or nuggets, breaded, regular | portion 3oz/85g | ☺ | ☺ ☺ | ☺ ☺ | 2 A 4 |
| Fish with breading | portion 3oz/85g | ☺ | ☺ ☺ | ☺ ☺ | ☺ ☺ |
| Gorton's® Battered Fish Fillets - Lemon Pepper | portion 3oz/85g | ☺ | ☺ ☺ | ☺ ☺ | ☺ ☺ |
| Gorton's® Popcorn Shrimp, Original | portion 3oz/85g | ☺ | ☺ ☺ | ☺ ☺ | 2 A 4 |
| Goulash, with beef, noodles or macaroni, tomato base | tbsp. 0.5ozfl/14.21ml | ☺ | ☺ ☺ | ☹ 4 | ☺ ☺ |
| Herring, pickled | portion 1.95oz/55g | ☺ | ☺ ☺ | ☺ ☺ | ☺ ☺ |
| Herring, pickled | portion 1.95oz/55g | ☺ | ☺ ☺ | ☺ ☺ | 6 12 |
| Liver pudding | portion 1.95oz/55g | ☺ | ☺ ☺ | ☺ ☺ | ☺ ☺ |
| Mrs. Paul's® Calamari Rings | portion 3oz/85g | ☺ | ☺ ☺ | ☺ ☺ | 2¼ A 4½ |
| Pickled beef | portion 1.95oz/55g | ☺ | ☺ ☺ | ☺ ☺ | ☺ ☺ |
| Pork cutlet (sirloin cutlet), visible fat eaten | portion 3oz/85g | ☺ | ☺ ☺ | ☺ ☺ | 1¼ A 2¾ |
| Ribs, beef, spare, visible fat eaten | portion 3oz/85g | ☺ | ☺ ☺ | ☺ ☺ | ☺ ☺ |
| Salami, beer or beerwurst, beef | portion 1.95oz/55g | ☺ | ☺+ ×1 unit ☺+ ×1 unit | ☺ ☺ | ☺ ☺ |
| Salmon, red (sockeye), smoked | portion 1.95oz/55g | ☺ | ☺ ☺ | ☺ ☺ | ☺ ☺ |
| Sauerbraten | portion 5.61oz/159g | ☺ | 34¾ 34¾ | ☺ ☺ | ☺ ☺ |
| Scallops | portion 3oz/85g | ☺ | ☺ ☺ | ☺ ☺ | ☺ ☺ |
| Sea Pak® Seasoned Shrimp, Roasted Garlic | portion 3oz/85g | ☺ | ☺ ☺ | ☺ ☺ | ☺ ☺ |
| Sea Pak® Shrimp Scampi in Italian Parmesan Sauce | portion 3oz/85g | ☺ | ☺ ☺ | ☺ ☺ | ☺ ☺ |
| Tuna, canned, light, oil pack, not drained | portion 1.95oz/55g | ☺ | ☺ ☺ | ☺ ☺ | ☺ ☺ |

| Meat and fish | Unit | Lactose ↓<br>+ unit/💊 | Fructose* ⊙↓<br>Fructose ⊙↓ | Sorbitol ⊙↓<br>Sorbitol ↓ | FrucGalactans ⊙↓<br>FrucGalactans ↓📖 |
|---|---|---|---|---|---|
| Venison or deer, stewed | portion<br>3oz/85g | ☺ | ☺<br>☺ | ☺<br>☺ | ☺<br>☺ |

## 3.5.3 Lactose hideouts

| Sauces and spices | Unit | Lactose ↓<br>+ unit/💊 | Fructose* ⊙↓<br>Fructose ⊙↓ | Sorbitol ⊙↓<br>Sorbitol ↓ | FrucGalactans ⊙↓<br>FrucGalactans ↓📖 |
|---|---|---|---|---|---|
| Casserole (hot dish), chicken with pasta, cream or white sauce, with cheese | portion<br>8.4oz/238g | ½<br>+½ unit | ☺<br>☺ | ☺<br>☺ | ☺<br>☺ |
| Chicken cake or patty | portion<br>3oz/85g | 1½<br>+1¼ unit | 14<br>14 | ☹<br>58¾ | 3¼ B<br>6½ |
| Chicken with cheese sauce, vegetables other than dark green | portion<br>7.62oz/216g | 1<br>+¾ unit | 5<br>23 | ☹<br>½ | ☺<br>☺ |
| Creamed chicken | portion<br>8.51oz/241g | ½<br>+¼ unit | ☺<br>☺ | ☹<br>13¾ | ☺<br>☺ |
| Fish croquette | portion<br>3oz/85g | 2¼<br>+1¾ unit | ☺<br>☺ | ☹<br>☺ | ☺<br>☺ |
| Fish or seafood with cream or white sauce | portion<br>6.39oz/181g | 1½<br>+1¼ unit | ☺<br>☺ | ☺<br>☺ | ☺<br>☺ |
| Ham croquette | portion<br>3oz/85g | 2¼<br>+1¾ unit | ☺<br>☺ | ☹<br>☺ | ☺<br>☺ |
| Loaf cold cut, spiced | portion<br>1.95oz/55g | 2¼<br>+1¾ unit | ☺+ ×¼ unit<br>☺+ ×¼ unit | ☺<br>☺ | ☺<br>☺ |
| Meatloaf, pork | portion<br>3oz/85g | 2¼<br>+2 unit | ☺+ ×¼ unit<br>☺+ ×¼ unit | ☹<br>3½ | ☺<br>☺ |
| Meatloaf, tuna | portion<br>3oz/85g | 5½<br>+4½ unit | ☺<br>☺ | ☹<br>14½ | ☺<br>☺ |
| Souffle, meat | portion<br>3.89oz/110g | 1¼<br>+1 unit | ☺+ ×½ unit<br>☺+ ×½ unit | ☹<br>☺ | 1¾ B<br>3¾ |
| Swedish Meatballs | portion<br>4.94oz/140g | 1½<br>+1¼ unit | ☺<br>☺ | ☹<br>71¼ | 9<br>18 |

⊙↓ *Level 0*: lactose measure ×½  
↓ *Level 1*: fructose measure ×2  
↓ *Level 2*: fructose-/sorbitol measure ×4. the rest ×2  
↓ *Level 3*: sorbitol measure ×7. the rest ×3  
📖: source of fruc/galactans data  

\+ Unit/💊: added tolerated amount of unit per strong lactase capsule  
Fructose*: fructose, sorbitol adjusted  

☺+ ×[Amount] unit: Per unit consumed you can additionally tolerate up to [amount] × fructose(*)-unit of another product.

☹: avoid;   ☹¹: ¼ at TL 1;   ☹²: ¼ at TL 2;   ☹³: ¼ at TL 3;   ☺: only contains traces;   ☺: is free from it

# 3.5.4 Sauces and spices

| Sauces and spices | Unit | Lactose<br>+ unit/ | Fructose*<br>Fructose | Sorbitol<br>Sorbitol | FrucGalactans<br>FrucGalactans |
|---|---|---|---|---|---|
| Arby's® ranch sauce | tbsp. | ☺ | ☺ | ☹ | ☺ |
| | 0.5oz/14.21ml | | ☺ | 18½ | ☺ |
| Balsamic vinegar | portion | ☺ | ☺ | ☹ | ☺ |
| | 0.53oz/15g | | ☺ | 23 | ☺ |
| Barbeque sauce (BBQ), store | pinch | ☺ | ☺ | ☹ | ☺ |
| bought | 0.04oz/1g | | ☺ | 76¾ | ☺ |
| Basil, fresh | pinch | ☺ | ☺ | ☺ | ☺ |
| | 0.04oz/1g | | ☺ | ☺ | ☺ |
| Beef gravy, canned | portion | ☺ | ☺ | ☹ | ☺ |
| | 2.05oz/58g | | ☺ | ☺ | ☺ |
| Bertolli® Classico Olive Oil | portion | ☺ | ☺ | ☺ | ☺ |
| | 0.46oz/13g | | ☺ | ☺ | ☺ |
| Black pepper, ground | pinch | ☺ | ☺ | ☺ | ☺ |
| | 0.04oz/1g | | ☺ | ☺ | ☺ |
| Bouillon, unprepared | portion | ☺ | ☺ | ☹ | ☺ |
| | 0.29oz/8g | | ☺ | ☺ | ☺ |
| Capers | pinch | ☺ | ☺ | ☹ | ☺ |
| | 0.04oz/1g | | ☺ | 70¼ | ☺ |
| Caramel sauce, store bought, | portion | 6 | ☺+ ×6 unit | ☺ | 33¾ |
| fat free | 1.45oz/41g | +5 unit | ☺+ ×6 unit | ☺ | 67¾ |
| Chili sauce, store bought | portion | ☺ | 2¾ | ☹ | ☺ |
| | 2.4oz/68g | | 2¾ | ¼ | ☺ |
| Chinese oyster sauce | portion | ☺ | ☺ | ☺ | ☺ |
| | 1.13oz/32g | | ☺ | ☺ | ☺ |
| Chives, raw | pinch | ☺ | ☺ | ☺ | ☺ B |
| | 0.04oz/1g | | ☺ | ☺ | ☺ |
| Chocolate sauce, syrup | tbsp. | ☺ | ☺+ ×1½ unit | ☹ | ☺ |
| | 0.5oz/14.21ml | | ☺+ ×1½ unit | ☺ | ☺ |
| Cider vinegar | portion | ☺ | 6¼ | ☹ | ☺ |
| | 0.5oz/14g | | 16½ | 1¾ | ☺ |
| Cilantro leaf, fresh | pinch | ☺ | ☺ | ☺ | ☺ |
| | 0.04oz/1g | | ☺ | ☺ | ☺ |
| Cocktail sauce | portion | ☺ | ☺+ ×2 unit | ☹ | ☺ |
| | 2.4oz/68g | | ☺+ ×2 unit | ¾ | ☺ |
| Coconut oil | pinch | ☺ | ☺ | ☺ | ☺ |
| | 0.04oz/1g | | ☺ | ☺ | ☺ |

| Sauces and spices | Unit | Lactose ☝<br>+ unit/ 💊 | Fructose* ☝<br>Fructose ☝ | Sorbitol ☝<br>Sorbitol ☝ | FrucGalactans ☝<br>FrucGalactans ☝ 📖 |
|---|---|---|---|---|---|
| Crisco® Pure Corn Oil | portion<br>0.46oz/13g | ☺ | ☺<br>☺ | ☺<br>☺ | ☺<br>☺ |
| Curry sauce, from cream | portion<br>2.09oz/59g | 2<br>+1½ unit | ☺<br>☺ | ☹<br>4 | 11¼<br>22½ |
| Dijon mustard | tbsp.<br>0.5oz/14.21ml | ☺ | ☺<br>☺ | ☹<br>☺ | ☺<br>☺ |
| Distilled vinegar | portion<br>0.5oz/14g | ☺ | ☺<br>☺ | ☺<br>☺ | ☺<br>☺ |
| Flax seed oil | portion<br>0.46oz/13g | ☺ | ☺<br>☺ | ☺<br>☺ | ☺<br>☺ |
| French onion soup, condensed | portion<br>4.45oz/126g | ☺ | ☺+ ×1½ unit<br>☺+ ×1½ unit | ☹<br>2 | ¼ CB<br>¾ |
| Gardenburger® Sun-Dried Tomato Basil | portion<br>3oz/85g | ☺ | 1¼<br>1¼ | ☹<br>1 | 7¾ B<br>15¾ |
| Garlic sauce | tbsp.<br>0.5oz/14.21ml | ☺ | ☺<br>☺ | ☺<br>☺ | ☹ FB<br>☹ |
| Garlic, powder | pinch<br>0.04oz/1g | ☺ | ☺<br>☺ | ☺<br>☺ | 3¼ FB<br>6½ |
| Ginger sauce, Asian style | portion<br>1.13oz/32g | ☺ | ☺<br>☺ | ☹<br>9¼ | ☺ B<br>☺ |
| Ginger, ground | pinch<br>0.04oz/1g | ☺ | 89¼<br>89¼ | ☺<br>☺ | ☺ B<br>☺ |
| Girard's® Wasabi and Ginger Vinaigrette | pinch<br>0.04oz/1g | ☺ | ☺<br>☺ | ☹<br>☺ | ☺ B<br>☺ |
| Hamburger gravy | portion<br>7.17oz/203g | ☺ | ☺<br>☺ | ☹<br>12¼ | ☺<br>☺ |
| Heinz® 57 sauce® | portion<br>0.53oz/15g | ☺ | ☺+ ×¼ unit<br>☺+ ×½ unit | ☹<br>3¾ | ☺<br>☺ |
| Hollandaise sauce, store bought | tbsp.<br>0.5oz/14.21ml | 5<br>+4¼ unit | ☺<br>☺ | ☺<br>☺ | 28½<br>57 |
| Horseradish | pinch<br>0.04oz/1g | ☺ | ☺<br>☺ | ☺<br>☺ | ☺<br>☺ |
| Ketchup | portion<br>0.53oz/15g | ☺ | ☺+ ×¼ unit<br>☺+ ×¼ unit | ☹<br>3¾ | ☺<br>☺ |

☝ *Level 0*: lactose measure ×½    + Unit/ 💊: added tolerated amount of unit per strong lactase capsule
☝ *Level 1*: fructose measure ×2    Fructose*: fructose, sorbitol adjusted
☝ *Level 2*: fructose-/sorbitol measure ×4. the rest ×2    ☺+ ×[Amount] unit: Per unit consumed you can
☝ *Level 3*: sorbitol measure ×7. the rest ×3    additionally tolerate up to [amount] ×
📖: source of fruc/galactans data    fructose(*)-unit of another product.
☹: avoid;    ☹¹: ¼ at TL 1;    ☹²: ¼ at TL 2;    ☹³: ¼ at TL 3;    ☺: only contains traces;    ☺: is free from it

| Sauces and spices | Unit | Lactose ☺ + unit/📖 | Fructose* ☺ Fructose ☺ | Sorbitol ☺ Sorbitol ☺ | FrucGalactans ☺ FrucGalactans ☺ |
|---|---|---|---|---|---|
| Ketchup, low sodium | portion 0.53oz/15g | ☺ | ☺+ ×¼ unit ☺+ ×¼ unit | ☹ 4¼ | ☺ ☺ |
| Kraft® Balsamic Vinaigrette | portion 1.06oz/30g | ☺ | ☺ ☺ | ☹ 22 | ☺ ☺ |
| Kraft® Classic Caesar Dressing | portion 1.06oz/30g | ☺ | ☺+ ×½ unit ☺+ ×½ unit | ☹ 12¼ | ☺ ☺ |
| Kraft® Creamy French Dressing | portion 1.06oz/30g | ☺ | 64 64 | ☹ ☺ | ☺ ☺ |
| Kraft® Creamy Italian Dressing | portion 1.06oz/30g | ☺ | ☺+ ×¾ unit ☺+ ×¾ unit | ☺ ☺ | ☺ ☺ |
| Kraft® Fat Free Mayonnaise | portion 0.53oz/15g | ☺ | ☺ ☺ | ☺ ☺ | ☺ ☺ |
| Kraft® Free Sour Cream & Onion Ranch Dressing, fat free | portion 1.06oz/30g | ☺ | 4½ 4½ | ☺ ☺ | ☺ ☺ |
| Kraft® Mayo with Olive Oil, Reduced Fat | portion 0.53oz/15g | ☺ | ☺ ☺ | ☺ ☺ | ☺ ☺ |
| Kraft® Miracle Whip® Free Nonfat Dressing | tbsp. 0.5oz/14.21ml | 80 +66½ unit | ☺ ☺ | ☺ ☺ | ☺ ☺ |
| Kraft® Miracle Whip® Light Dressing | tbsp. 0.5oz/14.21ml | ☺ | ☺ ☺ | ☺ ☺ | ☺ ☺ |
| Kraft® Miracle Whip® Salad Dressing | tbsp. 0.5oz/14.21ml | ☺ | ☺ ☺ | ☺ ☺ | ☺ ☺ |
| Kraft® Sandwich Spread | tbsp. 0.5oz/14.21ml | ☺ | ☺ ☺ | ☹ ☺ | ☺ ☺ |
| Kraft® Thousand Island Dressing® | tbsp. 0.5oz/14.21ml | ☺ | ☺+ ×¼ unit ☺+ ×¼ unit | ☺ ☺ | ☺ ☺ |
| Lemon butter sauce | tbsp. 0.5oz/14.21ml | ☺ | ☺ ☺ | ☹ 60½ | ☺ ☺ |
| Long John Silver's® tartar sauce | tbsp. 0.5oz/14.21ml | ☺ | ☺ ☺ | ☹ ☺ | ☺ ☺ |
| Mushroom gravy, canned | tbsp. 0.5oz/14.21ml | 75¼ +62¾ unit | ☺ ☺ | ☹ 2¼ | ☺ ☺ |
| Oregano, dried | pinch 0.04oz/1g | ☺ | ☺ ☺ | ☺ ☺ | ☺ ☺ |
| Palm kernel oil | tbsp. 0.5oz/14.21ml | ☺ | ☺ ☺ | ☺ ☺ | ☺ ☺ |
| Parsley, fresh | pinch 0.04oz/1g | ☺ | ☺ ☺ | ☹ ☺ | ☺ ☺ |
| Peanut sauce, store bought | portion 1.24oz/35g | ☺ | ☹ ☺ | ☹ 8¼ | ☺ G ☺ |

| Sauces and spices | Unit | Lactose ↓ + unit/🥛 | Fructose* ☺ Fructose ☺ | Sorbitol ☺ Sorbitol ↓ | FrucGalactans ☺ FrucGalactans ↓ 📖 |
|---|---|---|---|---|---|
| Peppermint, fresh | pinch 0.04oz/1g | ☺ | ☺ ☺ | ☺ ☺ | ☺ ☺ |
| Pesto sauce, store bought | portion 2.19oz/62g | ☺ | ☺ ☺ | ☺ ☺ | 1¾ A 3¾ |
| Pumpkin seed oil | portion 0.46oz/13g | ☺ | ☺ ☺ | ☺ ☺ | ☺ ☺ |
| Red pepper (cayenne), ground | pinch 0.04oz/1g | ☺ | 51 51 | ☺ ☺ | ☺ ☺ |
| Red wine vinegar | tbsp. 0.5oz/14.21ml | ☺ | ☺ ☺ | ☹ 20 | ☺ ☺ |
| Rosemary, dried | pinch 0.04oz/1g | ☺ | ☺ ☺ | ☺ ☺ | ☺ ☺ |
| Safflower oil | portion 0.46oz/13g | ☺ | ☺ ☺ | ☺ ☺ | ☺ ☺ |
| Salsa, store bought | tbsp. 0.5oz/14.21ml | ☺ | 6¼ 6¼ | ☹ 6¾ | 5½ 11¼ |
| Scallions or spring onions, raw or blanched, tops and bulbs, marinated in oil | piece 0.56oz/15.7g | ☺ | ☺+ ×¼ unit ☺+ ×¼ unit | ☹ 6 | ¼ G ¾ |
| Soy sauce | tbsp. 0.5oz/14.21ml | ☺ | ☺ ☺ | ☹ 4½ | 3 A 6 |
| Soybean oil, unhydrogenated | tbsp. 0.5oz/14.21ml | ☺ | ☺ ☺ | ☺ ☺ | ☺ ☺ |
| Subway® honey mustard sauce, fat free | portion 0.99oz/28g | ☺ | 4¾ 4¾ | ☺ ☺ | ☺ ☺ |
| Sunflower oil | tbsp. 0.5oz/14.21ml | ☺ | ☺ ☺ | ☺ ☺ | ☺ ☺ |
| Sweet and sour sauce, store bought | tbsp. 0.5oz/14.21ml | ☺ | ½ ½ | ☹ 83¼ | ☺ ☺ |
| Tabasco® sauce | tbsp. 0.5oz/14.21ml | ☺ | ☺ ☺ | ☺ ☺ | ☺ ☺ |
| Taco sauce, red | portion 1.13oz/32g | ☺ | 2¾ 2¾ | ☹ 3 | 11 22 |

☺ *Level 0*: lactose measure ×½  + Unit/🥛: added tolerated amount of unit per strong lactase capsule
↓ *Level 1*: fructose measure ×2  Fructose*: fructose, sorbitol adjusted
↓ *Level 2*: fructose-/sorbitol measure ×4. the rest ×2  ☺+ ×[Amount] unit: Per unit consumed you can
↓ *Level 3*: sorbitol measure ×7. the rest ×3  additionally tolerate up to [amount] ×
📖: source of fruc/galactans data  fructose(*)-unit of another product.
☹: avoid;   ☹1: ¼ at TL 1;   ☹2: ¼ at TL 2;   ☹3: ¼ at TL 3;   ☺: only contains traces;   ☺: is free from it

| Sauces and spices | Unit + unit/🥄 | Lactose | Fructose* / Fructose | Sorbitol / Sorbitol | FrucGalactans / FrucGalactans |
|---|---|---|---|---|---|
| Tahini (sesame butter) | portion 1.06oz/30g | ☺ | ☺ ☺ | ☺ ☺ | ☺ G ☺ |
| Thyme, dried | pinch 0.04oz/1g | ☺ | ☺ ☺ | ☺ ☺ | ☺ ☺ |
| Tomato sauce | portion 2.12oz/60g | ☺ | ☺+ ×¾ unit ☺+ ×¾ unit | ☹ ¾ | 9¼ B 18½ |
| Tzatziki sauce (yogurt and cucumber) | portion 1.06oz/30g | 4½ +3¾ unit | 38¾ 38¾ | ☹ 9¼ | 11½ FB 23¼ |
| Vanilla sauce | tbsp. 0.5oz/14.21ml | ☺ | ☺ ☺ | ☺ ☺ | ☺ ☺ |
| Walnut oil | tbsp. 0.5oz/14.21ml | ☺ | ☺ ☺ | ☺ ☺ | ☺ ☺ |
| Watercress, raw | pinch 0.04oz/1g | ☺ | ☺ ☺ | ☺ ☺ | ☺ ☺ |
| White sauce, store bought | tbsp. 0.5oz/14.21ml | 4 +3¼ unit | ☺ ☺ | ☺ ☺ | 22¼ 44½ |

# 3.5.5 Side dishes

| Side dishes | Unit | Lactose ☹ + unit/💊 | Fructose* ☹ Fructose ☹ | Sorbitol ☹ Sorbitol ☹ | FrucGalactans ☹ FrucGalactans ☹ 📖 |
|---|---|---|---|---|---|
| Au gratin potato, prepared from fresh | portion 4.94oz/140g | 1 +¾ unit | ☺ ☺ | ☹ 7¾ | 6¼ B 12½ |
| Basmati rice, cooked in unsalted water | portion 4.94oz/140g | ☺ | ☺ ☺ | ☺ ☺ | ☺ A ☺ |
| Boston Market® sweet corn | portion 3oz/85g | ☺ | ☺+ ×¼ unit ☺+ ×½ unit | ☹ 4 | ☺ B ☺ |
| Bulgur, home cooked | portion 4.94oz/140g | ☺ | ☺ ☺ | ☺ ☺ | ☺ ☺ |
| Cheese gnocchi | portion 2.47oz/70g | 28 +23¼ unit | ☺ ☺ | ☺ ☺ | 1 A 2¼ |
| Couscous, cooked | portion 4.94oz/140g | ☺ | ☺ ☺ | ☺ ☺ | ¼ A ¾ |
| Falafel | portion 1.95oz/55g | ☺ | ☺ ☺ | ☺ 1¾ | ☺ G ☺ |
| Fettuccini noodles, whole wheat, cooked in unsalted water | portion 4.94oz/140g | ☺ | ☺+ ×¼ unit ☺+ ×¼ unit | ☺ ☺ | 1 A 2 |
| Garbanzo beans (chickpeas), canned, drained | portion 3.18oz/90g | ☺ | ☺ ☺ | ☹ 1 | 1½ A 3 |
| Green peas, raw | tbsp. 0.5ozfl/14.21ml | ☺ | 9½ 12¼ | ☹ 3½ | 1¼ A 2½ |
| Kidney beans, cooked from dried | portion 3.18oz/90g | ☺ | ☺ ☺ | ☺ ☺ | ¼ A ½ |
| Lentils, cooked from dried | portion 3.18oz/90g | ☺ | ☺ ☺ | ☺ ☺ | ¾ A 1½ |
| Plain dumplings for stew, biscuit type | portion 1.95oz/55g | 1¾ +1½ unit | ☺ ☺ | ☺ ☺ | ½ A 1 |
| Polenta | portion 8.47oz/240g | ½ +½ unit | ☺+ ×¼ unit ☺+ ×¼ unit | ☹ 20¾ | 3¼ B 6¾ |
| Potato dumpling (Kartoffelkloesse) | portion 4.94oz/140g | 45½ +37¾ unit | ☺+ ×¼ unit ☺+ ×¼ unit | ☹ 35½ | ☺ C ☺ |

☹ Level 0: lactose measure ×½
☹ Level 1: fructose measure ×2
☹ Level 2: fructose-/sorbitol measure ×4. the rest ×2
☹ Level 3: sorbitol measure ×7. the rest ×3
📖: source of fruc/galactans data

+ Unit/💊: added tolerated amount of unit per strong lactase capsule
Fructose*: fructose, sorbitol adjusted
☺+ ×[Amount] unit: Per unit consumed you can additionally tolerate up to [amount] × fructose(*)-unit of another product.

☹: avoid;   ☹1: ¼ at TL 1;   ☹2: ¼ at TL 2;   ☹3: ¼ at TL 3;   ☺: only contains traces;   ☺: is free from it

| Side dishes | Unit | Lactose  + unit/ | Fructose*  Fructose | Sorbitol  Sorbitol | FrucGalactans  FrucGalactans |
|---|---|---|---|---|---|
| Potato gnocchi | portion 6.64oz/188g | 2½ +2 unit | ☺ ☺ | ☺ ☺ | 14 A 28¼ |
| Potato pancakes | portion 2.47oz/70g | ☺ | ☺+ ×½ unit ☺+ ×½ unit | ☹ 12¾ | ☺ B ☺ |
| Potato, boiled, with skin | portion 3.89oz/110g | ☺ | ☺ ☺ | ☹ 45¼ | ☺ B ☺ |
| Potato, boiled, without skin | portion 3.89oz/110g | ☺ | ☺ ☺ | ☹ 45¼ | ☺ B ☺ |
| Quinoa, cooked | portion 4.94oz/140g | ☺ | ☺+ ×1¾ unit ☺+ ×1¾ unit | ☺ ☺ | 2½ A 5 |
| Rice noodles, fried | portion 0.89oz/25g | ☺ | ☺ ☺ | ☺ ☺ | ☺ A ☺ |
| Spaetzle (spatzen) | portion 4.94oz/140g | 5¼ +4¼ unit | ☺+ ×¼ unit ☺+ ×¼ unit | ☺ ☺ | 1 A 2 |

# 3.6 Fast food chains

## 3.6.1 Burger King®

| Burger King® | Unit + unit/💊 | Lactose ↳ | Fructose* ↳ Fructose ↳ | Sorbitol ↳ Sorbitol ↳ | FrucGalactans ↳ FrucGalactans ↳📖 |
|---|---|---|---|---|---|
| Bacon EGG® and Cheese BK Muffin® | piece 4.63oz/131g | 11½ +9½ unit | ☺+ ×1 unit ☺+ ×1 unit | ☺ ☺ | ¼ A ¾ |
| Barbecue sauce | portion 1.1oz.fl/31ml | ☺ | ☺+ ×1¼ unit ☺+ ×1¼ unit | ☹ 2¼ | ☺ ☺ |
| BBQ roasted jalapeno sauce | portion 1.1oz.fl/31ml | ☺ | ☺+ ×1 unit ☺+ ×1 unit | ☹ 2¾ | ☺ ☺ |
| BK Big Fish® | piece 8.05oz/228g | ☺ | ☺ ☺ | ☹ 21¾ | ☹ A ¼ |
| BK Fresh Apple Slices | portion 4.94oz/140g | ☺ | ☹² ☹² | ☹ ☹² | ☺ ☺ |
| BLT Salad® with TenderCrisp chicken (no dressing or croutons) | portion 4.94oz/140g | 79¼ +66 unit | 5¾ 5¾ | ☹ 3 | ☺ ☺ |
| Caesar Salad (no dressing or croutons) | portion 3.53oz/100g | 26½ +22 unit | 1½ 1½ | ☹ 4¼ | ☺ ☺ |
| Cheeseburger | piece 4.27oz/121g | 11½ +9½ unit | 51½ 59 | ☹ 3¼ | ¼ A ¾ |
| French fries | portion 2.47oz/70g | ☺ | ☺ ☺ | ☹ 35½ | ☺ ☺ |
| Hamburger | piece 3.85oz/109g | ☺ | 57¼ 65½ | ☹ 3¼ | ½ A 1 |
| Ken's® Apple Cider Vinaigrette salad dressing | portion 1.06oz.fl/30ml | ☺ | ☺ ☺ | ☺ ☺ | ☺ ☺ |
| Onion rings | portion 2.47oz/70g | ☺ | ☺+ ×1½ unit ☺+ ×1½ unit | ☹ ¾ | ¼ AC ½ |
| Original Chicken Crisp® Sandwich | piece 5.26oz/149g | ☺ | 1½ 1½ | ☹ 67 | 5¾ A 11½ |
| Pancakes and syrup | piece 6.6oz/187g | ½ +½ unit | ☺+ ×6 unit ☺+ ×6 unit | ☺ ☺ | ¼ A ½ |

↳ *Level 0*: lactose measure ×½  
↳ *Level 1*: fructose measure ×2  
↳ *Level 2*: fructose-/sorbitol measure ×4, the rest ×2  
↳ *Level 3*: sorbitol measure ×7, the rest ×3  
📖: source of fruc/galactans data  

+ Unit/💊: added tolerated amount of unit per strong lactase capsule  
Fructose*: fructose, sorbitol adjusted  
☺+ ×[Amount] unit: Per unit consumed you can additionally tolerate up to [amount] × fructose(*)-unit of another product.

☹: avoid;   ☹¹: ¼ at TL 1;   ☹²: ¼ at TL 2;   ☹³: ¼ at TL 3;   ☺: only contains traces;   ☺: is free from it

| Burger King® | Unit | Lactose ↯<br>+ unit/💊 | Fructose* ☻↯<br>Fructose ☻↯ | Sorbitol ☻↯<br>Sorbitol ↯ | FrucGalactans ☻↯<br>FrucGalactans ↯📖 |
|---|---|---|---|---|---|
| Picante taco sauce sauce | portion<br>1.24oz.fl/35ml | ☻<br> | 2½<br>2½ | ☹<br>2¾ | ☻<br>☻ |
| Ranch Crispy Chicken Wrap | piece<br>4.84oz/137g | 5<br>+4¼ unit | ☹<br>☻ | ☹<br>36¼ | ¼ A<br>½ |
| Shake, chocolate | portion<br>8.15oz.fl/231ml | ☹²<br>+0.15 unit | ☻+ ×7¼ unit<br>☻+ ×7¼ unit | ☻<br>☻ | ½<br>1 |
| Shake, strawberry | portion<br>8.08oz.fl/229ml | ☹²<br>+0.15 unit | ☻+ ×5¼ unit<br>☻+ ×5¼ unit | ☹<br>3¼ | 1<br>2 |
| Shake, vanilla or other | portion<br>8.4oz.fl/238ml | ☹²<br>+0.13 unit | ☻+ ×5¾ unit<br>☻+ ×5¾ unit | ☻<br>☻ | ¾<br>1¾ |
| Sundaes®, caramel | portion<br>4.98oz.fl/141ml | ¼<br>+¼ unit | ☻+ ×8½ unit<br>☻+ ×8½ unit | ☻<br>☻ | 2<br>4 |
| Sundaes®, chocolate fudge | portion<br>4.98oz.fl/141ml | ¼<br>+¼ unit | ☻+ ×6¾ unit<br>☻+ ×6¾ unit | ☻<br>☻ | 1¾<br>3¾ |
| Sundaes®, mini M & M's® | portion<br>7.2oz.fl/204ml | ¼<br>+0.23 unit | ☻+ ×6¾ unit<br>☻+ ×6¾ unit | ☻<br>☻ | 1½<br>3 |
| Sundaes®, Oreo® | portion<br>7.2oz.fl/204ml | ¼<br>+¼ unit | ☻+ ×7¼ unit<br>☻+ ×7¼ unit | ☹<br>49 | 1¾<br>3¾ |
| Sundaes®, strawberry | portion<br>4.98oz.fl/141ml | ¼<br>+¼ unit | ☻+ ×2½ unit<br>☻+ ×2½ unit | ☹<br>2½ | 2¼<br>4¾ |
| Sweet and sour sauce | portion<br>1.06oz.fl/30ml | ☻<br> | ¼<br>¼ | ☹<br>41½ | ☻<br>☻ |
| TenderCrisp® Chicken Sandwich | piece<br>9.32oz/264g | ☻<br> | 8<br>8½ | ☹<br>2½ | ☹ A<br>¼ |
| Whopper® with cheese | piece<br>11.12oz/315g | 5¾<br>+4¾ unit | 2¾<br>2¾ | ☹<br>1 | ☹ A<br>¼ |
| Zesty onion ring sauce | portion<br>1.1oz.fl/31ml | ☻<br> | ☻<br>☻ | ☹<br>64½ | ☻<br>☻ |

# 3.6.2 KFC®

| KFC® | Unit | Lactose (1) + unit/capsule | Fructose* (0) Fructose (0) | Sorbitol (0) Sorbitol (1) | FrucGalactans (0) FrucGalactans (1) 📖 |
|---|---|---|---|---|---|
| Caesar salad dressing | portion | 4¾ | ☺ | ☺ | 26½ |
| | 1.06oz.fl/30ml | +3¾ unit | ☺ | ☺ | 53 |
| Chicken breast, spicy crispy | piece | ☺ | ☺ | ☺ | ¾ A |
| | 6.18oz/175g | | ☺ | ☺ | 1¾ |
| Chicken Littles with sauce | piece | ☺ | 3 | ☹ | ½ A |
| | 3.57oz/101g | | 3 | 33 | 1 |
| Cole slaw | portion | ☺ | ☺+ ×¼ unit | ☹ | 1 B |
| | 3.53oz/100g | | ☺+ ×¼ unit | 2¾ | 2 |
| Creamy buffalo sauce | portion | 6 | ☺+ ×1 unit | ☺ | 34½ |
| | 1.04ozfl/29.4ml | +5 unit | ☺+ ×1 unit | ☺ | 69 |
| Crispy Chicken Caesar Salad | portion | ☺ | 2¼ | ☹ | 1 A |
| | 4.94oz/140g | | 2¼ | 17¾ | 2¼ |
| Crispy Twister without sauce | piece | ☺ | 19 | ☹ | ☹ A |
| | 7.69oz/218g | | 20¾ | 2 | ¼ |
| Crispy Twister® with sauce | piece | ☺ | 17¼ | ☹ | ☹ A |
| | 8.47oz/240g | | 18¾ | 2 | ¼ |
| Extra Crispy Tenders | piece | ☺ | ☺ | ☺ | 3¼ A |
| | 1.84oz/52g | | ☺ | ☺ | 6½ |
| Honey BBQ sauce | portion | ☺ | ☺+ ×1¼ unit | ☹ | ☺ |
| | 1.1oz.fl/31ml | | ☺+ ×1¼ unit | 2¼ | ☺ |
| Hot wings | portion | ☺ | ☺ | ☺ | ☺ |
| | 3oz/85g | | ☺ | ☺ | ☺ |
| House side salad | portion | ☺ | 2 | ☹ | ☺ |
| | 3.53oz/100g | | 2 | 4 | ☺ |
| Mashed potatoes with gravy | portion | ½ | ☺ | ☹ | 4 |
| | 4.94oz/140g | +½ unit | ☺ | 35½ | 8¼ |
| Sweet and sour sauce | portion | ☺ | ¼ | ☹ | ☺ |
| | 1.06oz.fl/30ml | | ¼ | 37 | ☺ |
| Sweet corn | piece | ☺ | ☺ | ☹ | ☺ B |
| | 3.36oz/95g | | ☺ | 2½ | ☺ |

(0) *Level 0:* lactose measure ×½
(1) *Level 1:* fructose measure ×2
(2) *Level 2:* fructose-/sorbitol measure ×4. the rest ×2
(3) *Level 3:* sorbitol measure ×7. the rest ×3
📖: source of fruc/galactans data

+ Unit/capsule: added tolerated amount of unit per strong lactase capsule
Fructose*: fructose, sorbitol adjusted

☺+ ×[Amount] unit: Per unit consumed you can additionally tolerate up to [amount] × fructose(*)-unit of another product.

☹: avoid; ☹[1]: ¼ at TL 1; ☹[2]: ¼ at TL 2; ☹[3]: ¼ at TL 3; ☺: only contains traces; ☺: is free from it

# 3.6.3 McDonald's®

| | | Lactose | Fructose* | Sorbitol | FrucGalactans |
|---|---|---|---|---|---|
| **McDonald's®** | **Unit** | **+ unit/** | **Fructose** | **Sorbitol** | **FrucGalactans** |
| apple slices | piece | ☺ | ¼ | ☹ | ☺ |
| | 1.2oz/34g | | ½ | ¼ | ☺ |
| barbecue sauce | portion | ☺ | ☺+ ×1½ unit | ☹ | ☺ |
| | 1.1oz.fl/31ml | | ☺+ ×1½ unit | 1¾ | ☺ |
| Big Mac® | piece | 9¾ | 5 | ☹ | ¼ A |
| | 7.59oz/215g | +8¼ unit | 5 | 6½ | ½ |
| caramel sundae® | portion | ¼ | ☺+ ×6¾ unit | ☺ | 1¾ |
| | 6.42oz.fl/182ml | +¼ unit | ☺+ ×6¾ unit | ☺ | 3¾ |
| Cheeseburger | piece | 9¾ | 3¾ | ☹ | ¼ A |
| | 4.03oz/114g | +8¼ unit | 3¾ | 5 | ¾ |
| Chicken McNuggets® | piece | ☺ | ☺ | ☺ | 10¾ A |
| | 0.58oz/16.25g | | ☺ | ☺ | 21½ |
| chocolate chip cookies | piece | ☺ | ☺+ ×½ unit | ☹ | ¾ A |
| | 1.17oz/33g | | ☺+ ×½ unit | ☺ | 1½ |
| chocolate milk | cup | ¼ | ☺+ ×2 unit | ☺ | 1¾ |
| | 5.2oz.fl/150ml | +¼ unit | ☺+ ×2 unit | ☺ | 3¾ |
| Crispy Chicken Snack Wrap | piece | 62 | ☺ | ☹ | ¼ A |
| with ranch sauce | 4.17oz.fl/118ml | +51½ unit | ☺ | 84½ | ½ |
| Double Cheeseburger | piece | 4¾ | 4½ | ☹ | ¼ A |
| | 5.83oz/165g | +4 unit | 4½ | 4¼ | ½ |
| Filet-O-Fish® | piece | 19¾ | 2 | ☹ | ¼ A |
| | 5.01oz/142g | +16½ unit | 2 | 70¼ | ¾ |
| French fries | portion | ☺ | ☺ | ☹ | ☺ |
| | 2.47oz/70g | | ☺ | 35½ | ☺ |
| Hamburger | piece | ☺ | 3¾ | ☹ | ½ A |
| | 3.53oz/100g | | 4 | 5 | 1 |
| hot fudge sundae® | portion | ¼ | ☺+ ×7½ unit | ☹ | 1¼ G |
| | 6.32oz.fl/179ml | +¼ unit | ☺+ ×7½ unit | 55¾ | 2½ |
| hot mustard sauce | portion | ☺ | ☺+ ×1¼ unit | ☺ | ☺ |
| | 0.71oz.fl/20ml | | ☺+ ×1¼ unit | ☺ | ☺ |
| M & M's® McFlurry® | portion | ☹2 | ☺+ ×3½ unit | ☺ | 1 |
| | 8.05oz.fl/228ml | +0.18 unit | ☺+ ×3½ unit | ☺ | 2¼ |
| McCafe® shakes, chocolate | cup | ¼ | ☺+ ×4 unit | ☹ | 2¼ |
| flavors | 5.2oz.fl/150ml | +¼ unit | ☺+ ×4 unit | 22 | 4¾ |
| McCafe® shakes, vanilla or | cup | ¼ | ☺+ ×¼ unit | ☹ | 2¼ |
| other flavors | 5.2oz.fl/150ml | +¼ unit | ☺+ ×¼ unit | 16½ | 4½ |

| McDonald's® | Unit | Lactose ⌇ + unit/💊 | Fructose* ⌇ Fructose ⌇ | Sorbitol ⌇ Sorbitol ⌇ | FrucGalactans ⌇ FrucGalactans ⌇ 📖 |
|---|---|---|---|---|---|
| McChicken® | piece 5.05oz/143g | ☺ | 1½ 1½ | ☹ 69¾ | ¼ A ¾ |
| McDouble® | piece 5.33oz/151g | 9¾ +8¼ unit | 4¼ 4¼ | ☹ 4¼ | ¼ A ½ |
| McRib® | piece 7.34oz/208g | ☺ | ☺+ ×¾ unit ☺+ ×¾ unit | ☹ 1¾ | ¼ A ½ |
| Newman's Own® Creamy Caesar salad dressing | portion 1.06oz.fl/30ml | 18¼ +15¼ unit | 26¾ 79¼ | ☹ 7¼ | ☺ ☺ |
| Newman's Own® Low Fat Balsamic Vinaigrette salad dressing | portion 1.06oz.fl/30ml | ☺ | ☺ ☺ | ☺ ☺ | ☺ ☺ |
| Orange juice | glass 8.4oz.fl/240ml | ☺ | 1½ 1½ | ☹ ¼ | ☺ ☺ |
| Quarter Pounder | piece 6.11oz/173g | ☺ | 48 57¾ | ☹ 2½ | ¼ A ½ |
| Sausage & EGG® McMuffin® | piece 5.79oz/164g | 9¾ +8¼ unit | ☺+ ×1 unit ☺+ ×1 unit | ☺ ☺ | ¼ A ½ |
| Side salad | portion 3.53oz/100g | ☺ | 3¾ 3¾ | ☹ 2½ | ☺ ☺ |
| Smoothies, all flavors | glass 8.4oz.fl/240ml | 2¾ +2¼ unit | 3¾ 4¼ | ☹ 1¼ | 15½ 31 |
| Southwestern chipotle barbecue sauce | portion 1.1oz.fl/31ml | ☺ | ☺+ ×1¾ unit ☺+ ×1¾ unit | ☹ 2¾ | ☺ ☺ |
| Sweet and sour sauce | portion 1.06oz.fl/30ml | ☺ | ¼ ¼ | ☹ 41½ | ☺ ☺ |

⌇ *Level 0*: lactose measure ×½  + Unit/💊: added tolerated amount of unit per strong lactase capsule
⌇ *Level 1*: fructose measure ×2  Fructose*: fructose, sorbitol adjusted
⌇ *Level 2*: fructose-/sorbitol measure ×4. the rest ×2  ☺+ ×[Amount] unit: Per unit consumed you can
⌇ *Level 3*: sorbitol measure ×7. the rest ×3  additionally tolerate up to [amount] ×
📖: source of fruc/galactans data  fructose(*)-unit of another product.

☹: avoid;  ☹¹: ¼ at TL 1;  ☹²: ¼ at TL 2;  ☹³: ¼ at TL 3;  ☺: only contains traces;  ☺: is free from it

## 3.6.4 Subway®

| Subway® | Unit + unit/🥄 | Lactose ⚕ | Fructose* ⚕ Fructose ⚕ | Sorbitol ⚕ Sorbitol ⚕ | FrucGalactans ⚕ FrucGalactans ⚕ 📖 |
|---|---|---|---|---|---|
| 9-grain Wheat bread | piece 2.76oz/78g | | 1 1 | ☺ ☺ | ¼ A ¾ |
| American cheese | portion 1.06oz/30g | 4½ +3¾ unit | ☺ ☺ | ☺ ☺ | 25¾ 51½ |
| Bacon | portion 0.53oz/15g | ☺ | ☺ ☺ | ☺ ☺ | ☺ ☺ |
| Cheddar cheese | portion 1.06oz/30g | 43¼ +36 unit | ☺ ☺ | ☺ ☺ | ☺ ☺ |
| Chipotle southwest salad dressing | portion 1.06oz.fl/30ml | 7¼ +6 unit | ☺ ☺ | ☺ ☺ | 40½ 81 |
| Chocolate chip cookie | piece 1.59oz/45g | ☺ | ☺+ ×1 unit ☺+ ×1 unit | ☹ ☺ | ½ A 1 |
| Chocolate chunk cookie | piece 1.59oz/45g | ☺ | ☺+ ×1 unit ☺+ ×1 unit | ☹ ☺ | ½ A 1 |
| Ham Sandwich with Veggies, no mayo | piece 7.73oz/219g | 12½ +10½ unit | ¾ ¾ | ☹ 1¼ | ¼ A ½ |
| Honey mustard salad dressing | portion 1.06oz.fl/30ml | ☺ | 4½ 4½ | ☺ ☺ | ☺ ☺ |
| Honey Oat bread | piece 3.14oz/89g | ¾ +½ unit | 2½ 2½ | ☹ 6½ | ¼ A ¾ |
| Italian BMT® Sandwich with Veggies, no mayo | piece 7.98oz/226g | 12½ +10½ unit | ¾ ¾ | ☹ 1¼ | ¼ A ½ |
| M & M's® cookie | piece 1.59oz/45g | 9 +7½ unit | ☺+ ×½ unit ☺+ ×½ unit | ☹ ☺ | ½ A 1 |
| Mustard | portion 0.18oz/5g | ☺ | ☺ ☺ | ☺ ☺ | ☺ ☺ |
| Oven Roasted Chicken Sandwich with Veggies, no mayo | piece 8.22oz/233g | 12½ +10½ unit | 1¾ 1¾ | ☹ 1¼ | ☹ A ¼ |
| Parmesan Oregano bread | piece 2.65oz/75g | ☺ | ☺+ ×½ unit ☺+ ×½ unit | ☺ ☺ | ¾ A 1½ |
| Ranch salad dressing | portion 1.06oz.fl/30ml | ☺ | ☺ ☺ | ☹ ☺ | ☺ ☺ |
| Roast Beef Sandwich with Veggies, no mayo | piece 8.22oz/233g | 12½ +10½ unit | ¾ ¾ | ☹ 1¼ | ☹ A ¼ |
| Spicy Italian Sandwich with Veggies, no meat | piece 7.84oz/222g | 12½ +10½ unit | ¾ ¾ | ☹ 1¼ | ¼ A ½ |

| Subway® | Unit | Lactose [1]<br>+ unit/capsule | Fructose* [0]<br>Fructose [0] | Sorbitol [0]<br>Sorbitol [1] | FrucGalactans [0]<br>FrucGalactans [1] 📖 |
|---|---|---|---|---|---|
| Steak & Cheese Sandwich with Veggies, no mayo | piece<br>8.65oz/245g | ☺ | 1<br>1 | ☹<br>1¼ | ☹ A<br>¼ |
| Sweet Onion Chicken Teriyaki Sandwich with Veggies, no mayo | piece<br>9.74oz/276g | 12½<br>+10½ unit | 22½<br>25¾ | ☹<br>1¼ | ☹ A<br>¼ |
| Sweet onion salad dressing | portion<br>1.06oz.fl/30ml | ☺ | ☺+ ×1 unit<br>☺+ ×1 unit | ☹<br>55½ | ½<br>1¼ |
| Tuna Sandwich with Veggies, no mayo | piece<br>8.22oz/233g | 12½<br>+10½ unit | ¾<br>¾ | ☹<br>1¼ | ☹ A<br>¼ |
| Turkey Breast & Ham Sandwich with Veggies, no mayo | piece<br>7.73oz/219g | 12½<br>+10½ unit | ¾<br>¾ | ☹<br>1¼ | ¼ A<br>½ |
| Turkey Breast Sandwich with Veggies, no mayo | piece<br>7.73oz/219g | 12½<br>+10½ unit | ¾<br>¾ | ☹<br>1¼ | ¼ A<br>½ |
| Veggie Delite Salad, no dressing | portion<br>3.53oz/100g | 34¼<br>+28½ unit | 83¼<br>☺ | ☹<br>2¼ | ☺<br>☺ |
| Veggie Delite Sandwich, no mayo | piece<br>5.72oz/162g | 12½<br>+10½ unit | ¾<br>¾ | ☹<br>1½ | ¼ A<br>½ |

[0] *Level 0:* lactose measure ×½
[1] *Level 1:* fructose measure ×2
+ Unit/capsule: added tolerated amount of unit per strong lactase capsule
Fructose*: fructose, sorbitol adjusted

[2] *Level 2*: fructose-/sorbitol measure ×4. the rest ×2
[3] *Level 3:* sorbitol measure ×7. the rest ×3
📖: source of fruc/galactans data

☺+ ×[Amount] unit: Per unit consumed you can additionally tolerate up to [amount] × fructose(*)-unit of another product.

☹: avoid; ☹¹: ¼ at TL 1; ☹²: ¼ at TL 2; ☹³: ¼ at TL 3; ☺: only contains traces; ☺: is free from it

## 3.7 Fruit and vegetables

### 3.7.1 Fruit

| Fruit | Unit + unit/ | Lactose ☺ + unit/ | Fructose* ☹ Fructose ☺ | Sorbitol ☹ Sorbitol ☺ | FrucGalactans ☹ FrucGalactans ☺ |
|---|---|---|---|---|---|
| Apple, fresh, with skin | piece 6.42oz/182g | ☺ | ☹² ☹² | ☹² ☹² | 1¾ ᶜᴮ 3½ |
| Applesauce, canned, sweetened | tbsp. 0.5ozfl/14.21ml | ☺ | 1½ 1¾ | ☹ ¾ | 21½ ᶜᴮ 43 |
| Applesauce, canned, unsweetened | tbsp. 0.5ozfl/14.21ml | ☺ | ¾ ¾ | ☹ 1 | 21½ ᶜᴮ 43 |
| Apricot, dried, cooked, sweetened | piece 0.71oz/20g | ☺ | ☺+ ×1¼ unit ☺+ ×1½ unit | ☹ 1¼ | ☺ ☺ |
| Apricot, dried, uncooked | piece 0.71oz/20g | ☺ | ☺+ ×7¾ unit ☺+ ×8 unit | ☹ ¼ | ☺ ☺ |
| Apricot, fresh | piece 1.24oz/35g | ☺ | ☺+ ×¾ unit ☺+ ×1 unit | ☹ ¾ | ☺ ☺ |
| Banana, chips | portion 1.42oz/40g | ☺ | 3¾ 3¾ | ☹ 12½ | ½ ᶠᴮ 1¼ |
| Banana, fresh | piece 4.17oz/118g | ☺ | ☺+ ×¼ unit ☺+ ×¼ unit | ☹ 9¼ | ¾ ᶠᴮ 1½ |
| Blackberries, fresh | portion 4.94oz/140g | ☺ | 3¾ 3¾ | ☺ ☺ | 2¼ ᴮ 4½ |
| Blueberries, fresh | portion 4.94oz/140g | ☺ | 3¾ 3¾ | ☺ ☺ | ¾ ᴮ 1½ |
| Boysenberries, fresh | portion 0.29oz/8g | ☺ | 69¼ 69¼ | ☺ ☺ | ☺ ☺ |
| Cantaloupe, fresh | portion 4.94oz/140g | ☺ | 1 1 | ☹ 14¼ | 2 ᴮ 4¼ |
| Carambola (starfruit), fresh | piece 3.21oz/91g | ☺ | ☺+ ×¼ unit ☺+ ×¼ unit | ☹ 1¼ | ☺ ☺ |
| Clementine, fresh | portion 4.94oz/140g | ☺ | 7 7 | ☺ ☺ | 2¼ ᴮ 4½ |
| Cranberries, dried (Craisins®) | portion 1.42oz/40g | ☺ | ☺+ ×3¼ unit ☺+ ×3¼ unit | ☹ 41½ | ☺ ☺ |
| Cranberries, fresh | portion 1.95oz/55g | ☺ | ☺+ ×2¾ unit ☺+ ×2¾ unit | ☹ 45¼ | ☺ ☺ |
| Currants, fresh, black | portion 4.94oz/140g | ☺ | 1¼ 1¼ | ☺ ☺ | ☺ ☺ |

| Fruit | Unit | Lactose ☞ + unit/🔲 | Fructose* ☞ Fructose ☞ | Sorbitol ☞ Sorbitol ☞ | FrucGalactans ☞ FrucGalactans ☞ 📖 |
|---|---|---|---|---|---|
| Currants, fresh, red and white | portion<br>4.94oz/140g | ☺ | 1<br>1 | ☺<br>☺ | ☺<br>☺ |
| Dates | portion<br>1.42oz/40g | ☺ | ☺<br>☺ | ☺<br>☺ | ☺<br>☺ |
| Elderberries, fresh | portion<br>4.94oz/140g | ☺ | ¼<br>¼ | ☺<br>☺ | ☺<br>☺ |
| Figs, dried, cooked, sweetened | piece<br>1.77oz/50g | ☺ | ☺+ ×¾ unit<br>☺+ ×¾ unit | ☺<br>☺ | ☺<br>☺ |
| Figs, fresh | piece<br>1.77oz/50g | ☺ | ☺+ ×2 unit<br>☺+ ×2 unit | ☺<br>☺ | ☺<br>☺ |
| Gooseberries, fresh | portion<br>4.94oz/140g | ☺ | ☺+ ×1 unit<br>☺+ ×1 unit | ☺<br>☺ | ☺<br>☺ |
| Grapefruit, fresh, pink or red | portion<br>4.94oz/140g | ☺ | 2<br>2 | ☺<br>☺ | 1½ CB<br>3 |
| Grapes, fresh | portion<br>4.94oz/140g | ☺ | ¼<br>¼ | ☹<br>½ | 2¼ B<br>4½ |
| Guava (guayaba), fresh, common | piece<br>5.3oz/150g | ☺ | 2¼<br>2¼ | ☹<br>½ | ☺<br>☺ |
| Honeydew | portion<br>4.94oz/140g | ☺ | ¾<br>¾ | ☺<br>☺ | 1½ B<br>3¼ |
| Jackfruit, fresh | tbsp.<br>0.5ozfl/14.21ml | ☺ | ☺<br>☺ | ☹<br>½ | ☺<br>☺ |
| Kiwi fruit, gold | piece<br>3.04oz/86g | ☺ | 1<br>1 | ☺<br>☺ | ☺ B<br>☺ |
| Kiwi fruit, green | piece<br>2.44oz/69g | ☺ | 3<br>3 | ☺<br>☺ | ☺ B<br>☺ |
| Lemon, fresh | piece<br>2.05oz/58g | ☺ | ☺<br>☺ | ☺<br>☺ | 7¾ B<br>15½ |
| Lime, fresh | piece<br>2.37oz/67g | ☺ | ☺<br>☺ | ☺<br>☺ | 6¾ B<br>13½ |
| Loganberries, fresh | portion<br>4.94oz/140g | ☺ | ☺+ ×1½ unit<br>☺+ ×1½ unit | ☺<br>☺ | ☺<br>☺ |
| Lowbush cranberries (lingonberries) | portion<br>4.94oz/140g | ☺ | ☺+ ×9¼ unit<br>☺+ ×9¼ unit | ☹<br>35½ | ☺<br>☺ |

☞ *Level 0*: lactose measure ×½  
☞ *Level 1*: fructose measure ×2  
☞ *Level 2*: fructose-/sorbitol measure ×4. the rest ×2  
☞ *Level 3*: sorbitol measure ×7. the rest ×3  
📖: source of fruc/galactans data  

+ Unit/🔲: added tolerated amount of unit per strong lactase capsule  
Fructose*: fructose, sorbitol adjusted  
☺+ ×[Amount] unit: Per unit consumed you can additionally tolerate up to [amount] × fructose(*)-unit of another product.  

☹: avoid;   ☹¹: ¼ at TL 1;   ☹²: ¼ at TL 2;   ☹³: ¼ at TL 3;   ☺: only contains traces;   ☺: is free from it

| Fruit | Unit | Lactose + unit/ | Fructose* Fructose | Sorbitol Sorbitol | FrucGalactans FrucGalactans |
|---|---|---|---|---|---|
| Lychees (litchis), fresh | portion | ☺ | 1 | ☺ | ☺ B |
|  | 4.94oz/140g |  | 1 | ☺ | ☺ |
| lycium (wolf or goji berries) | portion | ☺ | ☺+ ×1 unit | ☺ | ☺ |
|  | 4.94oz/140g |  | ☺+ ×1 unit | ☺ | ☺ |
| Mandarin orange, fresh | portion | ☺ | 1¼ | ☺ | 2¼ B |
|  | 4.94oz/140g |  | 1¼ | ☺ | 4½ |
| Mango, fresh | tbsp. | ☺ | 1 | ☹ | ☺ B |
|  | 0.5ozfl/14.21ml |  | 1 | 4 | ☺ |
| Mangosteen, fresh | portion | ☺ | 35½ | ☺ | ☺ |
|  | 4.94oz/140g |  | 35½ | ☺ | ☺ |
| Mulberries | portion | ☺ | ½ | ☺ | ☺ |
|  | 4.94oz/140g |  | ½ | ☺ | ☺ |
| Muskmelon | portion | ☺ | 1¼ | ☺ | 1½ B |
|  | 4.94oz/140g |  | 1¼ | ☺ | 3¼ |
| Nectarine, fresh | tbsp. | ☺ | 8¼ | ☹ | 5½ B |
|  | 0.5ozfl/14.21ml |  | ☺ | 1 | 11¼ |
| Orange, fresh | portion | ☺ | 2¼ | ☺ | 2¼ B |
|  | 4.94oz/140g |  | 2¼ | ☺ | 4½ |
| Papaya, fresh | portion | ☺ | ☺+ ×1 unit | ☺ | ☺ |
|  | 4.94oz/140g |  | ☺+ ×1 unit | ☺ | ☺ |
| Passion fruit (maracuya), fresh | portion | ☺ | ☺+ ×2½ unit | ☺ | ☺ |
|  | 4.94oz/140g |  | ☺+ ×2½ unit | ☺ | ☺ |
| Peach, fresh | piece | ☺ | ☺+ ×½ unit | ☹ | ¾ B |
|  | 5.3oz/150g |  | ☺+ ×1¼ unit | ¼ | 1½ |
| Pear, fresh | tbsp. | ☺ | ½ | ☹ | ☺ B |
|  | 0.5ozfl/14.21ml |  | ¾ | ¼ | ☺ |
| Persimmon, fresh | piece | ☺ | 2¾ | ☺ | 1 C |
|  | 4.94oz/140g |  | 2¾ | ☺ | 2 |
| Pineapple, dried | portion | ☺ | ½ | ☹ | 2 CB |
|  | 1.42oz/40g |  | ½ | ½ | 4 |
| Pineapple, fresh | portion | ☺ | ¾ | ☹ | 2¼ CB |
|  | 4.94oz/140g |  | ¾ | ¾ | 4½ |
| Plantains, green, boiled | piece | ☺ | ¾ | ☺ | ¼ FB |
|  | 7.87oz/223g |  | ¾ | ☺ | ¾ |
| Plum, fresh | tbsp. | ☺ | ☺+ ×¼ unit | ☹ | 21½ C |
|  | 0.5ozfl/14.21ml |  | ☺+ ×½ unit | ¾ | 43 |
| Pomegranate, fresh (arils-seed/juice sacs) | tbsp. | ☺ | ☺+ ×½ unit | ☹ | ☺ |
|  | 0.5ozfl/14.21ml |  | ☺+ ×½ unit | 2 | ☺ |
| Quince, fresh | tbsp. | ☺ | 1¼ | ☺ | ☺ |
|  | 0.5ozfl/14.21ml |  | 1¼ | ☺ | ☺ |

| Fruit | Unit | Lactose 1<br>+ unit/capsule | Fructose* 0<br>Fructose 0 | Sorbitol 0<br>Sorbitol 1 | FrucGalactans 0<br>FrucGalactans 1 📖 |
|---|---|---|---|---|---|
| Raisins, uncooked | portion<br>1.42oz/40g | ☺ | ½<br>½ | ☹<br>½ | 2[B]<br>4 |
| Rambutan, canned in syrup | portion<br>4.94oz/140g | ☺ | 1¼<br>1¼ | ☺<br>☺ | ¾[CB]<br>1¾ |
| Raspberries, fresh, red | portion<br>4.94oz/140g | ☺ | ½<br>½ | ☹<br>1½ | 1[B]<br>2¼ |
| Rhubarb, fresh | portion<br>4.94oz/140g | ☺ | ☺<br>☺ | ☺<br>☺ | ☺<br>☺ |
| Rose hips | portion<br>4.94oz/140g | ☺ | ☺+ ×½ unit<br>☺+ ×½ unit | ☺<br>☺ | ☺<br>☺ |
| Santa Claus melon | portion<br>4.94oz/140g | ☺ | 1¼<br>1¼ | ☺<br>☺ | ☺<br>☺ |
| Sapodilla, fresh | portion<br>4.94oz/140g | ☺ | ☺+ ×3½ unit<br>☺+ ×3½ unit | ☺<br>☺ | ☺<br>☺ |
| Sour cherries, fresh | tbsp.<br>0.5ozfl/14.21ml | ☺ | 10<br>☺ | ☹<br>½ | ☺<br>☺ |
| Soursop (guanabana), fresh | portion<br>4.94oz/140g | ☺ | 1¼<br>1¼ | ☺<br>☺ | ☺<br>☺ |
| Strawberries, fresh | portion<br>4.94oz/140g | ☺ | ½<br>¾ | ☹<br>¼ | ☺[C]<br>☺ |
| Sweet cherries, fresh | tbsp.<br>0.5ozfl/14.21ml | ☺ | 3¾<br>☺+ ×¼ unit | ☹<br>¼ | ☺<br>☺ |
| Watermelon, fresh | tbsp.<br>0.5ozfl/14.21ml | ☺ | 1¾<br>1¾ | ☹<br>☺ | 10¼[B]<br>20¾ |

0 *Level 0:* lactose measure ×½
1 *Level 1:* fructose measure ×2
2 *Level 2:* fructose-/sorbitol measure ×4. the rest ×2
3 *Level 3:* sorbitol measure ×7. the rest ×3
📖: source of fruc/galactans data

+ Unit/capsule: added tolerated amount of unit per strong lactase capsule
Fructose*: fructose, sorbitol adjusted

☺+ ×[Amount] unit: Per unit consumed you can additionally tolerate up to [amount] × fructose(*)-unit of another product.

☹: avoid; ☹[1]: ¼ at TL 1; ☹[2]: ¼ at TL 2; ☹[3]: ¼ at TL 3; ☺: only contains traces; ☺: is free from it

## 3.7.2 Vegetables

| Vegetables | Unit | Lactose ↲ + unit/ 💊 | Fructose* ↺ Fructose ↲ | Sorbitol ↺ Sorbitol ↲ | FrucGalactans ↺ FrucGalactans ↲ 📖 |
|---|---|---|---|---|---|
| Alfalfa sprouts | portion | ☺ | 14½ | ☺ | ☺ G |
|  | 3oz/85g |  | 14½ | ☺ | ☺ |
| Artichoke, globe raw | tbsp. | ☺ | ☺ | ☹ | 1 FB |
|  | 0.5ozfl/14.21ml |  | ☺ | 23¾ | 2¼ |
| Asparagus, raw | portion | ☺ | 1½ | ☹ | ½ FB |
|  | 3oz/85g |  | 1½ | 9¾ | 1¼ |
| Avocado, green skin, Florida type | portion | ☺ | ☺+ ×1 unit | ☺ | ☺ B |
|  | 1.06oz/30g |  | ☺+ ×1 unit | ☺ | ☺ |
| Bamboo shoots, canned and drained | portion | ☺ | 19½ | ☺ | ☺ |
|  | 3oz/85g |  | 19½ | ☺ | ☺ |
| Beets, raw | portion | ☺ | 58¾ | ☹ | 1 CB |
|  | 3oz/85g |  | ☺ | 3¼ | 2 |
| Black olives | portion | ☺ | ☺ | ☹ | ☺ |
|  | 0.53oz/15g |  | ☺ | 33¼ | ☺ |
| Bok choy, raw | portion | ☺ | ☺+ ×¼ unit | ☹ | ☺ B |
|  | 3oz/85g |  | ☺+ ×¼ unit | 23½ | ☺ |
| Boston Market® sweet corn | portion | ☺ | ☺+ ×¼ unit | ☹ | ☺ B |
|  | 3oz/85g |  | ☺+ ×½ unit | 4 | ☺ |
| Broccoflower (green cauliflower), cooked from fresh | portion | ☺ | 1 | ☺ | ☺ B |
|  | 3oz/85g |  | 1 | ☺ | ☺ |
| Broccoli, raw | portion | 16¾ | 3 | ☺ | ½ B |
|  | 3oz/85g | +14 unit | 3 | ☺ | 1¼ |
| Brown mushrooms (Italian or Crimini mushrooms), raw | tbsp. | ☺ | ☺+ ×¼ unit | ☹ | 12¼ B |
|  | 0.5ozfl/14.21ml |  | ☺+ ×¼ unit | ¾ | 24½ |
| Brussels sprouts, cooked from fresh | portion | ☺ | ☺ | ☺ | 1 B |
|  | 3oz/85g |  | ☺ | ☺ | 2 |
| Butternut squash | portion | ☺ | ☺ | ☺ | ½ G |
|  | 4.59oz/130g |  | ☺ | ☺ | 1¼ |
| Cabbage, green, cooked | portion | ☺ | ☺+ ×¾ unit | ☹ | 1¼ B |
|  | 3oz/85g |  | ☺+ ×¾ unit | 58¾ | 2½ |
| Cabbage, red, cooked | portion | ☺ | ☺+ ×¼ unit | ☺ | 1¼ B |
|  | 3oz/85g |  | ☺+ ×¼ unit | ☺ | 2½ |
| Cabbage, savoy, raw | portion | ☺ | ☺ | ☹ | 1½ B |
|  | 3oz/85g |  | ☺ | 39 | 3 |
| Carrots, cooked from fresh | portion | ☺ | ☺ | ☹ | ☺ B |
|  | 3oz/85g |  | ☺ | ½ | ☺ |

| Vegetables | Unit | Lactose ☹/ + unit/🔵 | Fructose* ☹/ Fructose ☹/ | Sorbitol ☹/ Sorbitol ☹/ | FrucGalactans ☹/ FrucGalactans ☹/📖 |
|---|---|---|---|---|---|
| Carrots, raw | piece 2.16oz/61g | ☺ | ☺ ☺ | ☹ ¾ | ☺ᴮ ☺ |
| Cauliflower, cooked from frozen | portion 3oz/85g | ☺ | ☺ ☺ | ☹ 2½ | ☺ᶜᴮ ☺ |
| Celeriac (celery root), cooked from fresh | tbsp. 0.5ozfl/14.21ml | ☺ | 13¼ 13¼ | ☹ ¾ | ☺ ☺ |
| Celery, cooked | tbsp. 0.5ozfl/14.21ml | ☺ | ☺ ☺ | ☹ 1 | ☺ᶜ ☺ |
| Chard, raw or blanched, marinated in oil | portion 3oz/85g | ☺ | ☺+ ×½ unit ☺+ ×½ unit | ☺ ☺ | ☺ ☺ |
| Chayote squash, cooked | portion 4.59oz/130g | ☺ | 6¼ 6¼ | ☺ ☺ | ☺ᴮ ☺ |
| Chestnuts, boiled, steamed | portion 1.06oz/30g | ☺ | ☺ ☺ | ☹ 6 | ☺ ☺ |
| Chicory coffee powder, unprepared | portion 0.08oz/2g | ☺ | ☺ ☺ | ☹ 8¾ | ½ᴱ 1 |
| Chicory greens, raw | portion 3oz/85g | ☺ | 5¼ 5¼ | ☹ 39 | 2¼ᴮ 4½ |
| Coleslaw, with apples and raisins, mayo dressing | portion 3.53oz/100g | ☺ | ½ ½ | ☹ ½ | 1ᴮ 2 |
| Coleslaw, with pineapple, mayo dressing | portion 3.53oz/100g | ☺ | ☺+ ×¼ unit ☺+ ×¼ unit | ☹ 3¾ | ☺ᴮ ☺ |
| Collards, raw | portion 3oz/85g | ☺ | ☺ ☺ | ☺ ☺ | 1¼ᴮ 2½ |
| Cucumber, raw, with peel | portion 3oz/85g | ☺ | 5¼ 5¼ | ☹ 1 | ☺ᴮ ☺ |
| Cucumber, raw, without peel | portion 3oz/85g | ☺ | 4¾ 4¾ | ☹ 1 | ☺ᴮ ☺ |
| Eggplant, cooked | portion 3oz/85g | ☺ | 3½ 3½ | ☹ 2½ | ☺ᴮ ☺ |
| Endive, curly, raw | portion 3oz/85g | ☺ | ☺ ☺ | ☹ 3 | 3¾ᶜ 7½ |
| Enoki mushrooms, raw | tbsp. 0.5ozfl/14.21ml | ☺ | ☺ ☺ | ☹ ¾ | ☺ ☺ |

☹/ *Level 0*: lactose measure ×½  
☹/ *Level 1*: fructose measure ×2  
☹/ *Level 2*: fructose-/sorbitol measure ×4. the rest ×2  
☹/ *Level 3*: sorbitol measure ×7. the rest ×3  
📖: source of fruc/galactans data  

+ Unit/🔵: added tolerated amount of unit per strong lactase capsule  
Fructose*: fructose, sorbitol adjusted  

☺+ ×[Amount] unit: Per unit consumed you can additionally tolerate up to [amount] × fructose(*)-unit of another product.

☹: avoid;  ☹¹: ¼ at TL 1;  ☹²: ¼ at TL 2;  ☹³: ¼ at TL 3;  ☺: only contains traces;  ☺: is free from it

| Vegetables | Unit | Lactose  + unit/ | Fructose*  Fructose | Sorbitol  Sorbitol | FrucGalactans  FrucGalactans |
|---|---|---|---|---|---|
| Fennel bulb, raw | portion  3oz/85g | ☺ | ☺+ ×¾ unit  ☺+ ×¾ unit | ☹  2 | 1¼ B  2¾ |
| Garbanzo beans (chickpeas), canned, drained | portion  3.18oz/90g | ☺ | ☺  ☺ | ☹  1 | 1½ A  3 |
| Garlic, fresh | portion  0.15oz/4g | ☺ | ☺  ☺ | ☺  ☺ | ¾ FB  1½ |
| Ginger root, raw | portion  0.15oz/4g | ☺ | 89¼  89¼ | ☺  ☺ | ☺ B  ☺ |
| Green beans (string beans), cooked from fresh | portion  3oz/85g | ☺ | 4½  4½ | ☺  ☺ | ¼ A  ¾ |
| Green bell peppers | portion  3oz/85g | ☺ | ☺  ☺ | ☺  ☺ | ☺ B  ☺ |
| Green olives | portion  0.53oz/15g | ☺ | ☺  ☺ | ☹  18 | ☺  ☺ |
| Green tomato, raw | portion  3oz/85g | ☺ | 3  3¼ | ☹  ¾ | 6½ B  13 |
| Hot chili peppers, green, cooked from fresh | piece  1.52oz/43g | ☺ | 4½  4½ | ☺  ☺ | 2½ B  5¼ |
| Hot chili peppers, red, cooked from fresh | piece  1.52oz/43g | ☺ | 2¾  2¾ | ☺  ☺ | 2½ B  5¼ |
| Hubbard squash | portion  3oz/85g | ☺ | ☺  ☺ | ☺  ☺ | ☺ B  ☺ |
| Jerusalem artichoke (sunchoke), raw | pinch  0.04ozfl/1g | ☺ | ☺  ☺ | ☺  ☺ | 3¼ FB  6½ |
| Kale, raw | portion  3oz/85g | ☺ | ☺  ☺ | ☹  ¾ | ☺  ☺ |
| Kelp, raw | portion  3oz/85g | ☺ | ☺  ☺ | ☺  ☺ | ☺  ☺ |
| Kidney beans, cooked from dried | portion  3.18oz/90g | ☺ | ☺  ☺ | ☺  ☺ | ¼ A  ½ |
| Kohlrabi, cooked | portion  3oz/85g | ☺ | ☺+ ×¼ unit  ☺+ ×¼ unit | ☹  13 | ☺  ☺ |
| Leeks, leafs | portion  3oz/85g | ☺ | 3¼  3¼ | ☹  ¼ | ¾ G  1½ |
| Leeks, root | tbsp.  0.5ozfl/14.21ml | ☺ | 18½  18½ | ☹  2¼ | ¼ C  ¾ |
| Leeks, whole | portion  3oz/85g | ☺ | 3¼  3¼ | ☹  ¼ | ¼ C  ½ |

| Vegetables | Unit + unit/🗨 | Lactose 🌱 | Fructose* 🌱 Fructose 🌱 | Sorbitol 🌱 Sorbitol 🌱 | FrucGalactans 🌱 FrucGalactans 🌱 📖 |
|---|---|---|---|---|---|
| Lentils, cooked from dried | portion 3.18oz/90g | ☺ | ☺ ☺ | ☺ ☺ | ¾ A 1½ |
| Lettuce, boston, bibb or butterhead | portion 3oz/85g | ☺ | 7¼ 7¼ | ☹ 19½ | ☺ B ☺ |
| Lettuce, green leaf | portion 3oz/85g | ☺ | 8¼ 8¼ | ☹ 16¾ | ☺ CB ☺ |
| Lettuce, iceberg | portion 3oz/85g | ☺ | 6½ 6½ | ☹ 19½ | ☺ CB ☺ |
| Lettuce, red leaf | portion 3oz/85g | ☺ | 7¼ 7¼ | ☹ 19½ | ☺ B ☺ |
| Lettuce, romaine or cos | portion 3oz/85g | ☺ | 1¼ 1¼ | ☹ 16¾ | ☺ CB ☺ |
| Lima beans, cooked from dried | portion 3.18oz/90g | ☺ | ½ ½ | ☺ ☺ | ¼ A ½ |
| Lotus root, cooked | portion 3oz/85g | ☺ | ☺ ☺ | ☺ ☺ | ☺ ☺ |
| Maitake mushrooms, raw | tbsp. 0.5ozfl/14.21ml | 60½ +50½ unit | ☺+ ×½ unit ☺+ ×½ unit | ☹ ¾ | ☺ ☺ |
| Morel mushrooms, raw | tbsp. 0.5ozfl/14.21ml | ☺ | ☺ ☺ | ☹ ¾ | ☺ ☺ |
| Mung beans, cooked from dried | portion 3.18oz/90g | ☺ | ½ ½ | ☺ ☺ | ¾ A 1¾ |
| Mushrooms, batter dipped or breaded | portion 2.47oz/70g | ☺ | ☺ ☺ | ☹ ¼ | 2½ B 5¼ |
| Okra, raw | portion 3oz/85g | ☺ | 2¼ 2¼ | ☺ ☺ | 2 CB 4¼ |
| Onion, white, yellow or red, raw | tbsp. 0.5ozfl/14.21ml | ☺ | ☺ ☺ | ☹ 6 | 1 CB 2 |
| Oyster mushrooms, raw | portion 3oz/85g | ☺ | ☺+ ×1¾ unit ☺+ ×1¾ unit | ☹ ¼ | ☺ ☺ |
| Parsnip, cooked | portion 3oz/85g | ☺ | ☺+ ×¼ unit ☺+ ×¼ unit | ☺ ☺ | ☺ C ☺ |
| Pickled beets | portion 1.06oz/30g | ☺ | ☺ ☺ | ☹ 15 | 3 CB 6 |

🌱 *Level 0*: lactose measure ×½  
🌱 *Level 1*: fructose measure ×2  
🌱 *Level 2*: fructose-/sorbitol measure ×4. the rest ×2  
🌱 *Level 3*: sorbitol measure ×7. the rest ×3  
📖: source of fruc/galactans data  

+ Unit/🗨: added tolerated amount of unit per strong lactase capsule  
Fructose*: fructose, sorbitol adjusted  
☺+ ×[Amount] unit: Per unit consumed you can additionally tolerate up to [amount] × fructose(*)-unit of another product.  

☹: avoid; ☹¹: ¼ at TL 1; ☹²: ¼ at TL 2; ☹³: ¼ at TL 3; ☺: only contains traces; ☺: is free from it

| Vegetables | Unit | Lactose<br>+ unit/ | Fructose*<br>Fructose | Sorbitol<br>Sorbitol | FrucGalactans<br>FrucGalactans |
|---|---|---|---|---|---|
| Portabella mushrooms, cooked from fresh | tbsp.<br>0.5ozfl/14.21ml | ☺ | ☺+ ×½ unit<br>☺+ ×½ unit | ☹<br>½ | 12¼[B]<br>24½ |
| Purslane, raw | portion<br>3oz/85g | ☺ | 58¾<br>58¾ | ☺<br>☺ | ☺<br>☺ |
| Radicchio, raw | portion<br>3oz/85g | ☺ | 2¼<br>2¼ | ☺<br>☺ | ¾<br>1½ |
| Radish, raw | portion<br>3oz/85g | ☺ | ☺+ ×½ unit<br>☺+ ×½ unit | ☹<br>1 | ☺[C]<br>☺ |
| Rocket (arugula), raw | portion<br>3oz/85g | ☺ | 4¾<br>4¾ | ☺<br>☺ | ☺<br>☺ |
| Rutabaga, raw or blanched, marinated in oil mixture | portion<br>3oz/85g | ☺ | ☺+ ×1 unit<br>☺+ ×1 unit | ☺<br>☺ | ☺[CB]<br>☺ |
| Sauerkraut | tbsp.<br>0.5ozfl/14.21ml | ☺ | ☺<br>☺ | ☹<br>¾ | 7[B]<br>14¼ |
| Scallop squash | portion<br>3oz/85g | ☺ | 4<br>4 | ☺<br>☺ | ☺[CB]<br>☺ |
| Shallot, raw | tbsp.<br>0.5ozfl/14.21ml | ☺ | ☺<br>☺ | ☺<br>☺ | ¼[CB]<br>½ |
| Shiitake mushrooms, cooked | tbsp.<br>0.5ozfl/14.21ml | ☺ | ☺+ ×1 unit<br>☺+ ×1 unit | ☹<br>½ | ☺<br>☺ |
| Snow peas (edible pea pods), cooked from fresh | portion<br>3oz/85g | ☺ | ☺+ ×3½ unit<br>☺+ ×3½ unit | ☺<br>☺ | ¾[B]<br>1¾ |
| Sour pickles | portion<br>1.06oz/30g | ☺ | ☺+ ×¼ unit<br>☺+ ×¼ unit | ☹<br>4¼ | ☺[CB]<br>☺ |
| Soybean sprouts, raw | portion<br>3oz/85g | ☺ | ☺<br>☺ | ☹<br>½ | 3¾[CB]<br>7½ |
| Soybeans, cooked from dried | tbsp.<br>0.5oz/14.21ml | ☺ | 9<br>9 | ☹<br>3 | 3[A]<br>6 |
| Spaghetti squash | portion<br>3oz/85g | ☺ | ☺+ ×¼ unit<br>☺+ ×¼ unit | ☺<br>☺ | ☺[CB]<br>☺ |
| Spinach, cooked from fresh | portion<br>3oz/85g | ☺ | ☺<br>☺ | ☹<br>13 | 4[CB]<br>8¼ |
| Split pea sprouts, cooked | tbsp.<br>0.5ozfl/14.21ml | ☺ | ☺<br>☺ | ☺<br>☺ | 1¼[A]<br>2½ |
| Straw mushrooms, canned, drained | portion<br>3oz/85g | ☺ | ☺<br>☺ | ☹<br>¼ | ☺<br>☺ |
| Summer squash, cooked from fresh | portion<br>3oz/85g | ☺ | 2¼<br>2¼ | ☺<br>☺ | 2[CB]<br>4 |
| Sun-dried tomatoes, oil pack, drained | portion<br>1.06oz/30g | ☺ | ¼<br>¼ | ☹<br>¼ | 4½[B]<br>9¼ |

| Vegetables | Unit | Lactose 1↯<br>+ unit/capsule | Fructose* 0↯<br>Fructose 0↯ | Sorbitol 0↯<br>Sorbitol 1↯ | FrucGalactans 0↯<br>FrucGalactans 1↯ 🕮 |
|---|---|---|---|---|---|
| Tempeh | portion<br>3oz/85g | ☺ | 3¼<br>3¼ | ☹<br>½ | ½[A]<br>1 |
| Tomato, cooked from fresh | portion<br>3oz/85g | ☺ | 4¼<br>4½ | ☹<br>¾ | 6½[B]<br>13 |
| Turnip, cooked | portion<br>3oz/85g | ☺ | ☺+ ×½ unit<br>☺+ ×½ unit | ☹<br>2½ | ☺[CB]<br>☺ |
| Wax beans (yellow beans), canned, drained | portion<br>3oz/85g | ☺ | ☺<br>☺ | ☺<br>☺ | ¼[A]<br>¾ |
| Winter (dark green or orange) squash, cooked | portion<br>4.59oz/130g | ☺ | 1¾<br>1¾ | ☺<br>☺ | ☺[CB]<br>☺ |
| Winter melon (waxgourd or chinese preserving melon) | portion<br>3oz/85g | ☺ | ☺<br>☺ | ☺<br>☺ | ☺[CB]<br>☺ |
| Yams, sweet potato type, boiled | portion<br>3.89oz/110g | ☺ | ☺<br>☺ | ☺<br>☺ | ☺[B]<br>☺ |
| Yellow bell pepper, raw | portion<br>3oz/85g | ☺ | ½<br>½ | ☺<br>☺ | ☺[CB]<br>☺ |
| Yellow tomato, raw | portion<br>3oz/85g | ☺ | 4½<br>4¾ | ☹<br>1 | 6½[B]<br>13 |

0↯ *Level 0:* lactose measure ×½
1↯ *Level 1:* fructose measure ×2
2↯ *Level 2*: fructose-/sorbitol measure ×4. the rest ×2
3↯ *Level 3:* sorbitol measure ×7. the rest ×3
🕮: source of fruc/galactans data

+ Unit/capsule: added tolerated amount of unit per strong lactase capsule
Fructose*: fructose, sorbitol adjusted
☺+ ×[Amount] unit: Per unit consumed you can additionally tolerate up to [amount] × fructose(*)-unit of another product.

☹: avoid; ☹[1]: ¼ at TL 1; ☹[2]: ¼ at TL 2; ☹[3]: ¼ at TL 3; ☺: only contains traces; ☺: is free from it

## 3.8 Ice cream

| Ice cream | Unit | Lactose ↲ + unit/ | Fructose* ↲ Fructose ↲ | Sorbitol ↲ Sorbitol ↲ | FrucGalactans ↲ FrucGalactans ↲ |
|---|---|---|---|---|---|
| Ben & Jerry's® Ice Cream, Brownie Batter | portion 3.89oz/110g | ¼ +¼ unit | ☺+ ×3 unit ☺+ ×3 unit | ☹ ☺ | 1¼ 2¾ |
| Ben & Jerry's® Ice Cream, Chocolate Chip Cookie Dough | portion 3.67oz/104g | ½ +¼ unit | ☺+ ×4¾ unit ☺+ ×4¾ unit | ☺ ☺ | 3¼ 6½ |
| Ben & Jerry's® Ice Cream, Chubby Hubby® | portion 3.78oz/107g | ½ +½ unit | ☺+ ×5 unit ☺+ ×5 unit | ☺ ☺ | 3½ 7 |
| Ben & Jerry's® Ice Cream, Chunky Monkey® | portion 3.78oz/107g | ¼ +¼ unit | ☺+ ×2¾ unit ☺+ ×2¾ unit | ☹ ☺ | 2½ 5¼ |
| Ben & Jerry's® Ice Cream, Half Baked | portion 3.81oz/108g | ¼ +¼ unit | ☺+ ×2¼ unit ☺+ ×2¼ unit | ☺ ☺ | 2¼ 4¾ |
| Ben & Jerry's® Ice Cream, Karamel Sutra® | portion 3.74oz/106g | ½ +¼ unit | ☺+ ×4¾ unit ☺+ ×4¾ unit | ☺ ☺ | 3 6¼ |
| Ben & Jerry's® Ice Cream, New York Super Fudge Chunk® | portion 3.74oz/106g | ½ +½ unit | 67¼ 67¼ | ☹ ☺ | 3½ 7¼ |
| Ben & Jerry's® Ice Cream, One Sweet Whirled | portion 3.74oz/106g | ½ +¼ unit | ☺+ ×4¾ unit ☺+ ×4¾ unit | ☺ ☺ | 3 6¼ |
| Ben & Jerry's® Ice Cream, Peanut Butter Cup | portion 4.06oz/115g | ½ +¼ unit | ☺+ ×5¼ unit ☺+ ×5¼ unit | ☺ ☺ | 3¼ 6½ |
| Ben & Jerry's® Ice Cream, Phish Food® | portion 3.67oz/104g | ¼ +¼ unit | ☺+ ×2¼ unit ☺+ ×2¼ unit | ☺ ☺ | 2¼ 4¾ |
| Ben & Jerry's® Ice Cream, Vanilla For A Change | portion 3.64oz/103g | ½ +¼ unit | ☺+ ×4½ unit ☺+ ×4½ unit | ☺ ☺ | 3¼ 6½ |
| Breyers® Ice Cream, Natural Vanilla, Lactose Free | portion 2.3oz/65g | 4 +3¼ unit | ☺+ ×4¾ unit ☺+ ×4¾ unit | ☺ ☺ | 23¼ 46½ |
| Dreyer's® Grand Ice Cream, Chocolate | portion 2.3oz/65g | 1 +1 unit | ☺+ ×¾ unit ☺+ ×¾ unit | ☹ ☺ | 6¾ 13¾ |
| Dreyer's® No Sugar Added Ice Cream, Triple Chocolate | tsp. 0.16ozfl/4.74ml | 11½ +9½ unit | ¾ ☺ | ☹ ☹[2] | 64½ ☺ |
| Drumstick® (sundae cone) | piece 3.39oz/96g | 1 +¾ unit | ☺+ ×2¼ unit ☺+ ×2¼ unit | ☹ ☺ | 6¼ 12¾ |
| Frozen fruit juice bar | piece 2.72oz/77g | ☺ | ☺+ ×1¼ unit ☺+ ×1¼ unit | ☹ 4½ | ☺ ☺ |
| Haagen-Dazs® Desserts Extraordinaire Ice Cream, Crème Brûlée | portion 3.78oz/107g | ½ +¼ unit | ☺+ ×4¾ unit ☺+ ×4¾ unit | ☺ ☺ | 3 6¼ |

| Ice cream | Unit + unit/ 🥛 | Lactose ⚕ | Fructose* ⚕ Fructose ⚕ | Sorbitol ⚕ Sorbitol ⚕ | FrucGalactans ⚕ FrucGalactans ⚕ 📖 |
|---|---|---|---|---|---|
| Haagen-Dazs® Frozen Yogurt, chocolate or coffee flavors | portion 3.74oz/106g | ½ +½ unit | ☺+ ×¾ unit ☺+ ×¾ unit | ☹ ☺ | 1¾ 3½ |
| Haagen-Dazs® Frozen Yogurt, vanilla or other flavors | portion 3.74oz/106g | ½ +½ unit | ☺+ ×3 unit ☺+ ×3 unit | ☺ ☺ | 3½ 7 |
| Haagen-Dazs® Ice Cream, Bailey's Irish Cream | portion 3.6oz/102g | ½ +¼ unit | ☺+ ×2¾ unit ☺+ ×2¾ unit | ☹ ☺ | 1½ 3 |
| Haagen-Dazs® Ice Cream, Black Walnut | portion 3.74oz/106g | ½ +½ unit | ☺+ ×4¾ unit ☺+ ×4¾ unit | ☺ ☺ | 3½ 7 |
| Haagen-Dazs® Ice Cream, Butter Pecan | portion 3.74oz/106g | ½ +½ unit | ☺+ ×4¾ unit ☺+ ×4¾ unit | ☺ ☺ | 2¼ 4¾ |
| Haagen-Dazs® Ice Cream, Cherry Vanilla | portion 3.57oz/101g | ½ +½ unit | ☺+ ×4½ unit ☺+ ×4½ unit | ☺ ☺ | 3¼ 6½ |
| Haagen-Dazs® Ice Cream, Chocolate | portion 3.74oz/106g | ¼ +¼ unit | ☺+ ×2¾ unit ☺+ ×2¾ unit | ☹ ☺ | 1¼ 2¾ |
| Haagen-Dazs® Ice Cream, Coffee | portion 3.74oz/106g | ¼ +¼ unit | ☺+ ×2¾ unit ☺+ ×2¾ unit | ☹ ☺ | 2½ 5¼ |
| Haagen-Dazs® Ice Cream, Cookies & Cream | portion 3.6oz/102g | ½ +¼ unit | ☺+ ×4½ unit ☺+ ×4½ unit | ☺ ☺ | 3¼ 6½ |
| Haagen-Dazs® Ice Cream, Mango | portion 3.74oz/106g | ¼ +¼ unit | ☺+ ×2¼ unit ☺+ ×2¼ unit | ☺ ☺ | 2¼ 4¾ |
| Haagen-Dazs® Ice Cream, Pistachio | portion 3.74oz/106g | ½ +½ unit | ☺+ ×4¾ unit ☺+ ×4¾ unit | ☺ ☺ | ½ 1¼ |
| Haagen-Dazs® Ice Cream, Rocky Road | portion 3.67oz/104g | ¼ +¼ unit | ☺+ ×2¾ unit ☺+ ×2¾ unit | ☹ ☺ | 2½ 5¼ |
| Haagen-Dazs® Ice Cream, Strawberry | portion 3.74oz/106g | ½ +¼ unit | ☺+ ×4¾ unit ☺+ ×4¾ unit | ☺ ☺ | 3 6¼ |
| Haagen-Dazs® Ice Cream, Vanilla Chocolate Chip | portion 3.74oz/106g | ½ +½ unit | ☺+ ×4¾ unit ☺+ ×4¾ unit | ☺ ☺ | 3½ 7 |
| Ice cream sandwich | piece 2.54oz/72g | 1¼ +1 unit | ☺+ ×1½ unit ☺+ ×1½ unit | ☺ ☺ | 7½ 15¼ |
| Ice cream, light, no sugar added, with aspartame, vanilla or other flavors (include chocolate chip) | tsp. 0.16ozfl/4.74ml | 9¾ +8 unit | 2¼ ☺ | ☹ ¼ | 54¾ ☺ |

⚕ *Level 0:* lactose measure ×½   + Unit/ 🥛: added tolerated amount of unit per strong lactase capsule
⚕ *Level 1:* fructose measure ×2   Fructose*: fructose, sorbitol adjusted
⚕ *Level 2:* fructose-/sorbitol measure ×4. the rest ×2   ☺+ ×[Amount] unit: Per unit consumed you
⚕ *Level 3:* sorbitol measure ×7. the rest ×3   can additionally tolerate up to [amount] ×
📖: source of fruc/galactans data   fructose(*)-unit of another product.

☹: avoid;   ☹¹: ¼ at TL 1;   ☹²: ¼ at TL 2;   ☹³: ¼ at TL 3;   ☺: only contains traces;   ☺: is free from it

| Ice cream | Unit | Lactose 🌱 + unit/💊 | Fructose* 😊 Sorbitol 😊 FrucGalactans 😊 Fructose 🌱 Sorbitol 🌱 FrucGalactans 🌱 📖 | | |
|---|---|---|---|---|---|
| Sorbet, chocolate | portion | ☺ | ☺+ ×3¼ unit | ☺ | ☺ |
|  | 3.71oz/105g |  | ☺+ ×3¼ unit | ☺ | ☺ |
| Sorbet, coconut | portion | 18¾ | ☺+ ×5 unit | ☺ | 3¼ |
|  | 3.74oz/106g | +15½ unit | ☺+ ×5 unit | ☺ | 6½ |
| Sorbet, fruit | portion | ☺ | ☺+ ×5½ unit | ☺ | ☺ |
|  | 3.74oz/106g |  | ☺+ ×5½ unit | ☺ | ☺ |

# 3.9 Ingredients

| Ice cream | Unit | Lactose ☹<br>+ unit/ 💊 | Fructose* ☹<br>Fructose ☹ | Sorbitol ☹<br>Sorbitol ☹ | FrucGalactans ☹<br>FrucGalactans ☹ 📖 |
|---|---|---|---|---|---|
| Baking powder | sachet<br>0.22oz/6g | ☺ | ☺<br>☺ | ☺<br>☺ | ☺<br>☺ |
| Barley flour | portion<br>1.06oz/30g | ☺ | ☺<br>☺ | ☺<br>☺ | 6¼ AD<br>12¾ |
| Lemon peel | tbsp.<br>0.5oz/14.21ml | ☺ | ☺<br>☺ | ☺<br>☺ | ☺<br>☺ |
| Orange peel | tbsp.<br>0.5oz/14.21ml | ☺ | 3¼<br>3¼ | ☺<br>☺ | ☺<br>☺ |
| Rye flour, in recipes not containing yeast | portion<br>1.06oz/30g | ☺ | 27¾<br>27¾ | ☺<br>☺ | ¾ AD<br>1¾ |
| Semolina flour | portion<br>1.06oz/30g | ☺ | ☺<br>☺ | ☺<br>☺ | 1¼ AD<br>2¾ |
| Spelt flour | portion<br>1.06oz/30g | ☺ | ☺+ ×¼ unit<br>☺+ ×¼ unit | ☺<br>☺ | ☺ A<br>☺ |
| Streusel topping, crumb | portion<br>0.68oz/19g | 68¼<br>+57 unit | ☺<br>☺ | ☺<br>☺ | 2¾ A<br>5¾ |
| Wheat bran, unprocessed | tbsp.<br>0.5oz/14.21ml | ☺ | ☺<br>☺ | ☺<br>☺ | ☺<br>☺ |
| White all-purpose flour, unenriched | portion<br>1.06oz/30g | ☺ | ☺<br>☺ | ☺<br>☺ | 1 AD<br>2 |
| White whole wheat flour | portion<br>1.06oz/30g | ☺ | 33¼<br>33¼ | ☺<br>☺ | 1¼ AD<br>2¾ |

☹ *Level 0*: lactose measure ×½
☹ *Level 1*: fructose measure ×2
☹ *Level 2*: fructose-/sorbitol measure ×4. the rest ×2
☹ *Level 3*: sorbitol measure ×7. the rest ×3
📖: source of fruc/galactans data

+ Unit/ 💊: added tolerated amount of unit per strong lactase capsule
Fructose*: fructose, sorbitol adjusted
☺+ ×[Amount] unit: Per unit consumed you can additionally tolerate up to [amount] × fructose(*)-unit of another product.

☹: avoid;   ☹¹: ¼ at TL 1;   ☹²: ¼ at TL 2;   ☹³: ¼ at TL 3;   ☺: only contains traces;   ☺: is free from it

# SUGGESTIONS

I hope that the diet has been effective for you and increased the well-being of your tummy. This is the first edition and more are planned to follow. Each input can help to make the book even more practical for those that are affected by an intolerance or irritable bowel syndrome. Your suggestions and tips are therefore highly welcomed. Please tell me about your experiences and wishes. Grey areas remain and new foods arrive on the market continuously. In order to keep the brick dragons chained, it is important for us to create a current knowledgebase regarding the handling of the disease. You can also help others like you, by sharing your personal TLs so that we can improve the BTLs in future versions. To do so please visit www.Laxiba.co.uk/tls.

You want to hire a coach for you to learn and keep the diet strategy or want to book a workshop regarding healthy nutrition and stress management for your firm? Come visit us at www.Laxiba.co.uk. We look forward to getting to know you.

As a closing, I wish you cheerfulness and above all healthfulness.

Your author brightly greets you,

Henry S. Grant
Henry@AmericanDietPublishing.co.uk

*This page has been intentionally left blank.*

# Keyword Index

In the following index, you find the foods once more in alphabetical order. The abbreviations remain the same but the base has changed to TL 1 for all foods.

| Keyword Index | Unit | Lactose<br>+ unit/ | Fructose*<br>Fructose* | Sorbitol<br>Sorbitol | FrucGalactans<br>FrucGalactans |
|---|---|---|---|---|---|
| 3 Musketeers® | piece<br>2.14oz/60.4g | 1¾<br>+1½ unit | ☺+ ×3¾ unit<br>☺+ ×1¾ unit | ☺<br>☺ | 6¼<br>12½ |
| 7 UP® | glass<br>8.4ozfl/240ml | ☺ | ☹[2]<br>☹[2] | ☺<br>☺ | ☺<br>☺ |
| Advocaat, regular | glass<br>8.4ozfl/240ml | ¼<br>+0,24 unit | ☺+ ×4¾ unit<br>☺+ ×2¼ unit | ☺<br>☺ | 1½<br>3¼ |
| After Eight® Thin Chocolate Mints | piece<br>0.29oz/8g | 10¼<br>+8½ unit | ☺<br>☺ | ☺<br>☺ | 57¾<br>☺ |
| Ale | glass<br>8.4ozfl/240ml | ☺ | 50<br>☺ | ☹<br>10 | ☺<br>☺ |
| Alfalfa sprouts | portion<br>3oz/85g | ☺ | 14½<br>29¼ | ☺<br>☺ | ☺[G]<br>☺ |
| All-Bran® Original (Kellogg's®) | portion<br>1.06oz/30g | ☺ | ☺+ ×¼ unit<br>☺ | ☺<br>☺ | ¼[A]<br>¾ |
| Almond cookies | piece<br>0.44oz/12.4g | ☺ | ☺<br>☺ | ☺<br>☺ | 3[A]<br>6 |
| Almond milk, vanilla or other flavors, unsweetened | glass<br>8.4oz/240g | ☺ | ☺<br>☺ | ☺<br>☺ | ☹[A]<br>☹[2] |
| Almond paste (Marzipan) | portion<br>0.99oz/28g | ☺ | ☺<br>☺ | ☹<br>20½ | ½[G]<br>1¼ |
| Almonds, honey roasted | hand<br>1.06oz/30g | ☺ | 2<br>4¼ | ☹<br>5½ | ½[G]<br>1¼ |
| Almonds, raw | hand<br>1.06oz/30g | ☺ | ☺<br>☺ | ☺<br>☺ | ½[G]<br>1¼ |
| Alpine Lace 25% Reduced Fat, Mozzarella | portion<br>1.06oz/30g | 37¼<br>+31 unit | ☺<br>☺ | ☺<br>☺ | ☺<br>☺ |
| Amaranth Flakes (Arrowhead Mills) | portion<br>1.06oz/30g | ☺ | 3<br>6¼ | ☹<br>2½ | ¾[G]<br>1½ |
| Amaretto | glass<br>8.4ozfl/240ml | ☺ | ☺+ ×4½ unit<br>☺+ ×2½ unit | ☹<br>¼ | ☺<br>☺ |
| American cheese, processed | portion<br>1.06oz/30g | 4½<br>+3¾ unit | ☺<br>☺ | ☺<br>☺ | 25¾<br>51½ |

| KEYWORD INDEX | Unit | Lactose ↯ + unit/ 💊 | Fructose* ↯ Fructose* ↯ | Sorbitol ↯ Sorbitol ↯ | FrucGalactans ↯ FrucGalactans ↯ 📖 |
|---|---|---|---|---|---|
| Americano, decaf, without flavored syrup | cup 5.2ozfl/150ml | ☺ | ☺ ☺ | ☺ ☺ | ☺ ☺ |
| Americano, with flavored syrup | cup 5.2ozfl/150ml | ☺ | ☺ ☺ | ☺ ☺ | ☺ ☺ |
| Americano, without flavored syrup | cup 5.2ozfl/150ml | ☺ | ☺ ☺ | ☺ ☺ | ☺ ☺ |
| Apple banana strawberry juice | glass 8.4ozfl/240ml | ☺ | ☹¹ ¼ | ☹ ☹² | ¾ FB 1¾ |
| Apple cake, glazed | piece 1.59oz/45g | ☺ | ¾ 1¾ | ☹ ½ | 1¼ A 2½ |
| Apple grape juice | glass 8.4ozfl/240ml | ☺ | ☹² ☹² | ☹ ☹² | 1½ CB 3 |
| Apple strudel | piece 2.26oz/64g | ☺ | ¼ ½ | ☹ ¼ | ¾ A 1¾ |
| Apple, fresh, with skin | piece 6.42oz/182g | ☺ | ☹² ☹² | ☹ ☹² | 1¾ CB 3½ |
| Applejack liquor | glass 8.4ozfl/240ml | ☺ | ☺ ☺ | ☺ ☺ | ☺ ☺ |
| Applesauce, canned, sweetened | tbsp. 0.5ozfl/14.21ml | ☺ | 1½ 3 | ☹ ¾ | 21½ CB 43 |
| Applesauce, canned, unsweetened | tbsp. 0.5ozfl/14.21ml | ☺ | ¾ 1½ | ☹ 1 | 21½ CB 43 |
| Apricot nectar | glass 8.4ozfl/240ml | ☺ | ☺+ ×4¾ unit ☺+ ×2½ unit | ☹ ¼ | ☺ ☺ |
| Apricot, dried, cooked, sweetened | piece 0.71oz/20g | ☺ | ☺+ ×1¼ unit ☺+ ×¾ unit | ☹ 1¼ | ☺ ☺ |
| Apricot, dried, uncooked | piece 0.71oz/20g | ☺ | ☺+ ×7¾ unit ☺+ ×4 unit | ☹ ¼ | ☺ ☺ |
| Apricot, fresh | piece 1.24oz/35g | ☺ | ☺+ ×¾ unit ☺+ ×½ unit | ☹ ¾ | ☺ ☺ |
| Aquavit | glass 8.4ozfl/240ml | ☺ | ☺ ☺ | ☺ ☺ | ☺ ☺ |

↯ *Level 0*: lactose measure ×½  
↯ *Level 1*: fructose measure ×2  
↯ *Level 2*: fructose-/sorbitol measure ×4. the rest ×2  
↯ *Level 3*: sorbitol measure ×7. the rest ×3  
📖: source of fruc/galactans data  

+ Unit/💊: added tolerated amount of unit per strong lactase capsule  
Fructose*: fructose, sorbitol adjusted  
☺+ ×[Amount] unit: Per unit consumed you can additionally tolerate up to [amount] × fructose(*)-unit of another product.  

☹: avoid;  ☹¹: ¼ at TL 1;  ☹²: ¼ at TL 2;  ☹³: ¼ at TL 3;  ☺: only contains traces;  ☺: is free from it

| Keyword Index | Unit | Lactose 🡇 + unit/ | Fructose* 🡇 Fructose* 🡇 | Sorbitol 🡇 Sorbitol 🡇 | FrucGalactans 🡇 FrucGalactans 🡇 |
|---|---|---|---|---|---|
| Arby's® Chicken Cordon Bleu Sandwich, crispy | portion 4.94oz/140g | 32¼ +27 unit | 2 4¼ | ☺ ☺ | 1 A 2¼ |
| Arby's® macaroni and cheese | portion 7.66oz/217g | 21½ +18 unit | ☺ ☺ | ☺ ☺ | ½ A 1¼ |
| Arby's® orange juice | glass 8.4ozfl/240ml | ☺ | 1½ 3¼ | ☹ ¼ | ☺ B ☺ |
| Arby's® ranch sauce | tbsp. 0.5ozfl/14.21ml | ☺ | ☺ ☺ | ☹ 18½ | ☺ ☺ |
| Archway® Oatmeal Raisin Cookies | piece 0.92oz/26g | 23¾ +19¾ unit | ☺ ☺ | ☹ 10¼ | 2¼ A 4¾ |
| Archway® Peanut Butter Cookies | piece 1.2oz/34g | 23¾ +19¾ unit | 2 4 | ☹ 10¾ | 1½ A 3 |
| Artichoke, globe raw | tbsp. 0.5ozfl/14.21ml | ☺ | ☺ ☺ | ☹ 23¾ | 1 FB 2¼ |
| Asian noodle bowl, vegetables only | portion 7.06oz/200g | ☺ | ☺+ ×1 unit ☺+ ×½ unit | ☹ 10 | 1½ A 3¼ |
| Asparagus, raw | portion 3oz/85g | ☺ | 1½ 3¼ | ☹ 9¾ | ½ FB 1¼ |
| Au gratin potato, prepared from fresh | portion 4.94oz/140g | 1 +¾ unit | ☺ ☺ | ☹ 7¾ | 6¼ B 12½ |
| Avocado, green skin, Florida type | portion 1.06oz/30g | ☺ | ☺+ ×1 unit ☺+ ×½ unit | ☺ ☺ | ☺ B ☺ |
| Baby food, double baked (zwieback) | portion 0.25oz/7g | ☺ | ☺ ☺ | ☺ ☺ | 1½ A 3 |
| Baby food, Gerber Graduates® Organic Pasta Pick-Ups Three Cheese Ravioli | Portion 170 g | 88 | ☺ ☺ | ☺ ☺ | ¾ A 1½ |
| Baguette | slice 1.49oz/42g | ☺ | ☺ ☺ | ☺ ☺ | 1¾ A 3½ |
| Baking powder | sachet 0.22oz/6g | ☺ | ☺ ☺ | ☺ ☺ | ☺ ☺ |
| Balsamic vinegar | portion 0.53oz/15g | ☺ | ☺ ☺ | ☹ 23 | ☺ ☺ |
| Bamboo shoots, canned and drained | portion 3oz/85g | ☺ | 19½ 39 | ☺ ☺ | ☺ ☺ |
| Banana, chips | portion 1.42oz/40g | ☺ | 3¾ 7¾ | ☹ 12½ | ½ FB 1¼ |
| Banana, fresh | piece 4.17oz/118g | ☺ | ☺+ ×¼ unit ☺ | ☹ 9¼ | ¾ FB 1½ |

| Keyword Index | Unit | Lactose ☹ + unit/ 💊 | Fructose* ☹ Fructose* ☹ | Sorbitol ☹ Sorbitol ☹ | FrucGalactans ☹ FrucGalactans ☹ 📖 |
|---|---|---|---|---|---|
| Barbeque sauce (BBQ), store bought | pinch 0.04oz/1g | ☺ | ☺ ☺ | ☹ 76¾ | ☺ ☺ |
| Barley flour | portion 1.06oz/30g | ☺ | ☺ ☺ | ☺ ☺ | 6¼ [AD] 12¾ |
| Basil, fresh | pinch 0.04oz/1g | ☺ | ☺ ☺ | ☺ ☺ | ☺ ☺ |
| Basmati rice, cooked in unsalted water | portion 4.94oz/140g | ☺ | ☺ ☺ | ☺ ☺ | ☺ [A] ☺ |
| Beef bacon (kosher) | portion 0.53oz/15g | ☺ | ☺ ☺ | ☺ ☺ | ☺ ☺ |
| Beef gravy, canned | portion 2.05oz/58g | ☺ | ☺ ☺ | ☹ ☺ | ☺ ☺ |
| Beef steak, chuck, visible fat eaten | portion 3oz/85g | ☺ | ☺ ☺ | ☺ ☺ | ☺ ☺ |
| Beef with noodles soup, condensed | portion 4.45oz/126g | ☺ | ☺ ☺ | ☹ 4¼ | 4 [A] 8¼ |
| Beer | glass 8.4ozfl/240ml | ☺ | 50 ☺ | ☹ 10 | ☺ ☺ |
| Beer, low alcohol | glass 8.4ozfl/240ml | ☺ | ☺+ ×2¼ unit ☺+ ×1 unit | ☺ ☺ | ☺ ☺ |
| Beets, raw | portion 3oz/85g | ☺ | 58¾ ☺ | ☹ 3¼ | 1¼ [B] 2½ |
| Ben & Jerry's® Ice Cream, Brownie Batter | portion 3.89oz/110g | ¼ +¼ unit | ☺+ ×3 unit ☺+ ×1½ unit | ☹ ☺ | 1¼ 2¾ |
| Ben & Jerry's® Ice Cream, Chocolate Chip Cookie Dough | portion 3.67oz/104g | ½ +¼ unit | ☺+ ×4¾ unit ☺+ ×2¼ unit | ☺ ☺ | 3¼ 6½ |
| Ben & Jerry's® Ice Cream, Chubby Hubby® | portion 3.78oz/107g | ½ +½ unit | ☺+ ×5 unit ☺+ ×2½ unit | ☺ ☺ | 3½ 7 |
| Ben & Jerry's® Ice Cream, Chunky Monkey® | portion 3.78oz/107g | ¼ +¼ unit | ☺+ ×2¾ unit ☺+ ×1¼ unit | ☹ ☺ | 2½ 5¼ |
| Ben & Jerry's® Ice Cream, Half Baked | portion 3.81oz/108g | ¼ +¼ unit | ☺+ ×2¼ unit ☺+ ×1 unit | ☺ ☺ | 2¼ 4¾ |

☹ *Level 0*: lactose measure ×½   + Unit/ 💊: added tolerated amount of unit per strong lactase capsule
☹ *Level 1*: fructose measure ×2   Fructose*: fructose, sorbitol adjusted
☹ *Level 2*: fructose-/sorbitol measure ×4. the rest ×2   ☺+ ×[Amount] unit: Per unit consumed you can
☹ *Level 3*: sorbitol measure ×7. the rest ×3   additionally tolerate up to [amount] ×
📖: source of fruc/galactans data   fructose(*)-unit of another product.
☹: avoid;   ☹[1]: ¼ at TL 1;   ☹[2]: ¼ at TL 2;   ☹[3]: ¼ at TL 3;   ☺: only contains traces;   ☺: is free from it

| Keyword Index | Unit | Lactose ↓ + unit/🥛 | Fructose* ⚖ Fructose* ↓ | Sorbitol ⚖ Sorbitol ↓ | FrucGalactans ⚖ FrucGalactans ↓ 📖 |
|---|---|---|---|---|---|
| Ben & Jerry's® Ice Cream, Karamel Sutra® | portion 3.74oz/106g | ½ +¼ unit | ☺+ ×4¾ unit ☺+ ×2¼ unit | ☺ ☺ | 3 6¼ |
| Ben & Jerry's® Ice Cream, New York Super Fudge Chunk® | portion 3.74oz/106g | ½ +½ unit | 67¼ ☺ | ☹ ☺ | 3½ 7¼ |
| Ben & Jerry's® Ice Cream, One Sweet Whirled | portion 3.74oz/106g | ½ +¼ unit | ☺+ ×4¾ unit ☺+ ×2¼ unit | ☺ ☺ | 3 6¼ |
| Ben & Jerry's® Ice Cream, Peanut Butter Cup | portion 4.06oz/115g | ½ +¼ unit | ☺+ ×5¼ unit ☺+ ×2½ unit | ☺ ☺ | 3¼ 6½ |
| Ben & Jerry's® Ice Cream, Phish Food® | portion 3.67oz/104g | ¼ +¼ unit | ☺+ ×2¼ unit ☺+ ×1 unit | ☺ ☺ | 2¼ 4¾ |
| Ben & Jerry's® Ice Cream, Vanilla For A Change | portion 3.64oz/103g | ½ +¼ unit | ☺+ ×4½ unit ☺+ ×2¼ unit | ☺ ☺ | 3¼ 6½ |
| Bertolli® Classico Olive Oil | portion 0.46oz/13g | ☺ | ☺ ☺ | ☺ ☺ | ☺ ☺ |
| Biscotti, chocolate, nuts | piece 0.73oz/20.5g | ☺ | ☺ ☺ | ☹ ☺ | 2½ A 5 |
| Black cherry juice | glass 8.4ozfl/240ml | ☺ | ¼ ¾ | ☹ 2½ | ☺ ☺ |
| Black currant juice | glass 8.4ozfl/240ml | ☺ | ☺+ ×1½ unit ☺+ ×¾ unit | ☹ 1½ | ☺ ☺ |
| Black olives | portion 0.53oz/15g | ☺ | ☺ ☺ | ☹ 33¼ | ☺ ☺ |
| Black pepper, ground | pinch 0.04oz/1g | ☺ | ☺ ☺ | ☺ ☺ | ☺ ☺ |
| Black Russian | glass 8.4ozfl/240ml | ☺ | ☺ ☺ | ☹ 8¼ | ☺ ☺ |
| Blackberries, fresh | portion 4.94oz/140g | ☺ | 3¾ 7¾ | ☺ ☺ | 2¼ B 4½ |
| Blackberry juice | glass 8.4ozfl/240ml | ☺ | ¼ ½ | ☺ ☺ | ☺ ☺ |
| Bloody Mary | glass 8.4ozfl/240ml | ☺ | 1¾ 3½ | ☹ ½ | ☺ ☺ |
| Blue cheese | portion 1.06oz/30g | 20 +16½ unit | ☺ ☺ | ☺ ☺ | ☺ ☺ |
| Blueberries, fresh | portion 4.94oz/140g | ☺ | 3¾ 7¾ | ☺ ☺ | ¾ B 1½ |
| Bok choy, raw | portion 3oz/85g | ☺ | ☺+ ×¼ unit ☺ | ☹ 23½ | ☺ B ☺ |

| Keyword Index | Unit | Lactose ¹ + unit/capsule | Fructose* ⁰ / Fructose* ¹ | Sorbitol ⁰ / Sorbitol ¹ | FrucGalactans ⁰ / FrucGalactans ¹ 📖 |
|---|---|---|---|---|---|
| Bologna, beef ring | portion | ☺ | ☺+ ×5¾ unit | ☺ | ☺ |
| | 1.95oz/55g | | ☺+ ×2¾ unit | ☺ | ☺ |
| Bologna, combination of | portion | ☺ | ☺+ ×½ unit | ☺ | ☺ |
| meats, light (reduced fat) | 1.95oz/55g | | ☺+ ×¼ unit | ☺ | ☺ |
| Boston Market® 1/4 white | portion | ☺ | ☺ | ☺ | ☺ |
| rotisserie chicken, with skin | 3oz/85g | | ☺ | ☺ | ☺ |
| Boston Market® roasted | portion | ☺ | ☺ | ☺ | ☺ |
| turkey breast | 3oz/85g | | ☺ | ☺ | ☺ |
| Boston Market® sweet corn | portion | ☺ | ☺+ ×¼ unit | ☹ | ☺ B |
| | 3oz/85g | | ☺+ ×¼ unit | 4 | ☺ |
| Bouillon, unprepared | portion | ☺ | ☺ | ☹ | ☺ |
| | 0.29oz/8g | | ☺ | ☺ | ☺ |
| Bourbon | glass | ☺ | ☺ | ☺ | ☺ |
| | 8.4ozfl/240ml | | ☺ | ☺ | ☺ |
| Boysenberries, fresh | portion | ☺ | 69¼ | ☺ | ☺ |
| | 0.29oz/8g | | ☺ | ☺ | ☺ |
| Brandy | glass | ☺ | ☺ | ☺ | ☺ |
| | 8.4ozfl/240ml | | ☺ | ☺ | ☺ |
| Brandy, flavored | glass | ☺ | ☺+ ×4½ unit | ☹ | ☺ |
| | 8.4ozfl/240ml | | ☺+ ×2½ unit | ¼ | ☺ |
| Bratwurst | portion | ☺ | ☺+ ×¼ unit | ☺ | ☺ |
| | 1.95oz/55g | | ☺ | ☺ | ☺ |
| Bratwurst, beef | portion | ☺ | ☺+ ×1 unit | ☺ | ☺ |
| | 1.95oz/55g | | ☺+ ×½ unit | ☺ | ☺ |
| Bratwurst, light (reduced fat) | portion | ☺ | ☺+ ×2¾ unit | ☺ | ☺ |
| | 1.95oz/55g | | ☺+ ×1¼ unit | ☺ | ☺ |
| Bratwurst, made with beer | portion | ☺ | ☺+ ×¼ unit | ☹ | ☺ |
| | 1.95oz/55g | | ☺ | ☺ | ☺ |
| Bratwurst, made with beer, | portion | ☺ | ☺+ ×½ unit | ☹ | ☺ |
| cheese-filled | 1.95oz/55g | | ☺+ ×¼ unit | ☺ | ☺ |
| Bratwurst, turkey | portion | ☺ | ☺+ ×1½ unit | ☺ | ☺ |
| | 1.95oz/55g | | ☺+ ×¾ unit | ☺ | ☺ |

⁰ *Level 0:* lactose measure ×½
¹ *Level 1:* fructose measure ×2
+ Unit/capsule: added tolerated amount of unit per strong lactase capsule
Fructose*: fructose, sorbitol adjusted

² *Level 2*: fructose-/sorbitol measure ×4. the rest ×2
³ *Level 3:* sorbitol measure ×7. the rest ×3
📖: source of fruc/galactans data
☺+ ×[Amount] unit: Per unit consumed you can additionally tolerate up to [amount] × fructose(*)-unit of another product.

☹: avoid; ☹[1]: ¼ at TL 1; ☹[2]: ¼ at TL 2; ☹[3]: ¼ at TL 3; ☺: only contains traces; ☺: is free from it

| Keyword Index | Unit<br>+ unit/ | Lactose | Fructose*<br>Fructose* | Sorbitol<br>Sorbitol | FrucGalactans<br>FrucGalactans |
|---|---|---|---|---|---|
| Braunschweiger (liver sausage) | portion<br>1.95oz/55g | ☺ | ☺<br>☺ | ☺<br>☺ | ☺<br>☺ |
| Brazil nuts, unsalted | hand<br>1.06oz/30g | ☺ | ☺<br>☺ | ☺<br>☺ | ☺<br>☺ |
| Breath mint, regular | portion<br>0.08oz/2g | ☺ | ☺+ ×¼ unit<br>☺ | ☺<br>☺ | ☺<br>☺ |
| Breath mint, sugar free | portion<br>0.08oz/2g | ☺ | ¼<br>½ | ☹<br>☹³ | ☺<br>☺ |
| Breyers® Ice Cream, Natural Vanilla, Lactose Free | portion<br>2.3oz/65g | 4<br>+3¼ unit | ☺+ ×4¾ unit<br>☺+ ×2¼ unit | ☺<br>☺ | 23¼<br>46½ |
| Breyers® Light! Boosts Immunity Yogurt, all flavors | piece<br>4oz/114g | ½<br>+¼ unit | 28¾<br>57¾ | ☹<br>14¼ | 3<br>6 |
| Breyers® No Sugar Added Ice Cream, Vanilla | tbsp.<br>0.5ozfl/14.21ml | 3¼<br>+2½ unit | ¾<br>1½ | ☹<br>☹² | 18¼<br>36½ |
| Breyers® YoCrunch Light Nonfat Yogurt, with granola | piece<br>6.5oz/185g | ¼<br>+0,24 unit | ☺<br>☺ | ☹<br>6½ | 1½<br>3 |
| Brie cheese | portion<br>1.06oz/30g | 22<br>+18½ unit | ☺<br>☺ | ☺<br>☺ | ☺<br>☺ |
| Broccoflower (green cauliflower), cooked from fresh | portion<br>3oz/85g | ☺ | 1<br>2 | ☺<br>☺ | ☺ᴮ<br>☺ |
| Broccoli, raw | portion<br>3oz/85g | 16¾<br>+14 unit | 3<br>6 | ☺<br>☺ | ½ᴮ<br>1¼ |
| Brown mushrooms (Italian or Crimini mushrooms), raw | tbsp.<br>0.5ozfl/14.21ml | ☺ | ☺+ ×¼ unit<br>☺ | ☹<br>¾ | 12¼ᴮ<br>24½ |
| Brown sugar | tbsp.<br>0.5ozfl/14.21ml | ☺ | ☺<br>☺ | ☺<br>☺ | ☺<br>☺ |
| Brownie, chocolate, fat free | piece<br>1.56oz/44g | 3<br>+2½ unit | 71<br>☺ | ☹<br>☺ | 1ᴬ<br>2¼ |
| Brussels sprouts, cooked from fresh | portion<br>3oz/85g | ☺ | ☺<br>☺ | ☺<br>☺ | 1ᴮ<br>2 |
| Bulgur, home cooked | portion<br>4.94oz/140g | ☺ | ☺<br>☺ | ☺<br>☺ | ☺<br>☺ |
| Burger King® Ranch Crispy Chicken Wrap | piece<br>4.84oz/137g | 5<br>+4¼ unit | ☺<br>☺ | ☹<br>36¼ | ¼ᴬ<br>½ |
| Burger King® Bacon EGG® and Cheese BK Muffin® | piece<br>4.63oz/131g | 11½<br>+9½ unit | ☺+ ×1 unit<br>☺+ ×½ unit | ☺<br>☺ | ¼ᴬ<br>¾ |
| Burger King® barbecue sauce | portion<br>1.1ozfl/31ml | ☺ | ☺+ ×1¼ unit<br>☺+ ×½ unit | ☹<br>2¼ | ☺<br>☺ |
| Burger King® BBQ roasted jalapeno sauce | portion<br>1.1ozfl/31ml | ☺ | ☺+ ×1 unit<br>☺+ ×½ unit | ☹<br>2¾ | ☹<br>☺ |

| Keyword Index | Unit | Lactose ↡ + unit/ 💊 | Fructose* ↡ Fructose* ↡ | Sorbitol ↡ Sorbitol ↡ | FrucGalactans ↡ FrucGalactans ↡ 📖 |
|---|---|---|---|---|---|
| Burger King® BK Big Fish® | piece 8.05oz/228g | ☺ | ☺ | ☹ 21¾ | ☹ A ¼ |
| Burger King® BK Fresh Apple Slices | portion 4.94oz/140g | ☺ | ☹² ☹² | ☹ ☹² | ☺ ☺ |
| Burger King® BLT Salad® with TenderCrisp chicken (no dressing or croutons) | portion 4.94oz/140g | 79¼ +66 unit | 5¾ 11½ | ☹ 3 | ☺ ☺ |
| Burger King® Caesar Salad (no dressing or croutons) | portion 3.53oz/100g | 26½ +22 unit | 1½ 3¼ | ☹ 4¼ | ☺ ☺ |
| Burger King® Cheeseburger | piece 4.27oz/121g | 11½ +9½ unit | 51½ ☺ | ☹ 3¼ | ¼ A ¾ |
| Burger King® French fries | portion 2.47oz/70g | ☺ | ☺ ☺ | ☹ 35½ | ☺ ☺ |
| Burger King® Hamburger | piece 3.85oz/109g | ☺ | 57¼ ☺ | ☹ 3¼ | ½ A 1 |
| Burger King® Ken's® Apple Cider Vinaigrette salad dressing | portion 1.06ozfl/30ml | ☺ | ☺ ☺ | ☺ ☺ | ☺ ☺ |
| Burger King® onion rings | portion 2.47oz/70g | ☺ | ☺+ ×1½ unit ☺+ ×¾ unit | ☹ ¾ | ¼ AC ½ |
| Burger King® Original Chicken Crisp® Sandwich | piece 5.26oz/149g | ☺ | 1½ 3¼ | ☹ 67 | 5¾ A 11½ |
| Burger King® pancakes and syrup | piece 6.6oz/187g | ½ +½ unit | ☺+ ×6 unit ☺+ ×3 unit | ☺ ☺ | ¼ A ½ |
| Burger King® picante taco sauce sauce | portion 1.24ozfl/35ml | ☺ | 2½ 5¼ | ☹ 2¾ | ☺ ☺ |
| Burger King® shake, chocolate | portion 8.15ozfl/231ml | ☹² +0,15 unit | ☺+ ×7¼ unit ☺+ ×3½ unit | ☺ ☺ | ½ 1 |
| Burger King® shake, strawberry | portion 8.08ozfl/229ml | ☹² +0,15 unit | ☺+ ×5¼ unit ☺+ ×2½ unit | ☹ 3¼ | 1 2 |
| Burger King® shake, vanilla or other | portion 8.4ozfl/238ml | ☹² +0,13 unit | ☺+ ×5¾ unit ☺+ ×2¾ unit | ☺ ☺ | ¾ 1¾ |
| Burger King® sundaes®, caramel | portion 4.98ozfl/141ml | ¼ +¼ unit | ☺+ ×8½ unit ☺+ ×4¼ unit | ☺ ☺ | 2 4 |

↡ Level 0: lactose measure ×½   + Unit/ 💊: added tolerated amount of unit per strong lactase capsule
↡ Level 1: fructose measure ×2   Fructose*: fructose, sorbitol adjusted
↡ Level 2: fructose-/sorbitol measure ×4. the rest ×2   ☺+ ×[Amount] unit: Per unit consumed you can additionally tolerate up to [amount] × fructose(*)-unit of another product.
↡ Level 3: sorbitol measure ×7. the rest ×3
📖: source of fruc/galactans data

☹: avoid;   ☹¹: ¼ at TL 1;   ☹²: ¼ at TL 2;   ☹³: ¼ at TL 3;   ☺: only contains traces;   ☺: is free from it

| Keyword Index | Unit | Lactose ↳ + unit/⬤ | Fructose* ↻ Fructose* ↳ | Sorbitol ↻ Sorbitol ↳ | FrucGalactans ↻ FrucGalactans ↳ 📖 |
|---|---|---|---|---|---|
| Burger King® sundaes®, chocolate fudge | portion 4.98ozfl/141ml | ¼ +¼ unit | ☺+ ×6¾ unit ☺+ ×3¼ unit | ☺ ☺ | 1½ 3¼ |
| Burger King® sundaes®, mini M & M's® | portion 7.2ozfl/204ml | ¼ +0,23 unit | ☺+ ×6¾ unit ☺+ ×3¼ unit | ☺ ☺ | 1¼ 2¾ |
| Burger King® sundaes®, Oreo® | portion 7.2ozfl/204ml | ¼ +¼ unit | ☺+ ×7¼ unit ☺+ ×3½ unit | ☹ 49 | 1¾ 3½ |
| Burger King® sundaes®, strawberry | portion 4.98ozfl/141ml | ¼ +¼ unit | ☺+ ×2½ unit ☺+ ×1¼ unit | ☹ 2½ | 2¼ 4¾ |
| Burger King® sweet and sour sauce | portion 1.06ozfl/30ml | ☺ | ¼ ½ | ☹ 41½ | ☺ ☺ |
| Burger King® TenderCrisp® Chicken Sandwich | piece 9.32oz/264g | ☺ | 8 16¼ | ☹ 2½ | ☹ A ¼ |
| Burger King® Whopper® with cheese | piece 11.12oz/315g | 5¾ +4¾ unit | 2¾ 5¾ | ☹ 1 | ☹ A ¼ |
| Burger King® zesty onion ring sauce | portion 1.1ozfl/31ml | ☺ | ☺ ☺ | ☹ 64½ | ☺ ☺ |
| Burgundy wine, red | glass 8.4ozfl/240ml | ☺ | 17¾ 35½ | ☹ ½ | ☺ ☺ |
| Burgundy wine, white | glass 8.4ozfl/240ml | ☺ | 31¼ 62½ | ☹ ¾ | ☺ ☺ |
| Butter cracker | piece 0.15oz/4g | ☺ | ☺ ☺ | ☺ ☺ | 10 A 20 |
| Butter, light, salted | portion 0.5oz/14g | ☺ | ☺ ☺ | ☺ ☺ | ☺ ☺ |
| Butter, unsalted | portion 0.5oz/14g | ☺ | ☺ ☺ | ☺ ☺ | ☺ ☺ |
| Buttermels® (Switzer's®) | piece 0.25oz/6.9g | 8 +6½ unit | ☺+ ×½ unit ☺+ ×¼ unit | ☺ ☺ | 44¾ 89¾ |
| Butternut squash | portion 4.59oz/130g | ☺ | ☺ ☺ | ☺ ☺ | ½ G 1¼ |
| Butternut squash soup | portion 8.65oz/245g | 13½ +11¼ unit | ☺ ☺ | ☹ 2½ | ½ G 1 |
| Cabbage, green, cooked | portion 3oz/85g | ☺ | ☺+ ×¾ unit ☺+ ×¼ unit | ☹ 58¾ | 1¼ B 2½ |
| Cabbage, red, cooked | portion 3oz/85g | ☺ | ☺+ ×¼ unit ☺ | ☺ ☺ | 1¼ B 2½ |
| Cabbage, savoy, raw | portion 3oz/85g | ☺ | ☺ ☺ | ☹ 39 | 1½ B 3 |

| Keyword Index | Unit | Lactose ↯ + unit/ 💊 | Fructose* ☹ Fructose* ↯ | Sorbitol ☹ Sorbitol ↯ | FrucGalactans ☹ FrucGalactans ↯ 📖 |
|---|---|---|---|---|---|
| Cabot® Non Fat Yogurt, plain | piece 8.01oz/227g | ¼ +0,22 unit | ☺ ☺ | ☺ ☺ | 1¼ 2¾ |
| Cabot® Non Fat Yogurt, vanilla | piece 8.01oz/227g | ¼ +¼ unit | 30¼ 60½ | ☹ 13¼ | 2¼ 4½ |
| Cafe au lait, without flavored syrup | cup 5.2ozfl/150ml | 1 +¾ unit | ☺ ☺ | ☺ ☺ | 6½ 13 |
| Cafe latte, with flavored syrup | cup 5.2ozfl/150ml | ½ +¼ unit | ☺ ☺ | ☺ ☺ | 3 6 |
| Cafe latte, without flavored syrup | cup 5.2ozfl/150ml | ¼ +¼ unit | ☺ ☺ | ☺ ☺ | 2¾ 5½ |
| Calzone, cheese | piece 5.93oz/168g | 12¼ +10¼ unit | ☺ ☺ | ☹ 2¾ | ¼ ᴬ ½ |
| Camembert cheese | portion 1.06oz/30g | 21½ +18 unit | ☺ ☺ | ☺ ☺ | ☺ ☺ |
| Camomile tea | glass 8.5ozfl/242ml | ☺ | ☺ ☺ | ☺ ☺ | ½ ᴳ 1¼ |
| Campari® | glass 8.4ozfl/240ml | ☺ | ☺+ ×4½ unit ☺+ ×2½ unit | ☹ ¼ | ☺ ☺ |
| Candy necklace | piece 0.75oz/21g | ☺ | ☺+ ×3¼ unit ☺+ ×1½ unit | ☺ ☺ | ☺ ☺ |
| Cantaloupe, fresh | portion 4.94oz/140g | ☺ | 1 2 | ☹ 14¼ | 2 ᴮ 4¼ |
| Cape Cod | glass 8.4ozfl/240ml | ☺ | ☺+ ×5 unit ☺+ ×2½ unit | ☹ 25 | ☺ ☺ |
| Capers | pinch 0.04oz/1g | ☺ | ☺ ☺ | ☹ 70¼ | ☺ ☺ |
| Cappuccino, bottled or canned | cup 5.2ozfl/150ml | ½ +½ unit | ☺ ☺ | ☺ ☺ | 4 8 |
| Cappuccino, decaf, with flavored syrup | cup 5.2ozfl/150ml | ½ +¼ unit | ☺ ☺ | ☺ ☺ | 3 6¼ |
| Cappuccino, decaf, without flavored syrup | cup 5.2ozfl/150ml | ½ +¼ unit | ☺ ☺ | ☺ ☺ | 2¾ 5¾ |
| Capri Sun®, all flavors | glass 8.4ozfl/240ml | ☺ | ☺+ ×1 unit ☺+ ×½ unit | ☹ 2 | ☺ ☺ |

☹ *Level 0*: lactose measure ×½  + Unit/ 💊: added tolerated amount of unit per strong lactase capsule
↯ *Level 1*: fructose measure ×2  Fructose*: fructose, sorbitol adjusted
↯ *Level 2*: fructose-/sorbitol measure ×4. the rest ×2  ☺+ ×[Amount] unit: Per unit consumed you can
↯ *Level 3*: sorbitol measure ×7. the rest ×3  additionally tolerate up to [amount] ×
📖: source of fruc/galactans data  fructose(*)-unit of another product.

☹: avoid;  ☹¹: ¼ at TL 1;  ☹²: ¼ at TL 2;  ☹³: ¼ at TL 3;  ☺: only contains traces;  ☺: is free from it

| KEYWORD INDEX | Unit | Lactose ↯ +unit/ 🥛 | Fructose* ♀↯ Fructose* ↯ | Sorbitol ♀↯ Sorbitol ↯ | FrucGalactans ♀↯ FrucGalactans ↯ 📖 |
|---|---|---|---|---|---|
| Carambola (starfruit), fresh | piece 3.21oz/91g | ☺ | ☺+ ×¼ unit ☺ | ☹ 1¼ | ☺ ☺ |
| Caramel or sugar coated popcorn, store bought | hand 0.75oz/21g | ☺ | ☺+ ×1 unit ☺+ ×½ unit | ☺ ☺ | ☺ C ☺ |
| Caramel sauce, store bought, fat free | portion 1.45oz/41g | 6 +5 unit | ☺+ ×6 unit ☺+ ×3 unit | ☺ ☺ | 33¾ 67¾ |
| Carrot cake, glazed, homemade | piece 0.98oz/27.72g | ☺ | ☺+ ×¼ unit ☺ | ☹ 8 | 2 A 4 |
| Carrot juice | glass 8.4ozfl/240ml | ☺ | ☺+ ×1 unit ☺+ ×½ unit | ☹ 4 | ☺ B ☺ |
| Carrots, cooked from fresh | portion 3oz/85g | ☺ | ☺ ☺ | ☹ ½ | ☺ B ☺ |
| Carrots, raw | piece 2.16oz/61g | ☺ | ☺ ☺ | ☹ ¾ | ☺ B ☺ |
| Cascadian Farm® Organic Chewy Granola Bar, Trail Mix Dark Chocolate Cranberry | piece 1.24oz/35g | ☺ | ☺+ ×4¼ unit ☺+ ×2 unit | ☹ 71¼ | ½ A 1 |
| Cashews, raw | hand 1.06oz/30g | ☺ | ☺ ☺ | ☺ ☺ | ¼ G ¾ |
| Casserole (hot dish), chicken with pasta, cream or white sauce, with cheese | portion 8.4oz/238g | ½ +½ unit | ☺ ☺ | ☺ ☺ | ☺ ☺ |
| Casserole, pasta with turkey, gravy base, vegetables other than dark green, with cheese | portion 8.05oz/228g | 3¾ +3 unit | ☺ ☺ | ☹ 1¼ | ½ A 1 |
| Casserole, rice with beef, tomato base, vegetables other than dark green, with cheese | portion 8.61oz/244g | 9¾ +8¼ unit | ☺+ ×1 unit ☺+ ×½ unit | ☹ ¼ | ¼ A ¾ |
| Cauliflower, cooked from frozen | portion 3oz/85g | ☺ | ☺ ☺ | ☹ 2½ | ☺ CB ☺ |
| Caviar | tbsp. 0.5ozfl/14.21ml | ☺ | ☺ ☺ | ☺ ☺ | ☺ ☺ |
| Celeriac (celery root), cooked from fresh | tbsp. 0.5ozfl/14.21ml | ☺ | 13¼ 26½ | ☹ ¾ | ☺ ☺ |
| Celery, cooked | tbsp. 0.5ozfl/14.21ml | ☺ | ☺ ☺ | ☹ 1 | ☺ C ☺ |
| Champagne punch | glass 8.4ozfl/240ml | ☺ | ¾ 1½ | ☹ 1 | ☺ ☺ |
| Champagne, white | glass 8.4ozfl/240ml | ☺ | 31¼ 62½ | ☹ ¼ | ☺ ☺ |

| Keyword Index | Unit | Lactose + unit/💊 | Fructose* / Fructose* + unit | Sorbitol / Sorbitol | FrucGalactans / FrucGalactans 📖 |
|---|---|---|---|---|---|
| Chard, raw or blanched, marinated in oil | portion 3oz/85g | ☺ | ☺+ ×½ unit<br>☺+ ×¼ unit | ☺<br>☺ | ☺<br>☺ |
| Chardonnay | glass 8.4ozfl/240ml | ☺ | 31¼<br>62½ | ☹<br>¾ | ☺<br>☺ |
| Chayote squash, cooked | portion 4.59oz/130g | ☺ | 6¼<br>12¾ | ☺<br>☺ | ☺ B<br>☺ |
| Cheddar cheese, natural | portion 1.06oz/30g | 43¼<br>+36 unit | ☺<br>☺ | ☺<br>☺ | ☺<br>☺ |
| Cheese cracker | piece 0.11oz/3g | ☺ | ☺<br>☺ | ☺<br>☺ | 3½ A<br>7 |
| Cheese gnocchi | portion 2.47oz/70g | 28<br>+23¼ unit | ☺<br>☺ | ☺<br>☺ | 1 A<br>2¼ |
| Cheese sauce, store bought | portion 2.33oz/66g | ¼<br>+¼ unit | ☺<br>☺ | ☺<br>☺ | 1¾<br>3¾ |
| Cheesecake, plain or flavored, graham cracker crust, homemade | piece 7.77oz/220g | ½<br>+½ unit | ☺+ ×½ unit<br>☺+ ×¼ unit | ☺<br>☺ | ☹ A<br>¼ |
| Cherry Coke® | glass 8.4ozfl/240ml | ☺ | ½<br>1¼ | ☺<br>☺ | ☺<br>☺ |
| Cherry pie, bottom crust only | piece 4.31oz/122g | ☺ | 1<br>2¼ | ☹<br>☹2 | ¼ A<br>¾ |
| Chestnuts, boiled, steamed | portion 1.06oz/30g | ☺ | ☺<br>☺ | ☹<br>6 | ☺<br>☺ |
| Chestnuts, roasted | portion 1.06oz/30g | ☺ | ☺<br>☺ | ☹<br>3 | ☺<br>☺ |
| Chewing gum | piece 0.11oz/3g | ☺ | ☺<br>☺ | ☺<br>☺ | ☺<br>☺ |
| Chewing gum, sugar free | piece 0.08oz/2g | ☺ | ¼<br>¾ | ☹<br>☹2 | ☺<br>☺ |
| Chia seeds | hand 1.06oz/30g | ☺ | ☺<br>☺ | ☺<br>☺ | 1¼ G<br>2¾ |
| Chicken and dumplings soup, condensed | portion 4.45oz/126g | 7¼<br>+6 unit | ☺<br>☺ | ☹<br>2¼ | 2¼<br>4½ |

♀ *Level 0*: lactose measure ×½    + Unit/💊: added tolerated amount of unit per strong lactase capsule
♀ *Level 1*: fructose measure ×2    Fructose*: fructose, sorbitol adjusted
♀ *Level 2*: fructose-/sorbitol measure ×4. the rest ×2    ☺+ ×[Amount] unit: Per unit consumed you can
♀ *Level 3*: sorbitol measure ×7. the rest ×3    additionally tolerate up to [amount] ×
📖: source of fruc/galactans data    fructose(*)-unit of another product.

☹: avoid;    ☹¹: ¼ at TL 1;    ☹²: ¼ at TL 2;    ☹³: ¼ at TL 3;    ☺: only contains traces;    ☺: is free from it

| Keyword Index | Unit | Lactose ↓ + unit/ ⊙ | Fructose* ⊙ Fructose* ↓ | Sorbitol ⊙ Sorbitol ↓ | FrucGalactans ⊙ FrucGalactans ↓ |
|---|---|---|---|---|---|
| Chicken cake or patty | portion 3oz/85g | 1½ +1¼ unit | 14 28 | ☹ 58¾ | 3¼ [B] 6½ |
| Chicken fricassee with gravy, American style | portion 8.61oz/244g | ☺ | ☺ ☺ | ☺ ☺ | 5¾ [C] 11½ |
| Chicken noodle soup with vegetables, ready-to-serve can | portion 8.65oz/245g | ☺ | ☺ ☺ | ☹ 1 | 1¼ 2½ |
| Chicken with cheese sauce, vegetables other than dark green | portion 7.62oz/216g | 1 +¾ unit | 5 10 | ☹ ½ | ☺ ☺ |
| Chicken wonton soup, prepared from condensed can | portion 8.65oz/245g | ☺ | ☺ ☺ | ☹ 40¾ | ☺ ☺ |
| Chicory coffee | cup 5.2ozfl/150ml | ☺ | ☺ ☺ | ☹ 11 | ☹ [E] ☹ |
| Chicory coffee powder, unprepared | portion 0.08oz/2g | ☺ | ☺ ☺ | ☹ 8¾ | ½ [E] 1 |
| Chicory greens, raw | portion 3oz/85g | ☺ | 5¼ 10½ | ☹ 39 | 2¼ [B] 4½ |
| Chili sauce, store bought | portion 2.4oz/68g | ☺ | 2¾ 5½ | ☹ ¼ | ☺ ☺ |
| Chili with beans, beef, canned | tbsp. 0.5oz.fl/14.8ml | ☺ | ☺ ☺ | ☹ 55½ | 3 [AC] 6 |
| Chinese oyster sauce | portion 1.13oz/32g | ☺ | ☺ ☺ | ☺ ☺ | ☺ ☺ |
| Chips Ahoy!® Chewy Gooey Caramel Cookies (Nabisco®) | piece 0.55oz/15.5g | 12¼ +10¼ unit | ½ 1 | ☹ ☺ | 3 [A] 6¼ |
| Chives, raw | pinch 0.04oz/1g | ☺ | ☺ ☺ | ☺ ☺ | ☺ [B] ☺ |
| Chobani® Nonfat Greek Yogurt, Black Cherry | tbsp. 0.5ozfl/14.21ml | 5¼ +4½ unit | ☺ ☺ | ☹ 3¾ | 30¼ 60¾ |
| Chobani® Nonfat Greek Yogurt, Lemon | piece 6.04oz/171g | ½ +¼ unit | ☺+ ×½ unit ☺+ ×¼ unit | ☺ ☺ | 3 6 |
| Chobani® Nonfat Greek Yogurt, Peach | piece 6.04oz/171g | ¼ +¼ unit | ☺+ ×1 unit ☺+ ×½ unit | ☹ 4¼ | 1¾ 3½ |
| Chobani® Nonfat Greek Yogurt, Raspberry | piece 6.04oz/171g | ¼ +¼ unit | ☺+ ×¾ unit ☺+ ×¼ unit | ☹ 20 | 1¾ 3½ |
| Chobani® Nonfat Greek Yogurt, Strawberry | piece 6.04oz/171g | ¼ +¼ unit | ☺+ ×¾ unit ☺+ ×¼ unit | ☹ 3½ | 1¾ 3½ |
| Chocolate cake, glazed, store bought | piece 1.03oz/29g | ☺ | ☺+ ×½ unit ☺+ ×¼ unit | ☹ ☺ | 1¾ [A] 3¾ |

| Keyword Index | Unit | Lactose ↳ + unit/🥛 | Fructose* ↳ Fructose* ↳ | Sorbitol ↳ Sorbitol ↳ | FrucGalactans ↳ FrucGalactans ↳📖 |
|---|---|---|---|---|---|
| Chocolate Chex® (General Mills®) | tbsp. 0.5ozfl/14.21ml | ☺ | ¼ ½ | ☹ ☺ | 1¼ A 2¾ |
| Chocolate chip cookies, store bought | piece 0.36oz/10g | ☺ | ☺ ☺ | ☹ ☺ | 2½ A 5¼ |
| Chocolate cookies, iced, store bought | piece 0.36oz/10g | ☺ | ☺ ☺ | ☹ ☺ | 5 A 10¼ |
| Chocolate pudding, store bought | piece 3.5oz/98g | ¾ +½ unit | ☺ ☺ | ☹ 25 | 1 G 2¼ |
| Chocolate pudding, store bought, sugar free | tbsp. 0.5ozfl/14.21ml | 89¼ +74¼ unit | ¾ 1½ | ☹ ☹² | 21¼ G 42½ |
| Chocolate sandwich cookies, double filling | piece 0.52oz/14.5g | ☺ | ☺ ☺ | ☹ ☺ | 3½ A 7 |
| Chocolate sandwich cookies, sugar free | piece 0.43oz/12g | ☺ | 13¾ 27¾ | ☹ ☹ | 4¼ A 8½ |
| Chocolate sauce, syrup | tbsp. 0.5ozfl/14.21ml | ☺ | ☺+ ×1½ unit ☺+ ×¾ unit | ☹ ☺ | 3 G 6 |
| Chocolate truffles | piece 0.58oz/16.2g | 2½ +2 unit | ☺ ☺ | ☺ ☺ | 2¾ 5½ |
| Chop suey, chicken, no noodles | portion 5.86oz/166g | ☺ | ☺ ☺ | ☹ ¼ | ¼ AB ¾ |
| Chop suey, tofu, no noodles | portion 5.86oz/166g | ☺ | ☺ ☺ | ☹ ¼ | ☺ ☺ |
| Cider vinegar | portion 0.5oz/14g | ☺ | 6¼ 12½ | ☹ 1¾ | ☺ ☺ |
| Cilantro leaf, fresh | pinch 0.04oz/1g | ☺ | ☺ ☺ | ☺ ☺ | ☺ ☺ |
| Cinnamon Roll with Icing, all flavours | piece 1.56oz/44g | 9 +7½ unit | ☺+ ×8¼ unit ☺+ ×4 unit | ☺ ☺ | 1 A 2¼ |
| Cinnamon toast crunch® (General Mills®) | portion 1.06oz/30g | ☺ | ¼ ½ | ☺ ☺ | 1½ A 3 |
| Cinnamon Toasters® (Malt-O-Meal®) | portion 1.06oz/30g | ☺ | 2 4¼ | ☺ ☺ | 1½ A 3 |
| Clams, stuffed with mushroom, onions, and bread | portion 4.94oz/140g | 24½ +20½ unit | ☺ ☺ | ☹ ½ | 3¼ CB 6¾ |

↳ *Level 0*: lactose measure ×½  + Unit/🥛: added tolerated amount of unit per strong lactase capsule
↳ *Level 1*: fructose measure ×2  Fructose*: fructose, sorbitol adjusted
↳ *Level 2*: fructose-/sorbitol measure ×4. the rest ×2  ☺+ ×[Amount] unit: Per unit consumed you can
↳ *Level 3*: sorbitol measure ×7. the rest ×3  additionally tolerate up to [amount] ×
📖: source of fruc/galactans data  fructose(*)-unit of another product.

☹: avoid;   ☹¹: ¼ at TL 1;   ☹²: ¼ at TL 2;   ☹³: ¼ at TL 3;   ☺: only contains traces;   ☺: is free from it

| Keyword Index | Unit | Lactose ☻ + unit/☹ | Fructose* ☻ Fructose* ☻ | Sorbitol ☻ Sorbitol ☻ | FrucGalactans ☻ FrucGalactans ☻ |
|---|---|---|---|---|---|
| Classic Fruit Chocolates (Liberty Orchards®) | piece 0.53oz/15g | 56½ +47 unit | ☻+ ×¼ unit ☻ | ☹ 31½ | 5½ G 11¼ |
| Clementine, fresh | portion 4.94oz/140g | ☻ | 7 14¼ | ☻ ☻ | 2¼ B 4½ |
| Clif Bar®, Chocolate Chip | piece 2.4oz/68g | 9 +7½ unit | ☻+ ×10 unit ☻+ ×5 unit | ☹ 2¼ | ¾ 1½ |
| Clif Bar®, Crunchy Peanut Butter | piece 2.4oz/68g | ☻ | ☻+ ×10¼ unit ☻+ ×5 unit | ☹ 2½ | ☻ ☻ |
| Clif Bar®, Oatmeal Raisin Walnut | piece 2.4oz/68g | ☻ | ☻+ ×10¼ unit ☻+ ×5¼ unit | ☹ 1¾ | 1¾ AG 3½ |
| Club soda | glass 8.4ozfl/240ml | ☻ | ☻ ☻ | ☻ ☻ | ☻ ☻ |
| Cocktail sauce | portion 2.4oz/68g | ☻ | ☻+ ×2 unit ☻+ ×1 unit | ☹ ¾ | ☻ ☻ |
| Cocoa Krispies® (Kellogg's®) | portion 1.06oz/30g | ☻ | ☻ ☻ | ☹ ☻ | 1½ A 3 |
| Cocoa Puffs® (General Mills®) | portion 1.06oz/30g | ☻ | ☻+ ×2 unit ☻+ ×1 unit | ☹ ☻ | ½ A 1¼ |
| Coconut bars, nuts | piece 1.49oz/42g | 45¼ +37¾ unit | ☻ ☻ | ☻ ☻ | ☻ ☻ |
| Coconut cream (liquid from grated meat) | hand 1.06oz/30g | ☻ | 20¾ 41½ | ☻ ☻ | ☻ ☻ |
| Coconut milk, fresh (liquid from grated meat, water added) | glass 8.4oz/240g | ☻ | ☻+ ×1 unit ☻+ ×½ unit | ☻ ☻ | 1¾ G 3½ |
| Coconut oil | pinch 0.04oz/1g | ☻ | ☻ ☻ | ☻ ☻ | ☻ ☻ |
| Coconut, dried, shredded or flaked, unsweetened | hand 1.06oz/30g | ☻ | ☻+ ×¾ unit ☻+ ×¼ unit | ☻ ☻ | 12¼ 24½ |
| Coconut, fresh | portion 0.53oz/15g | ☻ | ☻+ ×¼ unit ☻ | ☻ ☻ | 24½ G 49 |
| Coffee substitute, prepared | cup 5.2ozfl/150ml | ☻ | ☻ ☻ | ☻ ☻ | ☻ ☻ |
| Coffee, prepared from flavored mix, sugar free | cup 5.2ozfl/150ml | ☻ | ☻ ☻ | ☹ 66½ | ☻ ☻ |
| Cognac | glass 8.4ozfl/240ml | ☻ | ☻ ☻ | ☻ ☻ | ☻ ☻ |
| Cointreau® | glass 8.4ozfl/240ml | ☻ | ☻+ ×4½ unit ☻+ ×2½ unit | ☹ ¼ | ☻ ☻ |
| Coke Zero® | glass 8.4ozfl/240ml | ☹ | ☹ ☻ | ☹ ☻ | ☹ ☻ |

| Keyword Index | Unit | Lactose ☹ + unit/ 💊 | Fructose* ☹ Fructose* ☹ | Sorbitol ☹ Sorbitol ☹ | FrucGalactans ☹ FrucGalactans ☹ 📖 |
|---|---|---|---|---|---|
| Coke® | glass 8.4ozfl/240ml | ☺ | ½ 1¼ | ☺ ☺ | ☺ ☺ |
| Coke® with Lime | glass 8.4ozfl/240ml | ☺ | ½ 1¼ | ☺ ☺ | ☺ ☺ |
| Colby Jack cheese | portion 1.06oz/30g | 27¼ +22¾ unit | ☺ ☺ | ☺ ☺ | ☺ ☺ |
| Coleslaw, with apples and raisins, mayo dressing | portion 3.53oz/100g | ☺ | ½ 1 | ☹ ½ | 1 B 2 |
| Coleslaw, with pineapple, mayo dressing | portion 3.53oz/100g | ☺ | ☺+ ×¼ unit ☺ | ☹ 3¾ | ☺ B ☺ |
| Collards, raw | portion 3oz/85g | ☺ | ☺ ☺ | ☺ ☺ | 1¼ B 2½ |
| Corn Chex® (General Mills®) | portion 1.06oz/30g | ☺ | ☺ ☺ | ☹ ☺ | ½ A 1¼ |
| Corn Flakes (Kellogg's®) | portion 1.06oz/30g | ☺ | ☺+ ×1½ unit ☺+ ×¾ unit | ☹ ☺ | 1½ A 3 |
| Cottage cheese, 1% fat, lactose reduced | portion 3.89oz/110g | 3¼ +2¾ unit | ☺+ ×1¾ unit ☺+ ×¾ unit | ☺ ☺ | 18¾ 37¾ |
| Cottage cheese, uncreamed dry curd | portion 1.95oz/55g | 3½ +2¾ unit | ☺ ☺ | ☺ ☺ | 19¾ 39½ |
| Couscous, cooked | portion 4.94oz/140g | ☺ | ☺ ☺ | ☺ ☺ | ¼ A ¾ |
| Cracked wheat bread, with raisins | slice 1.49oz/42g | ☺ | 1¼ 2¾ | ☹ 4¼ | 1¾ A 3½ |
| Cranberries, dried (Craisins®) | portion 1.42oz/40g | ☺ | ☺+ ×3¼ unit ☺+ ×1½ unit | ☹ 41½ | ☺ ☺ |
| Cranberries, fresh | portion 1.95oz/55g | ☺ | ☺+ ×2¾ unit ☺+ ×1¼ unit | ☹ 45¼ | ☺ ☺ |
| Cranberry juice cocktail, with apple juice | glass 8.4ozfl/240ml | ☺ | ☹¹ ¼ | ☹ ☹² | 1½ CB 3 |
| Cranberry juice cocktail, with blueberry juice | glass 8.4ozfl/240ml | ☺ | ☹¹ ¼ | ☹ ☹² | ☺ ☺ |
| Cream cheese spread | portion 1.06oz/30g | 2¾ +2¼ unit | ☺ ☺ | ☺ ☺ | 15¾ 31½ |

☹ *Level 0*: lactose measure ×½  
☹ *Level 1*: fructose measure ×2  
☹ *Level 2*: fructose-/sorbitol measure ×4. the rest ×2  
☹ *Level 3*: sorbitol measure ×7. the rest ×3  
📖: source of fruc/galactans data  

+ Unit/ 💊: added tolerated amount of unit per strong lactase capsule  
Fructose*: fructose, sorbitol adjusted  
☺+ ×[Amount] unit: Per unit consumed you can additionally tolerate up to [amount] × fructose(*)-unit of another product.  

☹: avoid;   ☹¹: ¼ at TL 1;   ☹²: ¼ at TL 2;   ☹³: ¼ at TL 3;   ☺: only contains traces;   ☺: is free from it

| Keyword Index | Unit + unit/🥄 | Lactose 🥛 | Fructose* 😊 Fructose* 🥛 | Sorbitol 😊 Sorbitol 🥛 | FrucGalactans 😊 FrucGalactans 🥛 📖 |
|---|---|---|---|---|---|
| Cream cheese, whipped, flavored | portion 1.06oz/30g | 2½ +2 unit | 😊 😊 | 😊 😊 | 14 28 |
| Cream cheese, whipped, plain | portion 1.06oz/30g | 3 +2½ unit | 😊 😊 | 😊 😊 | 17¼ 34½ |
| Cream of asparagus soup, prepared from condensed can | tbsp. 0.5ozfl/14.21ml | 6½ +5½ unit | 😊 😊 | ☹ 😊 | 1½ 3 |
| Cream of broccoli soup, condensed | portion 4.45oz/126g | 5 +4¼ unit | 😊 😊 | ☹ 19¾ | 1 ᶜ 2¼ |
| Cream of celery soup, homemade | portion 8.65oz/245g | ½ +½ unit | 😊 😊 | ☹ ¼ | ¼ ½ |
| Cream of chicken soup, condensed | portion 4.45oz/126g | 6½ +5½ unit | 😊 😊 | ☹ 26¼ | 37¼ ᶜᴮ 74¾ |
| Cream of mushroom soup, prepared from condensed can | portion 8.65oz/245g | 8½ +7 unit | 😊 😊 | ☹ ¼ | ½ 1 |
| Cream of potato soup mix, dry | portion 0.82oz/23g | 3¼ +2¾ unit | 😊 😊 | ☹ 3 | 5 10 |
| Cream of spinach soup mix, dry | portion 0.57oz/16g | 😊 | 😊+ ×¼ unit 😊 | ☹ 18¼ | 3¼ 6¾ |
| Creamed chicken | portion 8.51oz/241g | ½ +¼ unit | 😊 😊 | ☹ 13¾ | 😊 😊 |
| Creme de Cocoa | glass 8.4ozfl/240ml | 😊 | 😊 😊 | ☹ 2½ | 😊 😊 |
| Creme de menthe | glass 8.4ozfl/240ml | 😊 | 😊+ ×4½ unit 😊+ ×2½ unit | ☹ ¼ | 😊 😊 |
| Crepe, plain | piece 1.95oz/55g | 1¼ +1 unit | 😊 😊 | 😊 😊 | ¾ ᴬ 1¾ |
| Crisco® Pure Corn Oil | portion 0.46oz/13g | 😊 | 😊 😊 | 😊 😊 | 😊 😊 |
| Croissant, chocolate | piece 2.44oz/69g | 3½ +3 unit | 😊+ ×1 unit 😊+ ×½ unit | ☹ 😊 | ¾ ᴬ 1½ |
| Croissant, fruit | piece 2.62oz/74g | 3½ +3 unit | 😊+ ×2½ unit 😊+ ×1¼ unit | ☹ 2 | ½ ᴬ 1¼ |
| Crunchy Nut Roasted Nut & Honey (Kellogg's®) | portion 1.06oz/30g | 😊 | 23¾ 47½ | ☹ 15 | 1½ ᴬ 3 |
| Cucumber, raw, with peel | portion 3oz/85g | 😊 | 5¼ 10½ | ☹ 1 | 😊 ᴮ 😊 |
| Cucumber, raw, without peel | portion 3oz/85g | 😊 | 4¾ 9¾ | ☹ 1 | 😊 ᴮ 😊 |
| Curacao | glass 8.4ozfl/240ml | 😊 | 😊+ ×4½ unit 😊+ ×2½ unit | ☹ ¼ | 😊 😊 |

| Keyword Index | Unit + unit/🥛 | Lactose ᴸ | Fructose* ⁰ᶠ Fructose* ᶠ | Sorbitol ⁰ˢ Sorbitol ˢ | FrucGalactans ⁰ᶠᵍ FrucGalactans ᶠᵍ 📖 |
|---|---|---|---|---|---|
| Currants, fresh, black | portion 4.94oz/140g | ☺ | 1¼ 2½ | ☺ ☺ | ☺ ☺ |
| Currants, fresh, red and white | portion 4.94oz/140g | ☺ | 1 2¼ | ☺ ☺ | ☺ ☺ |
| Curry sauce, from cream | portion 2.09oz/59g | 2 +1½ unit | ☺ ☺ | ☹ 4 | 11¼ 22½ |
| Daiquiri | glass 8.4ozfl/240ml | ☺ | ☺ ☺ | ☺ ☺ | ☺ ☺ |
| Dairy Queen® Foot Long Hot Dog | piece 7.02oz/199g | ☺ | ☺+ ×1¾ unit ☺+ ×¾ unit | ☹ 8¼ | ¼ ᴬ ½ |
| Danish pastry, frosted or glazed, with cheese filling | piece 4.41oz/125g | 3 +2½ unit | ☺ ☺ | ☺ ☺ | ¼ ᴰ ½ |
| Danone® Activia® Light Yogurt, vanilla | piece 4oz/115g | ¼ +¼ unit | ¼ ¾ | ☺ ☺ | 2 4 |
| Danone® Activia® Yogurt, plain | piece 4oz/115g | ½ +¼ unit | ☺ ☺ | ☺ ☺ | 2¾ 5½ |
| Danone® Greek Yogurt, Honey | piece 5.3oz/150g | ½ +¼ unit | ¼ ½ | ☺ 3¼ | 2¾ 5¾ |
| Danone® Greek Yogurt, Plain | piece 5.3oz/150g | ½ +¼ unit | ☺ ☺ | ☺ ☺ | 1¼ 2½ |
| Danone® la Crème Yogurt, fruit flavors | piece 4oz/115g | ¼ +¼ unit | ¼ ½ | ☹ 10¾ | 2 4 |
| Dare Breaktime Ginger Cookies | piece 0.27oz/7.5g | ☺ | ☺ ☺ | ☺ ☺ | 8½ ᴬ 17¼ |
| Dare® Lemon Crème Cookies | piece 0.69oz/19.5g | 32½ +27 unit | ☺ ☺ | ☺ ☺ | 2½ ᴬ 5¼ |
| Dark chocolate bar 45%-59% cacoa | bar 4.77oz/135g | 1¼ +1 unit | ☺ ☺ | ☹ 8 | ¼ ¾ |
| Dark chocolate bar 60%-69% cacao | bar 4.77oz/135g | 7½ +6¼ unit | ☺ ☺ | ☹ 6½ | ¼ ¾ |
| Dark chocolate bar 70%-85% cacao | bar 4.77oz/135g | ☺ | ☺ ☺ | ☹ 5 | ¼ ¾ |
| Dark chocolate bar, sugar free | piece 0.43ozfl/12g | 26¾ +22¼ unit | 34 68¼ | ☹ ☹ | 4¼ 8¾ |

⁰ᶠ *Level 0*: lactose measure ×½
ᶠ *Level 1*: fructose measure ×2
²ᶠ *Level 2*: fructose-/sorbitol measure ×4. the rest ×2
³ᶠ *Level 3*: sorbitol measure ×7. the rest ×3
📖: source of fruc/galactans data
☹: avoid;   ☹¹: ¼ at TL 1;   ☹²: ¼ at TL 2;   ☹³: ¼ at TL 3;   ☺: only contains traces;   ☺: is free from it

+ Unit/🥛: added tolerated amount of unit per strong lactase capsule
Fructose*: fructose, sorbitol adjusted
☺+ ×[Amount] unit: Per unit consumed you can additionally tolerate up to [amount] × fructose(*)-unit of another product.

LAXIBA   The Nutrition Navigator

| Keyword Index | Unit | Lactose ⌘ + unit/ | Fructose* ⌘ Fructose* ⌘ | Sorbitol ⌘ Sorbitol ⌘ | FrucGalactans ⌘ FrucGalactans ⌘ |
|---|---|---|---|---|---|
| Dark Fruit Chocolates (Liberty Orchards®) | piece 0.53oz/15g | 56½ +47 unit | ☺+ ×¼ unit ☺ | ☹ 31½ | 5½ G 11¼ |
| Dark Fruit Chocolates, Sugar Free (Liberty Orchards®) | piece 0.6oz/17g | 37¾ +31¼ unit | ☹² ☹² | ☹ ☹ | 4¾ G 9¾ |
| Dates | portion 1.42oz/40g | ☺ | ☺ ☺ | ☺ ☺ | ☺ ☺ |
| Demitasse | cup 5.2ozfl/150ml | ☺ | ☺ ☺ | ☺ ☺ | ☺ ☺ |
| Diet 7 UP® | glass 8.4ozfl/240ml | ☺ | ☺ ☺ | ☺ ☺ | ☺ ☺ |
| Diet Coke® | glass 8.4ozfl/240ml | ☺ | ☺ ☺ | ☺ ☺ | ☺ ☺ |
| Diet Dr. Pepper® | glass 8.4ozfl/240ml | ☺ | ☺ ☺ | ☺ ☺ | ☺ ☺ |
| Diet Pepsi®, fountain | glass 8.4ozfl/240ml | ☺ | ☺ ☺ | ☺ ☺ | ☺ ☺ |
| Dijon mustard | tbsp. 0.5ozfl/14.21ml | ☺ | ☺ ☺ | ☹ ☺ | ☺ ☺ |
| Distilled vinegar | portion 0.5oz/14g | ☺ | ☺ ☺ | ☺ ☺ | ☺ ☺ |
| Doritos® Tortilla Chips, Nacho Cheese | hand 0.75oz/21g | ☺ | ☺ ☺ | ☹ ☺ | 10¾ A 21½ |
| Doughnut, raised, glazed, coconut topping | piece 2.79oz/79g | 4¾ +4 unit | ☺ ☺ | ☺ ☺ | ½ A 1¼ |
| Doughnut, raised, glazed, plain | piece 2.72oz/77g | 4¾ +4 unit | ☺ ☺ | ☺ ☺ | ½ A 1¼ |
| Doughnut, raised, sugared | piece 2.56oz/72.5g | 4¾ +4 unit | ☺ ☺ | ☺ ☺ | ¾ A 1½ |
| Dove® Promises, Milk Chocolate | cup 5.2ozfl/150ml | ¼ +0.21 unit | ☺ ☺ | ☹ ☺ | 1¾ 3¾ |
| Dreyer's® Grand Ice Cream, Chocolate | portion 2.3oz/65g | 1 +1 unit | ☺+ ×¾ unit ☺+ ×¼ unit | ☹ ☺ | 2¾ G 5¾ |
| Dreyer's® No Sugar Added Ice Cream, Triple Chocolate | tsp. 0.16ozfl/4.74ml | 11½ +9½ unit | ¾ 1¾ | ☹ ☹² | 32¾ G 65½ |
| Drumstick® (sundae cone) | piece 3.39oz/96g | 1 +¾ unit | ☺+ ×2¼ unit ☺+ ×1 unit | ☹ ☺ | 6¼ 12¾ |
| Earl Grey, strong | glass 8.4ozfl/240ml | ☺ | ½ 1¼ | ☺ ☺ | 1½ G 3 |
| Edam cheese | portion 1.06oz/30g | 6¾ +5¾ unit | ☹ ☺ | ☹ ☺ | 78¾ 77½ |

| KEYWORD INDEX | Unit | Lactose ☹/ Unit + unit/ 🗩 | Fructose* ☹/ Fructose* ☹ | Sorbitol ☹/ Sorbitol ☹ | FrucGalactans ☹/ FrucGalactans ☹ 📖 |
|---|---|---|---|---|---|
| EGG* bread roll | piece 1.24oz/35g | 5¼ +4¼ unit | ☺ ☺ | ☺ ☺ | 1½ A 3 |
| Eggplant, cooked | portion 3oz/85g | ☺ | 3½ 7¼ | ☹ 2½ | ☺ B ☺ |
| Elderberries, fresh | portion 4.94oz/140g | ☺ | ¼ ½ | ☺ ☺ | ☺ ☺ |
| Electrolyte replacement drink | glass 8.4oz/240g | ☺ | ☺+ ×9¾ unit ☺+ ×4¾ unit | ☺ ☺ | ☺ ☺ |
| Elephant ear (crispy) | piece 2.09oz/59g | 4¼ +3½ unit | ☺ ☺ | ☺ ☺ | 1 A 2 |
| Endive, curly, raw | portion 3oz/85g | ☺ | ☺ ☺ | ☹ 3 | 3¾ C 7½ |
| English muffin bread | slice 1.49oz/42g | ☺ | 38¼ 76¾ | ☺ ☺ | 1¾ A 3½ |
| English muffin, whole wheat, with raisins | piece 2.33oz/66g | 1¼ +1 unit | 2 4 | ☹ 2¼ | ¾ A 1½ |
| Enoki mushrooms, raw | tbsp. 0.5ozfl/14.21ml | ☺ | ☺ ☺ | ☹ ¾ | ☺ ☺ |
| Espresso, without flavored syrup | cup 5.2ozfl/150ml | ☺ | ☺ ☺ | ☺ ☺ | ☺ ☺ |
| Essentials Oat Bran cereal (Quaker*) | portion 1.95oz/55g | ☺ | ☺ ☺ | ☺ ☺ | 1¼ A 2¾ |
| Evaporated milk, diluted, 2% fat (reduced fat) | glass 8.4oz/240g | ¼ +0,22 unit | ☺ ☺ | ☺ ☺ | 1½ 3 |
| Evaporated milk, diluted, skim (fat free) | glass 8.4oz/240g | ¼ +0,21 unit | ☺ ☺ | ☺ ☺ | 1¼ 2¾ |
| Evaporated milk, diluted, whole | glass 8.4oz/240g | ¼ +0,24 unit | ☺ ☺ | ☺ ☺ | 1½ 3 |
| Falafel | portion 1.95oz/55g | ☺ | ☺ ☺ | ☹ 1¾ | ¾ G 1½ |
| Familia Swiss Muesli*, Original Recipe | portion 1.95oz/55g | ☺ | 1 2 | ☹ 1 | ¼ A ¾ |
| Fanta Zero*, fruit flavors | glass 8.4ozfl/240ml | ☺ | ☺ ☺ | ☺ ☺ | ☺ ☺ |

☹/ Level 0: lactose measure ×½   + Unit/ 🗩: added tolerated amount of unit per strong lactase capsule
☹/ Level 1: fructose measure ×2   Fructose*: fructose, sorbitol adjusted
☹/ Level 2: fructose-/sorbitol measure ×4. the rest ×2   ☺+ ×[Amount] unit: Per unit consumed you can
☹/ Level 3: sorbitol measure ×7. the rest ×3   additionally tolerate up to [amount] ×
📖: source of fruc/galactans data   fructose(*)-unit of another product.
☹: avoid;   ☹[1]: ¼ at TL 1;   ☹[2]: ¼ at TL 2;   ☹[3]: ¼ at TL 3;   ☺: only contains traces;   ☺: is free from it

| Keyword Index | Unit | Lactose ↳ + unit/ | Fructose* ☹ Fructose* ↳ | Sorbitol ☹ Sorbitol ↳ | FrucGalactans ☹ FrucGalactans ↳ |
|---|---|---|---|---|---|
| Fanta® Red | glass 8.4ozfl/240ml | ☺ | ☹[1] ¼ | ☺ ☺ | ☺ ☺ |
| Fanta®, fruit flavors | glass 8.4ozfl/240ml | ☺ | 8¼ 16½ | ☺ ☺ | ☺ ☺ |
| Fennel bulb, raw | portion 3oz/85g | ☺ | ☺+ ×¾ unit ☺+ ×¼ unit | ☹ 2 | 1¼ [B] 2¾ |
| Fennel tea | glass 8.6ozfl/247ml | ☺ | ☺ ☺ | ☺ ☺ | ½ [G] 1¼ |
| Feta cheese | portion 1.06oz/30g | 2¼ +2 unit | ☺ ☺ | ☺ ☺ | 13½ 27 |
| Feta cheese, fat free | portion 1.06oz/30g | ¾ +¾ unit | ☺ ☺ | ☺ ☺ | 5 10¼ |
| Fettuccini Alfredo®, no meat, vegetables other than dark green | tbsp. 0.5ozfl/14.21ml | 66¾ +55½ unit | ☺ ☺ | ☹ 2¾ | 81½ [A] ☺ |
| Fettuccini Alfredo®, no meat, with carrots or dark green vegetables | portion 7.06oz/200g | 5 +4 unit | ☺ ☺ | ☺ ☺ | 27¾ 55½ |
| Fettuccini noodles, whole wheat, cooked in unsalted water | portion 4.94oz/140g | ☺ | ☺+ ×¼ unit ☺ | ☺ ☺ | 1 [A] 2 |
| Fiber One Original® (General Mills®) | portion 1.06oz/30g | ☺ | 41½ 83¼ | ☺ ☺ | ½ [A] 1¼ |
| Fiber One® Nutty Clusters & Almonds (General Mills®) | portion 1.95oz/55g | ☺ | ☺ ☺ | ☺ ☺ | ¼ [A] ¾ |
| Fifty 50® Sugar Free Low Glycemic Butterscotch Hard Candy | piece 0.14oz/3.75g | ☺ | ☺ ☺ | ☹ ☹ | ☺ ☺ |
| Figs, dried, cooked, sweetened | piece 1.77oz/50g | ☺ | ☺+ ×¾ unit ☺+ ×¼ unit | ☺ ☺ | ☺ ☺ |
| Figs, fresh | piece 1.77oz/50g | ☺ | ☺+ ×2 unit ☺+ ×1 unit | ☺ ☺ | ☺ ☺ |
| Filberts, raw | hand 1.06oz/30g | ☺ | ☺ ☺ | ☹ 8¼ | 2¾ [G] 5¾ |
| Fish croquette | portion 3oz/85g | 2¼ +1¾ unit | ☺ ☺ | ☹ ☺ | 1¾ [A] 3½ |
| Fish or seafood with cream or white sauce | portion 6.39oz/181g | 1½ +1¼ unit | ☺ ☺ | ☺ ☺ | ☺ ☺ |
| Fish sticks, patties, or nuggets, breaded, regular | portion 3oz/85g | ☺ | ☺ ☺ | ☺ ☺ | 2 [A] 4 |
| Fish with breading | portion 3oz/85g | ☺ | ☹ ☺ | ☹ ☺ | ☹ ☺ |

| KEYWORD INDEX | Unit | Lactose ⍑<br>+ unit/💊 | Fructose* ⍑<br>Fructose* ⍑ | Sorbitol ⍑<br>Sorbitol ⍑ | FrucGalactans ⍑<br>FrucGalactans ⍑📖 |
|---|---|---|---|---|---|
| Flax seed oil | portion<br>0.46oz/13g | ☺<br> | ☺<br>☺ | ☺<br>☺ | ☺<br>☺ |
| Flax seeds, not fortifed | tbsp.<br>0.5ozfl/14.21ml | ☺<br> | ☺<br>☺ | ☺<br>☺ | 2<br>4¼ G |
| Fleischmann's® Move Over Butter Margarine, tub, whipped | portion<br>0.32oz/9g | 21¾<br>+18 unit | ☺<br>☺ | ☺<br>☺ | ☺<br>☺ |
| Focaccia bread | slice<br>1.49oz/42g | ☺ | ☺<br>☺ | ☺<br>☺ | 1¼ A<br>2½ |
| Fondue sauce | portion<br>1.87oz/53g | ☺ | ☺+ ×¼ unit<br>☺ | ☹<br>5 | ☺<br>☺ |
| Frappuccino® | cup<br>5.2ozfl/150ml | ½<br>+½ unit | ☺<br>☺ | ☺<br>☺ | 3¾<br>7½ |
| Frappuccino®, bottled or canned | cup<br>5.2ozfl/150ml | ½<br>+½ unit | ☺<br>☺ | ☺<br>☺ | 3½<br>7 |
| Frappuccino®, bottled or canned, light | cup<br>5.2ozfl/150ml | ½<br>+½ unit | ☺<br>☺ | ☺<br>☺ | 4<br>8 |
| French Burnt Peanuts | hand<br>1.06oz/30g | ☺ | ☺+ ×1¾ unit<br>☺+ ×¾ unit | ☺<br>☺ | ☺ G<br>☺ |
| French onion soup, condensed | portion<br>4.45oz/126g | ☺ | ☺+ ×1½ unit<br>☺+ ×¾ unit | ☹<br>2 | ¼ CB<br>¾ |
| French or Vienna roll | slice<br>1.49oz/42g | ☺ | ☺<br>☺ | ☺<br>☺ | 1¼ A<br>2½ |
| French toast, homemade, French bread | piece<br>4.63oz/131g | 1¼<br>+1 unit | ☺+ ×½ unit<br>☺+ ×¼ unit | ☺<br>☺ | ¼ A<br>¾ |
| Froot Loops® (Kellogg's®) | portion<br>1.06oz/30g | ☺ | ☺<br>☺ | ☺<br>☺ | ½ A<br>1¼ |
| Frosted Flakes® (Kellogg's®) | portion<br>1.06oz/30g | ☺ | ☺<br>☺ | ☹<br>☺ | 1½ A<br>3 |
| Frosted Flakes® Reduced Sugar (Kellogg's®) | portion<br>1.06oz/30g | ☺ | ☺+ ×¼ unit<br>☺ | ☺<br>☺ | 1½ A<br>3 |
| Frosted Mini-Wheats Big Bite® (Kellogg's®) | portion<br>1.95oz/55g | ☺ | ☺+ ×¼ unit<br>☺ | ☺<br>☺ | ¼ A<br>¾ |

⍑ *Level 0*: lactose measure ×½    + Unit/💊: added tolerated amount of unit per strong lactase capsule
⍑ *Level 1*: fructose measure ×2    Fructose*: fructose, sorbitol adjusted
⍑ *Level 2*: fructose-/sorbitol measure ×4. the rest ×2    ☺+ ×[Amount] unit: Per unit consumed you can additionally tolerate up to [amount] × fructose(*)-unit of another product.
⍑ *Level 3*: sorbitol measure ×7. the rest ×3
📖: source of fruc/galactans data

☹: avoid;   ☹[1]: ¼ at TL 1;   ☹[2]: ¼ at TL 2;   ☹[3]: ¼ at TL 3;   ☺: only contains traces;   ☺: is free from it

| Keyword Index | Unit + unit/ | Lactose ↓ | Fructose* ↓ Fructose* ↓ | Sorbitol ↓ Sorbitol ↓ | FrucGalactans ↓ FrucGalactans ↓ |
|---|---|---|---|---|---|
| Frozen custard, chocolate or coffee flavors | portion 3.09oz/87.5g | ½ +¼ unit | ☺+ ×2¼ unit ☺+ ×1 unit | ☹ ☺ | ½ A 1 |
| Frozen fruit juice bar | piece 2.72oz/77g | ☺ | ☺+ ×1¼ unit ☺+ ×½ unit | ☹ 4½ | ☺ ☺ |
| Fruit drink or punch, ready to drink | glass 8.4ozfl/240ml | ☺ | ☺+ ×1 unit ☺+ ×½ unit | ☹ 2 | 1½ C 3 |
| Fruit punch, alcoholic | glass 8.4ozfl/240ml | ☺ | ¾ 1½ | ☹ 1 | ☺ ☺ |
| Fruit sauce, jelly-based | portion 1.42oz/40g | ☺ | ☺+ ×5¼ unit ☺+ ×2½ unit | ☹ ¾ | ☺ ☺ |
| Garbanzo beans (chickpeas), canned, drained | portion 3.18oz/90g | ☺ | ☺ ☺ | ☹ 1 | 1½ A 3 |
| Gardenburger® Sun-Dried Tomato Basil | portion 3oz/85g | ☺ | 1¼ 2½ | ☹ 1 | 7¾ B 15¾ |
| Garlic sauce | tbsp. 0.5ozfl/14.21ml | ☺ | ☺ ☺ | ☺ ☺ | ☹ FB ☹ |
| Garlic, fresh | portion 0.15oz/4g | ☺ | ☺ ☺ | ☺ ☺ | ¾ FB 1½ |
| Garlic, powder | pinch 0.04oz/1g | ☺ | ☺ ☺ | ☺ ☺ | 3¼ FB 6½ |
| Gatorade®, all flavors | glass 8.4oz/240g | 7½ +6¼ unit | ☺+ ×1¼ unit ☺+ ×½ unit | ☺ ☺ | 41½ 83¼ |
| Gatorade®, from dry mix, all flavors | glass 8.4oz/240g | ☺ | ☺+ ×10½ unit ☺+ ×5¼ unit | ☺ ☺ | ☺ ☺ |
| Gelatin (jello) powder, flavored, sugar free | piece 0.18oz/5g | ☺ | ☺ ☺ | ☺ ☺ | ☺ ☺ |
| Gelatin (jello) powder, plain | piece 0.07oz/1.75g | ☺ | ☺ ☺ | ☺ ☺ | ☺ ☺ |
| German chocolate cake, glazed, homemade | piece 1.03oz/29g | ☺ | ☺+ ×½ unit ☺+ ×¼ unit | ☹ ☺ | 1¾ A 3¾ |
| German style potato salad, with bacon and vinegar dressing | portion 4.94oz/140g | ☺ | ☺+ ×¼ unit ☺ | ☹ 4¾ | 1 CB 2 |
| GG® Scandinavian Bran Crispbread (Health Valley®) | slice 1.49oz/42g | ☺ | ☺ ☺ | ☺ ☺ | ¼ A ½ |
| Gibson | glass 8.4ozfl/240ml | ☺ | ☺ ☺ | ☹ 3¼ | ☺ ☺ |
| Gin | glass 8.4ozfl/240ml | ☺ | ☺ ☺ | ☺ ☺ | ☺ ☺ |
| Ginger ale | glass 8.4ozfl/240ml | ☺ | ☹² ☹² | ☺ ☺ | ☺ ☺ |

| KEYWORD INDEX | Unit | Lactose ↳ + unit/ 💊 | Fructose* ☹ Fructose* ↳ | Sorbitol ☹ Sorbitol ↳ | FrucGalactans ☹ FrucGalactans ↳ 📖 |
|---|---|---|---|---|---|
| Ginger root, raw | portion 0.15oz/4g | ☺ | 89¼ ☺ | ☺ ☺ | ☺ B ☺ |
| Ginger sauce, Asian style | portion 1.13oz/32g | ☺ | ☺ ☺ | ☹ 9¼ | ☺ B ☺ |
| Ginger, ground | pinch 0.04oz/1g | ☺ | 89¼ ☺ | ☺ ☺ | ☺ B ☺ |
| Ginko nuts, dried | hand 1.06oz/30g | ☺ | ☺ ☺ | ☺ ☺ | ☺ ☺ |
| Girard's® Wasabi and Ginger Vinaigrette | pinch 0.04oz/1g | ☺ | ☺ ☺ | ☹ ☺ | ☺ B ☺ |
| Girl Scout® Lemonades | piece 0.55oz/15.5g | ☺ | ☺ ☺ | ☺ ☺ | 4 A 8¼ |
| Girl Scout® Peanut Butter Patties | piece 0.45oz/12.5g | ☺ | ☺ ☺ | ☹ ☺ | 4 A 8¼ |
| Girl Scout® Samoas® | piece 0.52oz/14.5g | 52¼ +43½ unit | 10¼ 20½ | ☹ ¾ | 3½ A 7 |
| Girl Scout® Shortbread® | piece 0.4oz/11.34g | 18½ +15½ unit | ☺ ☺ | ☺ ☺ | 3¼ A 6¾ |
| Girl Scout® Thin Mints | piece 0.29oz/8g | 32½ +27 unit | ☺ ☺ | ☹ ☺ | 6¼ A 12½ |
| Glaceau® Vitaminwater 10 | glass 8.4oz/240g | ☺ | ☹¹ ¼ | ☹ ☹² | ☺ ☺ |
| Glaceau® Vitaminwater Energy | glass 8.4oz/240g | ☺ | ☹² ☹² | ☺ ☺ | ☺ ☺ |
| Glaceau® Vitaminwater Essential | glass 8.4oz/240g | ☺ | ☹² ☹² | ☺ ☺ | ☺ ☺ |
| Glaceau® Vitaminwater Focus | glass 8.4oz/240g | ☺ | ☹² ☹² | ☺ ☺ | ☺ ☺ |
| Glaceau® Vitaminwater Power-C | glass 8.4oz/240g | ☺ | ☹² ☹² | ☺ ☺ | ☺ ☺ |
| Glaceau® Vitaminwater Revive | glass 8.4oz/240g | ☺ | ☹² ☹² | ☺ ☺ | ☺ ☺ |
| Gluten free bread | slice 1.49oz/42g | ☺ | ☺ ☺ | ☺ ☺ | 3½ A 7 |

☹ *Level 0*: lactose measure ×½  
↳ *Level 1*: fructose measure ×2  
↳ *Level 2*: fructose-/sorbitol measure ×4. the rest ×2  
↳ *Level 3*: sorbitol measure ×7. the rest ×3  
📖: source of fruc/galactans data  

\+ Unit/💊: added tolerated amount of unit per strong lactase capsule  
Fructose*: fructose, sorbitol adjusted  
☺+ ×[Amount] unit: Per unit consumed you can additionally tolerate up to [amount] × fructose(*)-unit of another product.  

☹: avoid;   ☹¹: ¼ at TL 1;   ☹²: ¼ at TL 2;   ☹³: ¼ at TL 3;   ☺: only contains traces;   ☺: is free from it

| Keyword Index | Unit | Lactose + unit/ | Fructose* Fructose* | Sorbitol Sorbitol | FrucGalactans FrucGalactans |
|---|---|---|---|---|---|
| GO Veggie!™ Rice Slices, all flavors | portion 1.06oz/30g | 12 +10 unit | ☺ ☺ | ☺ ☺ | 67¼ [A] ☺ |
| Goats cheese, hard | portion 1.06oz/30g | 4½ +3¾ unit | ☺ ☺ | ☺ ☺ | 25½ 51 |
| GoLEAN® Crisp! Cereal, Cinnamon Crumble (Kashi®) | portion 1.95oz/55g | ☺ | ☺+ ×1¼ unit ☺+ ×½ unit | ☹ 25¾ | ¼ [A] ¾ |
| GoLEAN® Crunch! Cereal, Honey Almond Flax (Kashi®) | portion 1.95oz/55g | ☺ | ☺+ ×1 unit ☺+ ×½ unit | ☹ 18 | ¼ [A] ¾ |
| Gooseberries, fresh | portion 4.94oz/140g | ☺ | ☺+ ×1 unit ☺+ ×½ unit | ☺ ☺ | ☺ ☺ |
| Gorgonzola cheese | portion 1.06oz/30g | 20 +16½ unit | ☺ ☺ | ☺ ☺ | ☺ ☺ |
| Gorton's® Battered Fish Fillets - Lemon Pepper | portion 3oz/85g | ☺ | ☺ ☺ | ☺ ☺ | ☺ ☺ |
| Gorton's® Popcorn Shrimp, Original | portion 3oz/85g | ☺ | ☺ ☺ | ☺ ☺ | 2 [A] 4 |
| Gouda cheese | portion 1.06oz/30g | 4½ +3¾ unit | ☺ ☺ | ☺ ☺ | 25 50 |
| Goulash, with beef, noodles or macaroni, tomato base | tbsp. 0.5ozfl/14.21ml | ☺ | ☺ ☺ | ☹ 4 | ☺ ☺ |
| Grand Marnier® | glass 8.4ozfl/240ml | ☺ | ☺+ ×4½ unit ☺+ ×2½ unit | ☹ ¼ | ☺ ☺ |
| Grapefruit juice, unsweetened, white | glass 8.4ozfl/240ml | ☺ | ☺+ ×5 unit ☺+ ×2½ unit | ☹ ¼ | 1 [CB] 2 |
| Grapefruit, fresh, pink or red | portion 4.94oz/140g | ☺ | 2 4¼ | ☺ ☺ | 1½ [CB] 3 |
| Grapes, fresh | portion 4.94oz/140g | ☺ | ¼ ½ | ☹ ½ | 2¼ [B] 4½ |
| Grasshopper | glass 8.4ozfl/240ml | 1¼ +1 unit | ☺+ ×1¼ unit ☺+ ×¾ unit | ☹ ¾ | 7 14 |
| Greek yogurt, plain, nonfat | piece 5.3oz/150g | ¼ +¼ unit | ☺ ☺ | ☺ ☺ | 2½ 5 |
| Green beans (string beans), cooked from fresh | portion 3oz/85g | ☺ | 4½ 9 | ☺ ☺ | ¼ [A] ¾ |
| Green bell peppers | portion 3oz/85g | ☺ | ☺ ☺ | ☺ ☺ | ☺ [B] ☺ |
| Green olives | portion 0.53oz/15g | ☺ | ☺ ☺ | ☹ 18 | ☺ ☺ |
| Green pea soup, prepared from condensed can | tbsp 0.5ozfl/14.21ml | ☹ | ☹ ☺ | ☹ 20 | 3¼ [AG] 6¾ |

| Keyword Index | Unit | Lactose ↓<br>+ unit/💊 | Fructose* ☹<br>Fructose* ↓ | Sorbitol ☹<br>Sorbitol ↓ | FrucGalactans ☹<br>FrucGalactans ↓ 📖 |
|---|---|---|---|---|---|
| Green tea, strong | glass<br>8.7ozfl/248ml | ☺ | ☺<br>☺ | ☺<br>☺ | ☺ G<br>☺ |
| Green tomato, raw | portion<br>3oz/85g | ☺ | 3<br>6¼ | ☹<br>¾ | 6½ B<br>13 |
| Guava (guayaba), fresh, common | piece<br>5.3oz/150g | ☺ | 2¼<br>5 | ☹<br>½ | ☺<br>☺ |
| Gum drops | hand<br>1.06oz/30g | ☺ | ☺+ ×2¼ unit<br>☺+ ×1 unit | ☺<br>☺ | ☺<br>☺ |
| Gum drops, sugar free | tsp.<br>0.16ozfl/4.74ml | ☺ | ☺<br>☺ | ☹<br>☹ | ☺<br>☺ |
| Gummi bears | hand<br>1.06oz/30g | ☺ | ☺+ ×3½ unit<br>☺+ ×1¾ unit | ☹<br>☺ | ☺<br>☺ |
| Gummi bears, sugar free | tsp.<br>0.16ozfl/4.74ml | ☺ | 10<br>20¼ | ☹<br>☹³ | ☺<br>☺ |
| Gummi dinosaurs | hand<br>1.06oz/30g | ☺ | ☺+ ×3½ unit<br>☺+ ×1¾ unit | ☹<br>☺ | ☺<br>☺ |
| Gummi dinosaurs, sugar free | tsp.<br>0.16ozfl/4.74ml | ☺ | 10<br>20¼ | ☹<br>☹³ | ☺<br>☺ |
| Gummi worms | hand<br>1.06oz/30g | ☺ | ☺+ ×3½ unit<br>☺+ ×1¾ unit | ☹<br>☺ | ☺<br>☺ |
| Gummi worms, sugar free | tsp.<br>0.16ozfl/4.74ml | ☺ | 10<br>20¼ | ☹<br>☹³ | ☺<br>☺ |
| Haagen-Dazs® Desserts Extraordinaire Ice Cream, Creme Brulee | portion<br>3.78oz/107g | ½<br>+¼ unit | ☺+ ×4¾ unit<br>☺+ ×2¼ unit | ☺<br>☺ | 3<br>6¼ |
| Haagen-Dazs® Frozen Yogurt, chocolate or coffee flavors | portion<br>3.74oz/106g | ½<br>+½ unit | ☺+ ×¾ unit<br>☺+ ×¼ unit | ☹<br>☺ | 1¾<br>3½ |
| Haagen-Dazs® Frozen Yogurt, vanilla or other flavors | portion<br>3.74oz/106g | ½<br>+½ unit | ☺+ ×3 unit<br>☺+ ×1½ unit | ☺<br>☺ | 3½<br>7 |
| Haagen-Dazs® Ice Cream, Bailey's Irish Cream | portion<br>3.6oz/102g | ½<br>+¼ unit | ☺+ ×2¾ unit<br>☺+ ×1¼ unit | ☹<br>☺ | 1½<br>3 |
| Haagen-Dazs® Ice Cream, Black Walnut | portion<br>3.74oz/106g | ½<br>+½ unit | ☺+ ×4¾ unit<br>☺+ ×2¼ unit | ☺<br>☺ | 1½<br>3 |

☹ *Level 0*: lactose measure ×½   + Unit/💊: added tolerated amount of unit per strong lactase capsule
↓ *Level 1*: fructose measure ×2   Fructose*: fructose, sorbitol adjusted
↓ *Level 2*: fructose-/sorbitol measure ×4. the rest ×2   ☺+ ×[Amount] unit: Per unit consumed you can additionally tolerate up to [amount] × fructose(*)-unit of another product.
↓ *Level 3*: sorbitol measure ×7. the rest ×3
📖: source of fruc/galactans data
☹: avoid;   ☹¹: ¼ at TL 1;   ☹²: ¼ at TL 2;   ☹³: ¼ at TL 3;   ☺: only contains traces;   ☺: is free from it

| Keyword Index | Unit + unit/ | Lactose | Fructose* / Fructose* | Sorbitol / Sorbitol | FrucGalactans / FrucGalactans |
|---|---|---|---|---|---|
| Haagen-Dazs® Ice Cream, Butter Pecan | portion 3.74oz/106g | ½ +½ unit | ☺+ ×4¾ unit ☺+ ×2¼ unit | ☺ ☺ | 2¼ 4¾ |
| Haagen-Dazs® Ice Cream, Cherry Vanilla | portion 3.57oz/101g | ½ +½ unit | ☺+ ×4½ unit ☺+ ×2¼ unit | ☺ ☺ | 3¼ 6½ |
| Haagen-Dazs® Ice Cream, Chocolate | portion 3.74oz/106g | ¼ +¼ unit | ☺+ ×2¾ unit ☺+ ×1¼ unit | ☹ ☺ | 1¼ 2¾ |
| Haagen-Dazs® Ice Cream, Coffee | portion 3.74oz/106g | ¼ +¼ unit | ☺+ ×2¾ unit ☺+ ×1¼ unit | ☹ ☺ | 2½ 5¼ |
| Haagen-Dazs® Ice Cream, Cookies & Cream | portion 3.6oz/102g | ½ +¼ unit | ☺+ ×4½ unit ☺+ ×2¼ unit | ☺ ☺ | 3¼ 6½ |
| Haagen-Dazs® Ice Cream, Mango | portion 3.74oz/106g | ¼ +¼ unit | ☺+ ×2¼ unit ☺+ ×1 unit | ☺ ☺ | 2¼ 4¾ |
| Haagen-Dazs® Ice Cream, Pistachio | portion 3.74oz/106g | ½ +½ unit | ☺+ ×4¾ unit ☺+ ×2¼ unit | ☺ ☺ | ½ 1¼ |
| Haagen-Dazs® Ice Cream, Rocky Road | portion 3.67oz/104g | ¼ +¼ unit | ☺+ ×2¾ unit ☺+ ×1¼ unit | ☹ ☺ | 2½ 5¼ |
| Haagen-Dazs® Ice Cream, Strawberry | portion 3.74oz/106g | ½ +¼ unit | ☺+ ×4¾ unit ☺+ ×2¼ unit | ☺ ☺ | 3 6¼ |
| Haagen-Dazs® Ice Cream, Vanilla Chocolate Chip | portion 3.74oz/106g | ½ +½ unit | ☺+ ×4¾ unit ☺+ ×2¼ unit | ☺ ☺ | 3½ 7 |
| Half and half | portion 1.06oz/30g | 2¼ +1¾ unit | ☺ ☺ | ☺ ☺ | 12¾ 25¾ |
| Halvah | portion 1.42oz/40g | ☺ | ☺+ ×1½ unit ☺+ ×¾ unit | ☺ ☺ | 1¼ [A] 2¾ |
| Ham croquette | portion 3oz/85g | 2¼ +1¾ unit | ☺ ☺ | ☹ ☺ | ☺ ☺ |
| Hamburger gravy | portion 7.17oz/203g | ☺ | ☺ ☺ | ☹ 12¼ | ☺ ☺ |
| Hard candy | piece 0.22oz/6g | ☺ | ☺+ ×¾ unit ☺+ ×¼ unit | ☺ ☺ | ☺ ☺ |
| Hard candy, sugar free | piece 0.11oz/3g | ☺ | ☹[1] ¼ | ☹ ☹ | ☺ ☺ |
| Hardee's® Loaded Omelet Biscuit | piece 5.58oz/158g | 12 +10 unit | ☺+ ×9¼ unit ☺+ ×4½ unit | ☺ ☺ | ¼ [A] ½ |
| Harvey Wallbanger | glass 8.4ozfl/240ml | ☺ | 16½ 33¼ | ☹ ¼ | ☺ ☺ |
| Health Valley® Multigrain Chewy Granola Bar, Chocolate Chip | piece 1.03oz/29g | 29½ +24¾ unit | ☺+ ×1 unit ☺+ ×½ unit | ☹ ☺ | ½ [A] 1¼ |

| Keyword Index | Unit | Lactose ☽ + unit/ 💊 | Fructose* ☽ Fructose* ☽ | Sorbitol ☽ Sorbitol ☽ | FrucGalactans ☽ FrucGalactans ☽ 📖 |
|---|---|---|---|---|---|
| Hershey's® Caramel Filled Chocolates Sugar Free | piece 0.31oz/8.6g | 74½ +62 unit | 21¾ 43½ | ☹ ☹ | ☺ ☺ |
| Hershey's® Milk Chocolate Bar | bar 4.77oz/135g | ¼ +¼ unit | ☺ ☺ | ☺ ☺ | ¼ G ¾ |
| Hickorynuts | hand 1.06oz/30g | ☺ | ☺ ☺ | ☺ ☺ | 2¾ G 5¾ |
| High-protein bar, generic | piece 2.3oz/65g | 39¼ +32¾ unit | ¾ 1¾ | ☹ 76¾ | ☺ ☺ |
| Hollandaise sauce, store bought | tbsp. 0.5ozfl/14.21ml | 5 +4¼ unit | ☺ ☺ | ☺ ☺ | 28½ 57 |
| Honey | tbsp. 0.5ozfl/14.21ml | ☺ | ½ 1¼ | ☹ 1¾ | ☺ ☺ |
| Honey Nut Chex® (General Mills®) | portion 1.06oz/30g | ☺ | ☺ ☺ | ☹ 37 | ½ A 1¼ |
| Honey Smacks® (Kellogg's®) | portion 1.06oz/30g | ☺ | ☺+ ×12 unit ☺+ ×6 unit | ☹ 83¼ | ½ A 1¼ |
| Honeydew | portion 4.94oz/140g | ☺ | ¾ 1½ | ☺ ☺ | 1½ B 3¼ |
| Horseradish | pinch 0.04oz/1g | ☺ | ☺ ☺ | ☺ ☺ | ☺ ☺ |
| Hot chili peppers, green, cooked from fresh | piece 1.52oz/43g | ☺ | 4½ 9¼ | ☺ ☺ | 2½ B 5¼ |
| Hot chili peppers, red, cooked from fresh | piece 1.52oz/43g | ☺ | 2¾ 5½ | ☺ ☺ | 2½ B 5¼ |
| Hot chocolate, homemade | cup 5.2ozfl/150ml | ¼ +¼ unit | 27¾ 27¾ | ☹ 66½ | 1¾ 3¾ |
| Hot dog, combination of meats, plain | portion 1.95oz/55g | ☺ | ☺+ ×3 unit ☺+ ×1½ unit | ☺ ☺ | ☺ ☺ |
| Hubbard squash | portion 3oz/85g | ☺ | ☺ ☺ | ☺ ☺ | ☺ B ☺ |
| Ice cream sandwich | piece 2.54oz/72g | 1¼ +1 unit | ☺+ ×1½ unit ☺+ ×¾ unit | ☺ ☺ | 6¼ 12½ |

☽ *Level 0:* lactose measure ×½
☽ *Level 1:* fructose measure ×2
☽ *Level 2:* fructose-/sorbitol measure ×4. the rest ×2
☽ *Level 3:* sorbitol measure ×7. the rest ×3
📖: source of fruc/galactans data

+ Unit/💊: added tolerated amount of unit per strong lactase capsule
Fructose*: fructose, sorbitol adjusted

☺+ ×[Amount] unit: Per unit consumed you can additionally tolerate up to [amount] × fructose(*)-unit of another product.

☹: avoid;   ☹¹: ¼ at TL 1;   ☹²: ¼ at TL 2;   ☹³: ¼ at TL 3;   ☺: only contains traces;   ☺: is free from it

LAXIBA® The Nutrition Navigator

| Keyword Index | Unit + unit/🥛 | Lactose ↳ | Fructose* ☺/Fructose* ↳ | Sorbitol ☺/Sorbitol ↳ | FrucGalactans ☺/FrucGalactans ↳ 📖 |
|---|---|---|---|---|---|
| Ice cream, light, no sugar added, with aspartame, vanilla or other flavors (include chocolate chip) | tsp. 0.16ozfl/4.74ml | 9¾ +8 unit | 2¼ 4¾ | ☹ ¼ | 54¾ ☺ |
| Instant coffee mix, unprepared | cup 5.2ozfl/150ml | ☺ | 8¼ 16½ | ☹ ☹² | ☺ ☺ |
| Irish coffee with alcohol and whipped cream | cup 5.2ozfl/150ml | 3¾ +3 unit | ☺ ☺ | ☺ ☺ | 21 42 |
| Jackfruit, fresh | tbsp. 0.5ozfl/14.21ml | ☺ | ☺ ☺ | ☺ ½ | ☺ ☺ |
| Jam or preserves | portion 0.71oz/20g | ☺ | ☺+ ×2¾ unit ☺+ ×1¼ unit | ☹ 1¾ | ☺ ☺ |
| Jam or preserves, reduced sugar | portion 0.71oz/20g | ☺ | 7 14 | ☹ 41½ | ☺ ☺ |
| Jam or preserves, sugar free with aspartame | portion 0.6oz/17g | ☺ | 15¾ 31¾ | ☹ 5¼ | ☺ ☺ |
| Jam or preserves, sugar free with saccharin | portion 0.5oz/14g | ☺ | 2¼ 4¾ | ☹ 19¼ | ☺ ☺ |
| Jam or preserves, sugar free with sucralose | portion 0.6oz/17g | ☺ | ☺ ☺ | ☹ 65¼ | ☺ ☺ |
| Jam or preserves, without sugar or artificial sweetener | tbsp. 0.5ozfl/14.21ml | ☺ | ¼ ½ | ☹ ☹² | ☺ ☺ |
| Jasmine tea | glass 8.4ozfl/240ml | ☺ | ☺ ☺ | ☺ ☺ | ☺ ☺ |
| Jelly beans* | hand 1.06oz/30g | ☺ | ☺+ ×9¾ unit ☺+ ×4¾ unit | ☺ ☺ | ☺ ☺ |
| Jelly beans*, sugar free | tsp. 0.16ozfl/4.74ml | ☺ | 12¼ 24½ | ☹ ☹ | ☺ ☺ |
| Jerusalem artichoke (sunchoke), raw | pinch 0.04ozfl/1g | ☺ | ☺ ☺ | ☺ ☺ | 3¼ [FB] 6½ |
| Jujyfruits* | hand 1.06oz/30g | ☺ | ☺+ ×12¼ unit ☺+ ×6 unit | ☺ ☺ | ☺ ☺ |
| Kale, raw | portion 3oz/85g | ☺ | ☺ ☺ | ☹ ¾ | ☺ ☺ |
| Kamikaze | glass 8.4ozfl/240ml | ☺ | ☺+ ×1½ unit ☺+ ×¾ unit | ☹ 1 | ☺ ☺ |
| Kashi* Chewy Granola Bar, Cherry Dark Chocolate | piece 1.24oz/35g | ☺ | ☺+ ×1 unit ☺+ ×½ unit | ☹ 1 | ½ [A] 1 |
| Kefir | portion 8.65oz/245g | ¼ +¼ unit | ☺ ☺ | ☺ ☺ | 1¾ 3¾ |

| Keyword Index | Unit | Lactose ↓ + unit/💊 | Fructose* ☺ Fructose* ↓ | Sorbitol ☺ Sorbitol ↓ | FrucGalactans ☺ FrucGalactans ↓ 📖 |
|---|---|---|---|---|---|
| Kelp, raw | portion 3oz/85g | ☺ | ☺ ☺ | ☺ ☺ | ☺ ☺ |
| Kern's® Mango-Orange Nectar | glass 8.4ozfl/240ml | ☺ | ☹¹ ¼ | ☹ 2 | 3 [B] 6¼ |
| Kern's® Strawberry Nectar | glass 8.4ozfl/240ml | ☺ | ☹¹ ¼ | ☹ ¾ | ☺ [C] ☺ |
| Ketchup | portion 0.53oz/15g | ☺ | ☺+ ×¼ unit ☺ | ☹ 3¾ | ☺ ☺ |
| Ketchup, low sodium | portion 0.53oz/15g | ☺ | ☺+ ×¼ unit ☺ | ☹ 4¼ | ☺ ☺ |
| KFC® honey BBQ sauce | portion 1.1ozfl/31ml | ☺ | ☺+ ×1¼ unit ☺+ ×½ unit | ☹ 2¼ | ☺ ☺ |
| KFC® Caesar salad dressing | portion 1.06ozfl/30ml | 4¾ +3¾ unit | ☺ ☺ | ☺ ☺ | 26½ 53 |
| KFC® chicken breast, spicy crispy | piece 6.18oz/175g | ☺ | ☺ ☺ | ☺ ☺ | ¾ [A] 1¾ |
| KFC® Chicken Littles with sauce | piece 3.57oz/101g | ☺ | 3 6¼ | ☹ 33 | ½ [A] 1 |
| KFC® cole slaw | portion 3.53oz/100g | ☺ | ☺+ ×¼ unit ☺ | ☹ 2¾ | 1 [B] 2 |
| KFC® creamy buffalo sauce | portion 1.04ozfl/29.4ml | 6 +5 unit | ☺+ ×1 unit ☺+ ×½ unit | ☺ ☺ | 34½ 69 |
| KFC® Crispy Chicken Caesar Salad | portion 4.94oz/140g | ☺ | 2¼ 4½ | ☹ 17¾ | 1 [A] 2¼ |
| KFC® Crispy Twister without sauce | piece 7.69oz/218g | ☺ | 19 38 | ☹ 2 | ☹ [A] ¼ |
| KFC® Crispy Twister® with sauce | piece 8.47oz/240g | ☺ | 17¼ 34½ | ☹ 2 | ☹ [A] ¼ |
| KFC® hot wings | portion 3oz/85g | ☺ | ☺ ☺ | ☺ ☺ | ☺ ☺ |
| KFC® house side salad | portion 3.53oz/100g | ☺ | 2 4¼ | ☹ 4 | ☺ ☺ |

☺ *Level 0*: lactose measure ×½  + Unit/💊: added tolerated amount of unit per strong lactase capsule
↓ *Level 1*: fructose measure ×2  Fructose*: fructose, sorbitol adjusted
↓↓ *Level 2*: fructose-/sorbitol measure ×4. the rest ×2  ☺+ ×[Amount] unit: Per unit consumed you can
↓↓↓ *Level 3*: sorbitol measure ×7. the rest ×3  additionally tolerate up to [amount] ×
📖: source of fruc/galactans data  fructose(*)-unit of another product.
☹: avoid;   ☹¹: ¼ at TL 1;   ☹²: ¼ at TL 2;   ☹³: ¼ at TL 3;   ☺: only contains traces;   ☺: is free from it

| Keyword Index | Unit | Lactose ⅃ + unit/ | Fructose* ☹ Fructose* ⅃ | Sorbitol ☹ Sorbitol ⅃ | FrucGalactans ☹ FrucGalactans ⅃ |
|---|---|---|---|---|---|
| KFC® mashed potatoes with gravy | portion 4.94oz/140g | ½ +½ unit | ☺ ☺ | ☹ 35½ | 4 8¼ |
| KFC® sweet and sour sauce | portion 1.06ozfl/30ml | ☺ | ¼ ½ | ☹ 37 | ☺ ☺ |
| KFC® sweet corn | piece 3.36oz/95g | ☺ | ☺ ☺ | ☹ 2½ | 1¼ G 2½ |
| KFC®, Extra Crispy Tenders | piece 1.84oz/52g | ☺ | ☺ ☺ | ☺ ☺ | 3¼ A 6½ |
| Kidney beans, cooked from dried | portion 3.18oz/90g | ☺ | ☺ ☺ | ☺ ☺ | ¼ A ½ |
| Kirsch | glass 8.4ozfl/240ml | ☺ | ☺+ ×4½ unit ☺+ ×2½ unit | ☹ ¼ | ☺ ☺ |
| Kit Kat® | piece 1.52oz/43g | 2 +1¾ unit | ☺ ☺ | ☹ ☺ | 2 A 4¼ |
| Kit Kat® White | piece 1.49oz/42g | ¾ +½ unit | ☺ ☺ | ☺ ☺ | 1½ A 3¼ |
| Kiwi fruit, gold | piece 3.04oz/86g | ☺ | 1 2¼ | ☺ ☺ | ☺ B ☺ |
| Kiwi fruit, green | piece 2.44oz/69g | ☺ | 3 6 | ☺ ☺ | ☺ B ☺ |
| Kohlrabi, cooked | portion 3oz/85g | ☺ | ☺+ ×¼ unit ☺ | ☹ 13 | ☺ ☺ |
| Kraft® Balsamic Vinaigrette | portion 1.06oz/30g | ☺ | ☺ ☺ | ☹ 22 | ☺ ☺ |
| Kraft® Cheese Spread, Roka Blue | portion 1.06oz/30g | 1¾ +1¼ unit | ☺ ☺ | ☺ ☺ | 9¾ 19½ |
| Kraft® Classic Caesar Dressing | portion 1.06oz/30g | ☺ | ☺+ ×½ unit ☺+ ×¼ unit | ☹ 12¼ | ☺ ☺ |
| Kraft® Creamy French Dressing | portion 1.06oz/30g | ☺ | 64 ☺ | ☹ ☺ | ☺ ☺ |
| Kraft® Creamy Italian Dressing | portion 1.06oz/30g | ☺ | ☺+ ×¾ unit ☺+ ×¼ unit | ☺ ☺ | ☺ ☺ |
| Kraft® Fat Free Mayonnaise | portion 0.53oz/15g | ☺ | ☺ ☺ | ☺ ☺ | ☺ ☺ |
| Kraft® Free Sour Cream & Onion Ranch Dressing, fat free | portion 1.06oz/30g | ☺ | 4½ 9 | ☺ ☺ | ☺ ☺ |
| Kraft® Mayo with Olive Oil, Reduced Fat | portion 0.53oz/15g | ☺ | ☺ ☺ | ☺ ☺ | ☺ ☺ |
| Kraft® Miracle Whip® Free Nonfat Dressing | tbsp. 0.5ozfl/14.21ml | 80 +66½ unit | ☺ ☺ | ☺ ☺ | ☺ ☺ |

| KEYWORD INDEX | Unit | Lactose ☞ + unit/💊 | Fructose* ☞ Fructose* ☞ | Sorbitol ☞ Sorbitol ☞ | FrucGalactans ☞ FrucGalactans ☞📖 |
|---|---|---|---|---|---|
| Kraft® Miracle Whip® Light Dressing | tbsp. 0.5ozfl/14.21ml | ☺ | ☺ ☺ | ☺ ☺ | ☺ ☺ |
| Kraft® Miracle Whip® Salad Dressing | tbsp. 0.5ozfl/14.21ml | ☺ | ☺ ☺ | ☺ ☺ | ☺ ☺ |
| Kraft® Sandwich Spread | tbsp. 0.5ozfl/14.21ml | ☺ | ☺ ☺ | ☹ ☺ | ☺ ☺ |
| Kraft® Thousand Island Dressing® | tbsp. 0.5ozfl/14.21ml | ☺ | ☺+ ×¼ unit ☺ | ☺ ☺ | ☺ ☺ |
| Lasagna, homemade, beef | portion 4.94oz/140g | 23¼ +19¼ unit | ☺+ ×¼ unit ☺ | ☹ 1 | ¾ A 1½ |
| Lasagna, homemade, cheese, no vegetables | portion 4.94oz/140g | 25¾ +21½ unit | 11 22¼ | ☹ ¾ | ¾ A 1½ |
| Lasagna, homemade, spinach, no meat | portion 4.94oz/140g | 8½ +7 unit | 9¾ 19¾ | ☹ ½ | ¾ A 1½ |
| Laughing Cow® Mini Babybel®, Cheddar | piece 0.75oz/21g | ☺ | ☺ ☺ | ☺ ☺ | ☺ ☺ |
| Laughing Cow® Mini Babybel®, Original | piece 0.75oz/21g | 12¾ +10½ unit | ☺ ☺ | ☺ ☺ | 70¾ ☺ |
| Lay's® Potato Chips, Classic | hand 0.75oz/21g | ☺ | 41¾ 83½ | ☹ 79¼ | 10¾ A 21½ |
| Lay's® Potato Chips, Salt & Vinegar | hand 0.75oz/21g | ☺ | 41¾ 83½ | ☹ 79¼ | 10¾ A 21½ |
| Lay's® Potato Chips, Sour Cream & Onion | hand 0.75oz/21g | ☺ | 41¾ 83½ | ☹ 79¼ | 10¾ A 21½ |
| Lay's® Stax Potato Crisps, Cheddar | hand 0.75oz/21g | ☺ | 41¾ 83½ | ☹ 79¼ | 10¾ A 21½ |
| Lay's® Stax Potato Crisps, Hot 'n Spicy Barbecue | hand 0.75oz/21g | ☺ | 54 ☺ | ☹ ☺ | 10¾ A 21½ |
| Lebkuchen | piece 1.15oz/32.4g | ☺ | 6¼ 12¾ | ☹ 6½ | 2 A 4 |
| Leeks, leafs | piece 3.14oz/89g | ☺ | 3 6 | ☹ ¼ | ¾ G 1½ |
| Leeks, root | tbsp. 0.5ozfl/14.21ml | ☺ | 18½ 37 | ☹ 2¼ | ¼ C ¾ |

☞ *Level 0:* lactose measure ×½    + Unit/💊: added tolerated amount of unit per strong lactase capsule
☞ *Level 1:* fructose measure ×2    Fructose*: fructose, sorbitol adjusted
☞ *Level 2:* fructose-/sorbitol measure ×4. the rest ×2    ☺+ ×[Amount] unit: Per unit consumed you can additionally tolerate up to [amount] ×
☞ *Level 3:* sorbitol measure ×7. the rest ×3    fructose(*)-unit of another product.
📖: source of fruc/galactans data

☹: avoid;    ☹¹: ¼ at TL 1;    ☹²: ¼ at TL 2;    ☹³: ¼ at TL 3;    ☺: only contains traces;    ☺: is free from it

| KEYWORD INDEX | Unit + unit/ | Lactose ↳ | Fructose* ☹ Fructose* ↳ | Sorbitol ☹ Sorbitol ↳ | FrucGalactans ☹ FrucGalactans ↳ |
|---|---|---|---|---|---|
| Leeks, whole | piece 3.14oz/89g | ☺ | 3 6 | ☹ ¼ | ¼ C ½ |
| Lemon butter sauce | tbsp. 0.5ozfl/14.21ml | ☺ | ☺ ☺ | ☹ 60½ | ☺ ☺ |
| Lemon juice, fresh | glass 8.4ozfl/240ml | ☺ | 2¼ 5 | ☹ 1½ | 2¼ B 4½ |
| Lemon peel | tbsp. 0.5ozfl/14.21ml | ☺ | ☺ ☺ | ☺ ☺ | ☺ ☺ |
| Lemon, fresh | piece 2.05oz/58g | ☺ | ☺ ☺ | ☺ ☺ | 7¾ B 15½ |
| Lentil soup, condensed | portion 4.45oz/126g | ☺ | ☺ ☺ | ☹ 1 | 5½ AC 11¼ |
| Lentils, cooked from dried | portion 3.18oz/90g | ☺ | ☺ ☺ | ☺ ☺ | ¾ A 1½ |
| Lettuce, boston, bibb or butterhead | portion 3oz/85g | ☺ | 7¼ 14½ | ☹ 19½ | ☺ B ☺ |
| Lettuce, green leaf | portion 3oz/85g | ☺ | 8¼ 16¾ | ☹ 16¾ | ☺ CB ☺ |
| Lettuce, iceberg | portion 3oz/85g | ☺ | 6½ 13 | ☹ 19½ | ☺ CB ☺ |
| Lettuce, red leaf | portion 3oz/85g | ☺ | 7¼ 14½ | ☹ 19½ | ☺ B ☺ |
| Lettuce, romaine or cos | portion 3oz/85g | ☺ | 1¼ 2¾ | ☹ 16¾ | ☺ CB ☺ |
| Libby's® Apricot Nectar | glass 8.4ozfl/240ml | ☺ | ☹1 ¼ | ☹ ¼ | ☺ ☺ |
| Libby's® Banana Nectar | glass 8.4ozfl/240ml | ☺ | ☹1 ¼ | ☹ 25 | ½ FB 1 |
| Libby's® Juicy Juice®, Apple Grape | glass 8.4ozfl/240ml | ☺ | ☹1 ¼ | ☹ ¼ | 1½ CB 3 |
| Libby's® Juicy Juice®, Grape | glass 8.4ozfl/240ml | ☺ | ☹1 ¼ | ☹ ¼ | 1½ CB 3 |
| Libby's® Pear Nectar | glass 8.4ozfl/240ml | ☺ | ☹2 ☹2 | ☹ ☹2 | ☺ B ☺ |
| Licorice | piece 0.39oz/11g | ☺ | ☺+ ×1½ unit ☺+ ×¾ unit | ☺ ☺ | ☺ ☺ |
| Licuado, mango | glass 8.4oz/240g | ¼ +¼ unit | ¼ ½ | ☹ 1 | 2½ 5 |
| Light cream | portion 0.53ozfl/15ml | 5¼ +4½ unit | ☺ ☺ | ☺ ☺ | 30¼ 60½ |

| Keyword Index | Unit | Lactose ⚡<br>+ unit/ 💊 | Fructose* ⚡<br>Fructose* ⚡ | Sorbitol ⚡<br>Sorbitol ⚡ | FrucGalactans ⚡<br>FrucGalactans ⚡ 📖 |
|---|---|---|---|---|---|
| Lima beans, cooked from dried | portion<br>3.18oz/90g | ☺ | ½<br>1¼ | ☺<br>☺ | ¼ A<br>½ |
| Limburger cheese | portion<br>1.06oz/30g | 20¼<br>+17 unit | ☺<br>☺ | ☺<br>☺ | ☺<br>☺ |
| Lime juice, fresh | glass<br>8.4ozfl/240ml | ☺ | ☺+ ×¾ unit<br>☺+ ×¼ unit | ☺<br>☺ | 2¼ B<br>4½ |
| Lime, fresh | piece<br>2.37oz/67g | ☺ | ☺<br>☺ | ☺<br>☺ | 6¾ B<br>13½ |
| Lipton® Iced Tea Mix, sweetened with sugar, prepared | glass<br>8.4ozfl/240ml | ☺ | ☺<br>☺ | ☺<br>☺ | ☺<br>☺ |
| Lipton® Instant 100% Tea, unsweetened, prepared | glass<br>8.4ozfl/240ml | ☺ | ☺<br>☺ | ☺<br>☺ | ☺<br>☺ |
| Liqueur, coffee flavored | glass<br>8.4ozfl/240ml | ☺ | ☺<br>☺ | ☹<br>2½ | ☺<br>☺ |
| Little Debbie® Coffee Cake, Apple Streusel | piece<br>1.84oz/52g | ☺ | ☺+ ×5¼ unit<br>☺+ ×2½ unit | ☺<br>☺ | 1 A<br>2 |
| Little Debbie® Fudge Brownies with English Walnuts | piece<br>1.08oz/30.5g | ☺ | ☺+ ×4¼ unit<br>☺+ ×2 unit | ☹<br>☺ | 1¾ A<br>3½ |
| Little Debbie® Nutty Bars | piece<br>1.01oz/28.5g | ☺ | ☺+ ×13¾ unit<br>☺+ ×6¾ unit | ☹<br>☺ | 4¼ A<br>8½ |
| Liver pudding | portion<br>1.95oz/55g | ☺ | ☺<br>☺ | ☺<br>☺ | ☺<br>☺ |
| Loaf cold cut, spiced | portion<br>1.95oz/55g | 2¼<br>+1¾ unit | ☺+ ×¼ unit<br>☺ | ☺<br>☺ | ☺<br>☺ |
| Loganberries, fresh | portion<br>4.94oz/140g | ☺ | ☺+ ×1½ unit<br>☺+ ×¾ unit | ☺<br>☺ | ☺<br>☺ |
| Long Island iced tea | glass<br>8.4ozfl/240ml | ☺ | ¾<br>1¾ | ☹<br>16½ | ☺<br>☺ |
| Long John or bismarck, glazed, cream or custard filled, with nuts | piece<br>3.71oz/105g | 2¼<br>+2 unit | ☺<br>☺ | ☺<br>☺ | ½ A<br>1 |
| Long John Silver's® tartar sauce | tbsp.<br>0.5ozfl/14.21ml | ☺ | ☺<br>☺ | ☹<br>☺ | ☺<br>☺ |

⚡ *Level 0*: lactose measure ×½    + Unit/💊: added tolerated amount of unit per strong lactase capsule
⚡ *Level 1*: fructose measure ×2    Fructose*: fructose, sorbitol adjusted
⚡ *Level 2*: fructose-/sorbitol measure ×4. the rest ×2    ☺+ ×[Amount] unit: Per unit consumed you can additionally tolerate up to [amount] × fructose(*)-unit of another product.
⚡ *Level 3*: sorbitol measure ×7. the rest ×3
📖: source of fruc/galactans data

☹: avoid;   ☹¹: ¼ at TL 1;   ☹²: ¼ at TL 2;   ☹³: ¼ at TL 3;   ☺: only contains traces;   ☺: is free from it

| Keyword Index | Unit<br>+ unit/ | Lactose | Fructose*<br>Fructose* | Sorbitol<br>Sorbitol | FrucGalactans<br>FrucGalactans |
|---|---|---|---|---|---|
| Long John Silver's® tartar sauce | tbsp.<br>0.5ozfl/14.21ml | ☺ | ☺<br>☺ | ☹<br>☺ | ☺<br>☺ |
| Lotus root, cooked | portion<br>3oz/85g | ☺ | ☺<br>☺ | ☺<br>☺ | ☺<br>☺ |
| Lowbush cranberries (lingonberries) | portion<br>4.94oz/140g | ☺ | ☺+ ×9¼ unit<br>☺+ ×4½ unit | ☹<br>35½ | ☺<br>☺ |
| Lychees (litchis), fresh | portion<br>4.94oz/140g | ☺ | 1<br>2¼ | ☺<br>☺ | ☺ B<br>☺ |
| lycium (wolf or goji berries) | portion<br>4.94oz/140g | ☺ | ☺+ ×1 unit<br>☺+ ×½ unit | ☺<br>☺ | ☺<br>☺ |
| Lyonnaise (potatoes and onions) | portion<br>2.47oz/70g | ☺ | ☺<br>☺ | ☹<br>15¾ | ☺<br>☺ |
| M & M's® Peanut | portion<br>1.42oz/40g | 2½<br>+2 unit | ☺<br>☺ | ☺<br>☺ | 8¾<br>17¾ |
| Macadamia nuts, raw | hand<br>1.06oz/30g | ☺ | ☺<br>☺ | ☺<br>☺ | ☺<br>☺ |
| Macaroni or pasta salad, with meat, egg, mayo dressing | portion<br>4.94oz/140g | ☺ | ☺+ ×¼ unit<br>☺+ ×¼ unit | ☹<br>1¼ | 1½ A<br>3 |
| Mai Tai | glass<br>8.4ozfl/240ml | ☺ | ☺+ ×½ unit<br>☺+ ×¼ unit | ☹<br>1¾ | ☺<br>☺ |
| Maitake mushrooms, raw | tbsp.<br>0.5ozfl/14.21ml | 60½<br>+50½ unit | ☺+ ×½ unit<br>☺+ ×¼ unit | ☹<br>¾ | ☺<br>☺ |
| Malt liquor | glass<br>8.4ozfl/240ml | ☺ | 50<br>☺ | ☹<br>10 | ☺<br>☺ |
| Mamba® Fruit Chews | portion<br>1.42oz/40g | ☺ | ☺<br>☺+ ×11 unit | ☹<br>☹ | ☺<br>☺ |
| Mamba® Sour Fruit Chews | portion<br>1.42oz/40g | ☺ | ☹²<br>☹² | ☹<br>☹ | ☺<br>☺ |
| Mandarin orange, fresh | portion<br>4.94oz/140g | ☺ | 1¼<br>2½ | ☺<br>☺ | 2¼ B<br>4½ |
| Mango nectar | glass<br>8.4ozfl/240ml | ☺ | 1<br>2 | ☹<br>1¼ | ☺ B<br>☺ |
| Mango, fresh | tbsp.<br>0.5ozfl/14.21ml | ☺ | 1<br>2¼ | ☹<br>4 | ☺ B<br>☺ |
| Mangosteen, fresh | portion<br>4.94oz/140g | ☺ | 35½<br>71¼ | ☺<br>☺ | ☺<br>☺ |
| Manhattan | glass<br>8.4ozfl/240ml | ☺ | ½<br>1 | ☹<br>2 | ☺<br>☺ |
| Maple syrup, pure | tbsp.<br>0.5ozfl/14.21ml | ☺ | ☺+ ×¼ unit<br>☺ | ☺<br>☺ | ☺<br>☺ |

| Keyword Index | Unit | Lactose ⌇ + unit/ 💊 | Fructose* ⌇ Fructose* ⌇ | Sorbitol ⌇ Sorbitol ⌇ | FrucGalactans ⌇ FrucGalactans ⌇📖 |
|---|---|---|---|---|---|
| Margarine, diet, fat free | portion 0.5oz/14g | 15½ +13 unit | ☺ ☺ | ☺ ☺ | 86¾ ☺ |
| Margarine, tub, salted, sunflower oil | portion 0.5oz/14g | 30 +25 unit | ☺ ☺ | ☺ ☺ | ☺ ☺ |
| Margarita, frozen | glass 8.4ozfl/240ml | ☺ | ☺+ ×¼ unit ☺ | ☹ 7 | ☺ ☺ |
| Marmalade, sugar free with aspartame | portion 0.6oz/17g | ☺ | 15¾ 31¾ | ☹ 5¼ | ☺ ☺ |
| Marmalade, sugar free with saccharin | portion 0.57oz/16g | ☺ | 2 4¼ | ☹ 16¾ | ☺ ☺ |
| Marmalade, sugar free with sucralose | portion 0.6oz/17g | ☺ | ☺ ☺ | ☹ 65¼ | ☺ ☺ |
| Marshmallow | portion 1.06oz/30g | ☺ | ☺+ ×4½ unit ☺+ ×2¼ unit | ☺ ☺ | ☺ ☺ |
| Martini* | glass 8.4ozfl/240ml | ☺ | 83¼ ☺ | ☹ 3¼ | ☺ ☺ |
| Mascarpone | portion 1.06oz/30g | 2½ +2 unit | ☺ ☺ | ☺ ☺ | 13¾ 27¾ |
| McDonald's® apple slices | piece 1.2oz/34g | ☺ | ¼ ¾ | ☹ ¼ | ☺ ☺ |
| McDonald's® barbecue sauce | portion 1.1ozfl/31ml | ☺ | ☺+ ×1½ unit ☺+ ×¾ unit | ☹ 1¾ | ☺ ☺ |
| McDonald's® Big Mac® | piece 7.59oz/215g | 9¾ +8¼ unit | 5 10¼ | ☹ 6½ | ¼ A ½ |
| McDonald's® caramel sundae® | portion 6.42ozfl/182ml | ¼ +¼ unit | ☺+ ×6¾ unit ☺+ ×3¼ unit | ☺ ☺ | 1¾ 3¾ |
| McDonald's® Cheeseburger | piece 4.03oz/114g | 9¾ +8¼ unit | 3¾ 7¾ | ☹ 5 | ¼ A ¾ |
| McDonald's® Chicken McNuggets® | piece 0.58oz/16.25g | ☺ | ☺ ☺ | ☺ ☺ | 10¾ A 21½ |
| McDonald's® chocolate chip cookies | piece 1.17oz/33g | ☺ | ☺+ ×½ unit ☺+ ×¼ unit | ☹ ☺ | ¾ A 1½ |

⌇ *Level 0*: lactose measure ×½    + Unit/💊: added tolerated amount of unit per strong lactase capsule
⌇ *Level 1*: fructose measure ×2    Fructose*: fructose, sorbitol adjusted
⌇ *Level 2*: fructose-/sorbitol measure ×4. the rest ×2    ☺+ ×[Amount] unit: Per unit consumed you can additionally tolerate up to [amount] × fructose(*)-unit of another product.
⌇ *Level 3*: sorbitol measure ×7. the rest ×3
📖: source of fruc/galactans data

☹: avoid;   ☹¹: ¼ at TL 1;   ☹²: ¼ at TL 2;   ☹³: ¼ at TL 3;   ☺: only contains traces;   ☺: is free from it

| KEYWORD INDEX | Unit | Lactose ☺ + unit/🥛 | Fructose* ☺ Fructose* ☹ | Sorbitol ☺ Sorbitol ☹ | FrucGalactans ☺ FrucGalactans ☹ |
|---|---|---|---|---|---|
| McDonald's® chocolate milk | cup 5.2ozfl/150ml | ¼ +¼ unit | ☺+ ×2 unit ☺+ ×1 unit | ☺ ☺ | 1¾ 3¾ |
| McDonald's® Crispy Chicken Snack Wrap with ranch sauce | piece 4.17ozfl/118ml | 62 +51½ unit | ☺ ☺ | ☹ 84½ | ¼ A ½ |
| McDonald's® Double Cheeseburger | piece 5.83oz/165g | 4¾ +4 unit | 4½ 9 | ☹ 4¼ | ¼ A ½ |
| McDonald's® Filet-O-Fish® | piece 5.01oz/142g | 19¾ +16½ unit | 2 4 | ☹ 70¼ | ¼ A ¾ |
| McDonald's® French fries | portion 2.47oz/70g | ☺ | ☺ ☺ | ☹ 35½ | ☺ ☺ |
| McDonald's® Hamburger | piece 3.53oz/100g | ☺ | 3¾ 7¾ | ☹ 5 | ½ A 1 |
| McDonald's® hot fudge sundae® | portion 6.32ozfl/179ml | ¼ +¼ unit | ☺+ ×7½ unit ☺+ ×3¾ unit | ☹ 55¾ | 1¼ G 2½ |
| McDonald's® hot mustard sauce | portion 0.71ozfl/20ml | ☺ | ☺+ ×1¼ unit ☺+ ×½ unit | ☺ ☺ | ☺ ☺ |
| McDonald's® M & M's® McFlurry® | portion 8.05ozfl/228ml | ☹² +0,18 unit | ☺+ ×3½ unit ☺+ ×1¾ unit | ☺ ☺ | 1 2¼ |
| McDonald's® McCafe® shakes, chocolate flavors | portion 7.41ozfl/210ml | ¼ +¼ unit | ☺+ ×5¾ unit ☺+ ×2¾ unit | ☹ 15¾ | 1½ 3¼ |
| McDonald's® McCafe® shakes, vanilla or other flavors | portion 7.27ozfl/206ml | ¼ +¼ unit | ☺+ ×¼ unit ☺ | ☹ 12 | 1½ 3¼ |
| McDonald's® McChicken® | piece 5.05oz/143g | ☺ | 1½ 3 | ☹ 69¾ | ¼ A ¾ |
| McDonald's® McDouble® | piece 5.33oz/151g | 9¾ +8¼ unit | 4¼ 8¾ | ☹ 4¼ | ¼ A ½ |
| McDonald's® McRib® | piece 7.34oz/208g | ☺ | ☺+ ×¾ unit ☺+ ×¼ unit | ☹ 1¾ | ¼ A ½ |
| McDonald's® Newman's Own® Creamy Caesar salad dressing | portion 1.06oz/30g | 18¼ +15¼ unit | 26¾ 53¾ | ☹ 7¼ | ☺ ☺ |
| McDonald's® Newman's Own® Low Fat Balsamic Vinaigrette salad dressing | portion 1.06ozfl/30ml | ☺ | ☺ ☺ | ☺ ☺ | ☺ ☺ |
| McDonald's® orange juice | glass 8.4ozfl/240ml | ☺ | 1½ 3¼ | ☹ ¼ | ☺ ☺ |
| McDonald's® Quarter Pounder | piece 6.11oz/173g | ☺ | 48 ☺ | ☹ 2½ | ¼ A ½ |
| McDonald's® Sausage & EGG® McMuffin® | piece 5.79oz/164g | 9¾ +8¼ unit | ☺+ ×1 unit ☺+ ×½ unit | ☺ ☺ | ¼ A ½ |

| Keyword Index | Unit | Lactose ↧ + unit/⊙ | Fructose* ⊙ Fructose* ↧ | Sorbitol ⊙ Sorbitol ↧ | FrucGalactans ⊙ FrucGalactans ↧ 📖 |
|---|---|---|---|---|---|
| McDonald's® side salad | portion 3.53oz/100g | ☺ | 3¾ 7½ | ⊙ 2½ | ☺ ☺ |
| McDonald's® smoothies, all flavors | glass 8.4oz/240g | 2¾ +2¼ unit | 3¾ 7¾ | ☹ 1¼ | 15½ 31 |
| McDonald's® Southwestern chipotle barbecue sauce | portion 1.1ozfl/31ml | ☺ | ☺+ ×1¾ unit ☺+ ×¾ unit | ☹ 2¾ | ☺ ☺ |
| McDonald's® sweet and sour sauce | portion 1.06ozfl/30ml | ☺ | ¼ ¾ | ☹ 41½ | ☺ ☺ |
| Meat ravioli, with tomato sauce | portion 8.82oz/250g | ☺ | ☺+ ×½ unit ☺+ ×¼ unit | ☹ ½ | ¼ A ¾ |
| Meatloaf, pork | portion 3oz/85g | 2¼ +2 unit | ☺+ ×¼ unit ☺ | ☹ 3½ | ☺ ☺ |
| Meatloaf, tuna | portion 3oz/85g | 5½ +4½ unit | ☺ ☺ | ☹ 14½ | ☺ ☺ |
| Melba Toast®, Classic (Old London®) | portion 0.53oz/15g | ☺ | ☺+ ×¼ unit ☺ | ☹ ☺ | ½ A 1¼ |
| Mentos® | piece 0.11oz/3g | ☺ | ☺ ☺ | ☺ ☺ | ☺ ☺ |
| Merlot, red | glass 8.4ozfl/240ml | ☺ | 17¾ 35½ | ☹ ½ | ☺ ☺ |
| Merlot, white | glass 8.4ozfl/240ml | ☺ | ¾ 1¾ | ☺ ☺ | ☺ ☺ |
| Milk chocolate bar, cereal | bar 4.77oz/135g | ½ +½ unit | ☺ ☺ | ☹ 40 | ¼ A ¾ |
| Milk chocolate bar, cereal, sugar free | piece 0.43ozfl/12g | 26½ +22 unit | 80 ☺ | ☹ ☹ | 4½ A 9 |
| Milk chocolate bar, sugar free | piece 0.43ozfl/12g | 32½ +27 unit | 80 ☺ | ☹ ☹ | 4½ 9 |
| Milk Chocolate covered raisins | hand 1.06oz/30g | 2¾ +2¼ unit | ☺+ ×¼ unit ☺ | ☹ 3¼ | 3¼ G 6½ |
| Milk, lactose reduced (Lactaid®), skim (fat free) | glass 8.4oz/240g | ☺ | ☺+ ×10 unit ☺+ ×5 unit | ☺ ☺ | ☺ ☺ |
| Milk, lactose reduced (Lactaid®), whole | cup 5.2ozfl/150ml | ☺ | ☺+ ×7½ unit ☺+ ×3¾ unit | ☺ ☺ | ☺ ☺ |

⊙ *Level 0*: lactose measure ×½    + Unit/⊙: added tolerated amount of unit per strong lactase capsule
↧ *Level 1*: fructose measure ×2    Fructose*: fructose, sorbitol adjusted
↯ *Level 2*: fructose-/sorbitol measure ×4. the rest ×2    ☺+ ×[Amount] unit: Per unit consumed you can additionally tolerate up to [amount] × fructose(*)-unit of another product.
↯ *Level 3*: sorbitol measure ×7. the rest ×3
📖: source of fruc/galactans data

☹: avoid;   ☹¹: ¼ at TL 1;   ☹²: ¼ at TL 2;   ☹³: ¼ at TL 3;   ☺: only contains traces;   ☺: is free from it

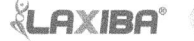 The Nutrition Navigator

| Keyword Index | Unit | Lactose ↲ + unit/🥛 | Fructose* ↲ Fructose* ↲ | Sorbitol ↲ Sorbitol ↲ | FrucGalactans ↲ FrucGalactans ↲ |
|---|---|---|---|---|---|
| Milk, lactose reduced, skim (fat free), fortified with calcium (Lactaid®) | glass 8.4ozfl/240g | ☺ | ☺+ ×10 unit ☺+ ×5 unit | ☺ ☺ | ☺ ☺ |
| Milk, unprepared dry powder, nonfat, instant | portion 0.78ozfl/22ml | ¼ +0,21 unit | ☺ ☺ | ☺ ☺ | 1¼ 2¾ |
| Mineral Water | glass 8.4ozfl/240ml | ☺ | ☺ ☺ | ☺ ☺ | ☺ ☺ |
| Minestrone soup, condensed | portion 4.45oz/126g | ☺ | ☺ ☺ | ☹ ¾ | ½ 1 |
| Minestrone soup, homemade | portion 8.65oz/245g | ☺ | ☺ ☺ | ☹ 1 | ¼ ½ |
| Mint Julep | glass 8.4ozfl/240ml | ☺ | ☺ ☺ | ☺ ☺ | ☺ ☺ |
| Mocha, without flavored syrup | cup 5.2ozfl/150ml | ½ +¼ unit | ☺+ ×1¾ unit ☺+ ×¾ unit | ☺ ☺ | 3 6 |
| Mojito | glass 8.4ozfl/240ml | ☺ | ☺ ☺ | ☺ ☺ | ☺ ☺ |
| Molasses cookies, store bought | piece 0.53oz/15g | ☺ | ☺ ☺ | ☺ ☺ | 3¼ ᴬ 6¾ |
| Molasses, dark | tbsp. 0.5ozfl/14.21ml | ☺ | 3¾ 7½ | ☺ ☺ | ☺ ☺ |
| Monster® Energy® | glass 8.4ozfl/240ml | ☺ | ☺+ ×17½ unit ☺+ ×8¾ unit | ☺ ☺ | ☺ ☺ |
| Monster® Khaos | portion 8.47oz/240g | ☺ | ☺+ ×9 unit ☺+ ×4¾ unit | ☹ ¼ | ☺ ☺ |
| Morel mushrooms, raw | tbsp. 0.5ozfl/14.21ml | ☺ | ☺ ☺ | ☹ ¾ | ☺ ☺ |
| Mortadella | portion 1.95oz/55g | ☺ | ☺+ ×¼ unit ☺ | ☺ ☺ | ☺ ☺ |
| Mountain Dew® | glass 8.4ozfl/240ml | ☺ | ☹¹ ¼ | ☺ ☺ | ☺ ☺ |
| Mountain Dew® Code Red | glass 8.4ozfl/240ml | ☺ | ☹¹ ¼ | ☺ ☺ | ☺ ☺ |
| Mozzarella cheese, fat free | portion 1.06oz/30g | ½ +½ unit | ☺ ☺ | ☺ ☺ | 3½ 7¼ |
| Mozzarella cheese, whole milk | portion 1.06oz/30g | 9¾ +8¼ unit | ☺ ☺ | ☺ ☺ | 55 ☺ |
| Mrs. Paul's® Calamari Rings | portion 3oz/85g | ☺ | ☺ ☺ | ☺ ☺ | 2¼ ᴬ 4½ |

| Keyword Index | Unit | Lactose ☺/ + unit/📖 | Fructose* ☺/ Fructose* ☺/ | Sorbitol ☺/ Sorbitol ☺/ | FrucGalactans ☺/ FrucGalactans ☺/📖 |
|---|---|---|---|---|---|
| Muenster cheese, natural | portion 1.06oz/30g | 8¾ +7¼ unit | ☺ ☺ | ☺ ☺ | 49½ ☺ |
| Mueslix® (Kellogg's®) | portion 1.95oz/55g | ☺ | ☺+ ×¾ unit ☺+ ×¼ unit | ☹ 2¾ | ¼ A ¾ |
| Muffins, banana | piece 3.99oz/113g | 2½ +2 unit | ☺+ ×¼ unit ☺ | ☹ 29¼ | ¼ A ¾ |
| Muffins, blueberry, store bought | piece 3.99oz/113g | 1½ +1¼ unit | ☺ ☺ | ☺ ☺ | ¼ A ¾ |
| Muffins, carrot, homemade, with nuts | piece 3.99oz/113g | 1½ +1¼ unit | ☺ ☺ | ☹ 3¼ | ¼ A ¾ |
| Muffins, oat bran or oatmeal, store bought | piece 3.99oz/113g | 1¼ +1 unit | ☺+ ×¼ unit ☺ | ☺ ☺ | ½ A 1 |
| Muffins, pumpkin, store bought | piece 3.99oz/113g | 1¾ +1¼ unit | ☺+ ×¼ unit ☺ | ☹ 14½ | ¼ A ¾ |
| Mulberries | portion 4.94oz/140g | ☺ | ½ 1¼ | ☺ ☺ | ☺ ☺ |
| Mung beans, cooked from dried | portion 3.18oz/90g | ☺ | ½ 1¼ | ☺ ☺ | ¾ A 1¾ |
| Murray® Sugar Free Oatmeal Cookies | piece 0.39oz/11g | ☺ | ½ 1¼ | ☹ ☹² | 4½ A 9 |
| Murray® Sugar Free Shortbread | piece 0.14oz/3.75g | ☺ | 1½ 3¼ | ☹ ☹² | 10½ A 21¼ |
| Muscatel | glass 8.4ozfl/240ml | ☺ | ☹² ☹² | ☹ ½ | ☺ ☺ |
| Mushroom gravy, canned | tbsp. 0.5ozfl/14.21ml | 75¼ +62¾ unit | ☺ ☺ | ☹ 2¼ | ☺ ☺ |
| Mushrooms, batter dipped or breaded | portion 2.47oz/70g | ☺ | ☺ ☺ | ☹ ¼ | 2½ B 5¼ |
| Muskmelon | portion 4.94oz/140g | ☺ | 1¼ 2½ | ☺ ☺ | 1½ B 3¼ |
| Nabisco® 100 Calorie Packs, Honey Maid Cinnamon Roll Thin Crisps | piece 0.46oz/13g | ☺ | ☺ ☺ | ☹ 42½ | 4¾ A 9¾ |

☺/ Level 0: lactose measure ×½    + Unit/📖: added tolerated amount of unit per strong lactase capsule
☺/ Level 1: fructose measure ×2    Fructose*: fructose, sorbitol adjusted

☺/ Level 2: fructose-/sorbitol measure ×4. the rest ×2    ☺+ ×[Amount] unit: Per unit consumed you can
☺/ Level 3: sorbitol measure ×7. the rest ×3    additionally tolerate up to [amount] ×
📖: source of fruc/galactans data    fructose(*)-unit of another product.

☹: avoid;    ☹¹: ¼ at TL 1;    ☹²: ¼ at TL 2;    ☹³: ¼ at TL 3;    ☺: only contains traces;    ☺: is free from it

| Keyword Index | Unit | Lactose 🠗 + unit/ | Fructose* 🠗 Fructose* 🠗 | Sorbitol 🠗 Sorbitol 🠗 | FrucGalactans 🠗 FrucGalactans 🠗 |
|---|---|---|---|---|---|
| Nectarine, fresh | tbsp. 0.5ozfl/14.21ml | ☺ | 8¼ 16½ | ☹ 1 | 5½ [B] 11¼ |
| Nestea® 100% Tea, unsweetened, dry | glass 8.4ozfl/240ml | ☺ | ☺+ ×22 unit ☺+ ×11 unit | ☺ ☺ | ☺ ☺ |
| Nestea® Iced Tea, Sugar Free, dry | glass 8.4ozfl/240ml | ☺ | ☺+ ×11½ unit ☺+ ×5¾ unit | ☺ ☺ | ☺ ☺ |
| Nestea® Iced Tea, Sugar Free, prepared | glass 8.4ozfl/240ml | ☺ | ☺ ☺ | ☺ ☺ | ☺ ☺ |
| Nestea® Iced Tea, sweetened with sugar, dry | glass 8.4ozfl/240ml | ☺ | ☺ ☺ | ☺ ☺ | ☺ ☺ |
| Nestle® Hot Cocoa Dark Chocolate, prepared | cup 5.2ozfl/150ml | ¼ +¼ unit | ☺+ ×½ unit ☺+ ×¼ unit | ☹ ☺ | 1¾ 3¾ |
| Nestle® Hot Cocoa Rich Milk Chocolate, prepared | cup 5.2ozfl/150ml | ¼ +¼ unit | ☺ ☺ | ☺ ☺ | 1¾ 3¾ |
| Newman's Own® Organic Pretzels, Spelt | slice 1.49oz/42g | ☺ | ☺+ ×½ unit ☺+ ×¼ unit | ☺ ☺ | ¾ [A] 1½ |
| Nilla Wafers® (Nabisco®) | piece 0.14oz/3.75g | 32½ +27 unit | ☺ ☺ | ☺ ☺ | 12¼ [A] 24¾ |
| No Fear® | glass 8.4ozfl/240ml | ☺ | ☺+ ×6¼ unit ☺+ ×3 unit | ☹ 50 | ☺ ☺ |
| No Fear® Sugar Free | glass 8.4ozfl/240ml | ☺ | ☺ ☺ | ☺ ☺ | ☺ ☺ |
| Non-alcoholic wine | glass 8.4ozfl/240ml | ☺ | 2¼ 4½ | ☹ 50 | ☺ ☺ |
| Noodle soup mix, dry | portion 0.57oz/16g | ☺ | ☺+ ×¼ unit ☺ | ☺ ☺ | 6¼ [CB] 12½ |
| Northland® Cranberry Juice, all flavors | glass 8.4ozfl/240ml | ☺ | ☺+ ×7¼ unit ☺+ ×3½ unit | ☹ 25 | ☺ ☺ |
| Nougat | bar 4.77oz/135g | ☺ | ☺+ ×18 unit ☺+ ×9 unit | ☺ ☺ | ¼ ¾ |
| Nutella® (filbert spread) | portion 1.31oz/37g | 32¼ +27 unit | 67½ ☺ | ☹ 20¾ | 1¼ [G] 2¾ |
| Nutter Butter® Cookies (Nabisco®) | portion 0.5oz/14g | ☺ | ☺ ☺ | ☺ ☺ | 3½ [A] 7¼ |
| Oat milk | glass 8.4oz/240g | ☺ | ☺ ☺ | ☺ ☺ | ¼ [A] ¾ |

| Keyword Index | Unit | Lactose ↳<br>+ unit/ 💊 | Fructose* ♀<br>Fructose* ↳ | Sorbitol ♀<br>Sorbitol ↳ | FrucGalactans ♀<br>FrucGalactans ↳ 📖 |
|---|---|---|---|---|---|
| Oatmeal cookies, store bought | piece<br>0.46oz/13g | 45¾<br>+38 unit | ☺<br>☺ | ☺<br>☺ | 3¾ A<br>7½ |
| Okra, raw | portion<br>3oz/85g | ☺ | 2¼<br>4½ | ☺<br>☺ | 2 CB<br>4¼ |
| Old Dutch® Crunch Curls | hand<br>0.75oz/21g | 4<br>+3¼ unit | ☺<br>☺ | ☹<br>☺ | 7¼ A<br>14½ |
| Omelet, made with bacon | portion<br>3.89oz/110g | 34¾<br>+29 unit | ☺+ ×1¾ unit<br>☺+ ×¾ unit | ☺<br>☺ | ☺<br>☺ |
| Omelet, made with sausage, potatoes, onions, cheese | portion<br>3.89oz/110g | 52¼<br>+43½ unit | ☺+ ×1 unit<br>☺+ ×½ unit | ☹<br>6¾ | ¼ CB<br>½ |
| Onion, white, yellow or red, raw | tbsp.<br>0.5ozfl/14.21ml | ☺ | ☺<br>☺ | ☹<br>6 | 1 CB<br>2 |
| Orange kiwi passion juice | glass<br>8.4ozfl/240ml | ☺ | ☺<br>☺ | ☹<br>¾ | ☺ B<br>☺ |
| Orange peel | tbsp.<br>0.5ozfl/14.21ml | ☺ | 3¼<br>6½ | ☺<br>☺ | ☺<br>☺ |
| Orange, fresh | portion<br>4.94oz/140g | ☺ | 2¼<br>4¾ | ☺<br>☺ | 2¼ B<br>4½ |
| Oregano, dried | pinch<br>0.04oz/1g | ☺ | ☺<br>☺ | ☺<br>☺ | ☺<br>☺ |
| Oreo® Brownie Cookies (Nabisco®) | piece<br>1.5oz/42.5g | ☺ | ¼<br>¾ | ☹<br>☺ | 1 A<br>2¼ |
| Oreo® Cookies (Nabisco®) | piece<br>0.43oz/12g | ☺ | ☺<br>☺ | ☹<br>☺ | 4¼ A<br>8½ |
| Oreo® Cookies, Sugar Free (Nabisco®) | piece<br>0.43oz/12g | ☺ | 13¾<br>27¾ | ☹<br>☹ | 4¼ A<br>8½ |
| Ouzo | glass<br>8.4ozfl/240ml | ☺ | ☺+ ×4½ unit<br>☺+ ×2½ unit | ☹<br>¼ | ☺<br>☺ |
| Oyster mushrooms, raw | portion<br>3oz/85g | ☺ | ☺+ ×1¾ unit<br>☺+ ×¾ unit | ☹<br>¼ | ☺<br>☺ |
| Pad thai, without meat | portion<br>4.94oz/140g | ☺ | ☺<br>☺ | ☹<br>3¾ | ☺ A<br>☺ |

♀ *Level 0*: lactose measure ×½  
↳ *Level 1*: fructose measure ×2  
↳ *Level 2*: fructose-/sorbitol measure ×4. the rest ×2  
↳ *Level 3*: sorbitol measure ×7. the rest ×3  
📖: source of fruc/galactans data  
☹: avoid;   ☹¹: ¼ at TL 1;   ☹²: ¼ at TL 2;   ☹³: ¼ at TL 3;   ☺: only contains traces;   ☺: is free from it

+ Unit/💊: added tolerated amount of unit per strong lactase capsule  
Fructose*: fructose, sorbitol adjusted  
☺+ ×[Amount] unit: Per unit consumed you can additionally tolerate up to [amount] × fructose(*)-unit of another product.

| Keyword Index | Unit | Lactose<br>+ unit/ | Fructose*<br>Fructose* | Sorbitol<br>Sorbitol | FrucGalactans<br>FrucGalactans |
|---|---|---|---|---|---|
| Paella | portion<br>8.47oz/240g | ☺ | 2¼<br>4½ | ☹<br>2¼ | 1<br>2 |
| Palm kernel oil | tbsp.<br>0.5ozfl/14.21ml | ☺ | ☺<br>☺ | ☺<br>☺ | ☺<br>☺ |
| Pancake, buckwheat, from mix, add water only | piece<br>1.56oz/44g | ☺ | ☺<br>☺ | ☹<br>3¾ | 1¼ A<br>2½ |
| Pancake, whole wheat, homemade | piece<br>1.56oz/44g | 2½<br>+2 unit | ☺<br>☺ | ☺<br>☺ | 1 A<br>2¼ |
| Papaya, fresh | portion<br>4.94oz/140g | ☺ | ☺+ ×1 unit<br>☺+ ×½ unit | ☺<br>☺ | ☺<br>☺ |
| Parmesan cheese, dry (grated) | portion<br>0.18oz/5g | ☺ | ☺<br>☺ | ☺<br>☺ | ☺<br>☺ |
| Parmesan cheese, dry (grated), nonfat | portion<br>0.18oz/5g | ☺<br>+75¾ unit | ☺<br>☺ | ☺<br>☺ | ☺<br>☺ |
| Parsley, fresh | pinch<br>0.04oz/1g | ☺ | ☺<br>☺ | ☹<br>☺ | ☺<br>☺ |
| Parsnip, cooked | portion<br>3oz/85g | ☺ | ☺+ ×¼ unit<br>☺ | ☺<br>☺ | ☺ C<br>☺ |
| Passion fruit (maracuya), fresh | portion<br>4.94oz/140g | ☺ | ☺+ ×2½ unit<br>☺+ ×1¼ unit | ☺<br>☺ | ☺<br>☺ |
| Passion fruit juice | glass<br>8.4ozfl/240ml | ☺ | ☺+ ×3¾ unit<br>☺+ ×1¾ unit | ☺<br>☺ | ☺<br>☺ |
| Pasta salad with vegetables, Italian dressing | portion<br>4.94oz/140g | ☺ | 3¾<br>7½ | ☹<br>1½ | 1½ A<br>3¼ |
| Peach juice | glass<br>8.4ozfl/240ml | ☺ | ¾<br>1½ | ☹<br>¾ | ½ B<br>1¼ |
| Peach pie, bottom crust only | piece<br>4.31oz/122g | ☺ | 2¾<br>5½ | ☹<br>1 | ¼ A<br>¾ |
| Peach, fresh | portion<br>4.94oz/140g | ☺ | ☺+ ×½ unit<br>☺+ ×½ unit | ☹<br>¼ | 2¼ B<br>4½ |
| Peanut butter, unsalted | portion<br>1.13oz/32g | ☺ | ☺+ ×¼ unit<br>☺ | ☺<br>☺ | ☺ G<br>☺ |
| Peanut sauce, store bought | portion<br>1.24oz/35g | ☺ | ☺<br>☺ | ☹<br>8¼ | ☺ G<br>☺ |
| Peanuts, dry roasted, salted | hand<br>1.06oz/30g | ☺ | ☺<br>☺ | ☺<br>☺ | ☺ G<br>☺ |
| Pear juice | glass<br>8.4ozfl/240ml | ☺ | ☹ 2<br>☹ 2 | ☹<br>☹ 3 | 1½ C<br>3 |
| Pear, fresh | tbsp<br>0.5ozfl/14.21ml | ☺ | ½<br>1 | ☹<br>¼ | ☺ B<br>☺ |

| KEYWORD INDEX | Unit | Lactose ☺ + unit/ 💊 | Fructose* ☺ Fructose* ☻ | Sorbitol ☺ Sorbitol ☻ | FrucGalactans ☺ FrucGalactans ☻ 📖 |
|---|---|---|---|---|---|
| Pecan praline | piece<br>1.95oz/55g | 3½<br>+2¾ unit | ☺+ ×1¼ unit<br>☺+ ×½ unit | ☺<br>☺ | 1¼ ᴳ<br>2¾ |
| Pepperidge Farm® Sweet & Simple, Soft Baked Sugar Cookies | piece<br>0.48oz/13.5g | ☺ | ☻¹<br>¼ | ☺<br>☺ | 4¾ ᴬ<br>9½ |
| Pepperidge Farm® Turnover, Apple | piece<br>3.14oz/89g | 9<br>+7½ unit | ½<br>1¼ | ☻<br>¼ | ½ ᴬ<br>1¼ |
| Peppermint, fresh | pinch<br>0.04oz/1g | ☺ | ☺<br>☺ | ☺<br>☺ | ☺<br>☺ |
| Pepsi® | glass<br>8.4ozfl/240ml | ☺ | ½<br>1¼ | ☺<br>☺ | ☺<br>☺ |
| Pepsi® Max | glass<br>8.4ozfl/240ml | ☺ | ☺<br>☺ | ☺<br>☺ | ☺<br>☺ |
| Pepsi® Twist | glass<br>8.4ozfl/240ml | ☺ | ½<br>1¼ | ☺<br>☺ | ☺<br>☺ |
| Persimmon, fresh | piece<br>4.94oz/140g | ☺ | 2¾<br>5¾ | ☺<br>☺ | 1 ᶜ<br>2 |
| Pesto sauce, store bought | portion<br>2.19oz/62g | ☺ | ☺<br>☺ | ☺<br>☺ | 1¾ ᴬ<br>3¾ |
| Pho soup (Vietnamese noodle soup) | portion<br>8.65oz/245g | ☺ | ☺<br>☺ | ☻<br>6¾ | ¾<br>1¾ |
| Pickled beef | portion<br>1.95oz/55g | ☺ | ☺<br>☺ | ☺<br>☺ | ☺<br>☺ |
| Pickled beets | portion<br>1.06oz/30g | ☺ | ☺<br>☺ | ☻<br>15 | 3 ᶜᴮ<br>6 |
| Pillsbury® Big Deluxe White Chunk Macadamia Nut Cookies | piece<br>1.35oz/38g | 6¾<br>+5½ unit | ☺<br>☺ | ☺<br>☺ | ½ ᴬ<br>1¼ |
| Pina colada | glass<br>8.4ozfl/240ml | ☺ | ☺+ ×1¼ unit<br>☺+ ×½ unit | ☻<br>4 | ☺<br>☺ |
| Pine nuts, pignolias | hand<br>1.06oz/30g | ☺ | ☺<br>☺ | ☺<br>☺ | 2¾ ᴳ<br>5¾ |
| Pineapple juice | glass<br>8.4ozfl/240ml | ☺ | ☺+ ×3¼ unit<br>☺+ ×1½ unit | ☻<br>1¾ | 1½ ᶜᴮ<br>3 |

☺ *Level 0*: lactose measure ×½   + Unit/ 💊: added tolerated amount of unit per strong lactase capsule
☻ *Level 1*: fructose measure ×2   Fructose*: fructose, sorbitol adjusted
☻ *Level 2*: fructose-/sorbitol measure ×4. the rest ×2   ☺+ ×[Amount] unit: Per unit consumed you can
☻ *Level 3*: sorbitol measure ×7. the rest ×3   additionally tolerate up to [amount] ×
📖: source of fruc/galactans data   fructose(*)-unit of another product.
☻: avoid;   ☻¹: ¼ at TL 1;   ☻²: ¼ at TL 2;   ☻³: ¼ at TL 3;   ☺: only contains traces;   ☺: is free from it

| Keyword Index | Unit + unit/ | Lactose | Fructose* / Fructose* | Sorbitol / Sorbitol | FrucGalactans / FrucGalactans |
|---|---|---|---|---|---|
| Pineapple orange drink | glass<br>8.4ozfl/240ml | ☺ | ¾<br>1½ | ☺<br>☺ | 1½ CB<br>3 |
| Pineapple, dried | portion<br>1.42oz/40g | ☺ | ½<br>1¼ | ☹<br>½ | 2 CB<br>4 |
| Pineapple, fresh | portion<br>4.94oz/140g | ☺ | ¾<br>1¾ | ☹<br>¾ | 2¼ CB<br>4½ |
| Pistachio nuts, raw | hand<br>0.75oz/21g | ☺ | ☺<br>☺ | ☺<br>☺ | ¼ G<br>¾ |
| Pizza Hut® cheese bread stick | piece<br>1.98oz/56g | 61½<br>+51¼ unit | ☺+ ×¼ unit<br>☺ | ☺<br>☺ | 1¼ A<br>2½ |
| Pizza Hut® Pepperoni Lover's pizza, stuffed crust | portion<br>4.94oz/140g | 30<br>+25 unit | ☺<br>☺ | ☹<br>1 | ¾ A<br>1½ |
| Pizza Hut® Personal Pan, supreme | piece<br>9.03oz/256g | 16¾<br>+14 unit | ☺<br>☺ | ☹<br>¼ | 4¾ A<br>9½ |
| Pizza, homemade or restaurant, cheese, thin crust | piece<br>7.38oz/209g | 12¼<br>+10¼ unit | ☺+ ×¾ unit<br>☺+ ×¼ unit | ☹<br>¾ | ½ A<br>1 |
| Plain dumplings for stew, biscuit type | portion<br>1.95oz/55g | 1¾<br>+1½ unit | ☺<br>☺ | ☺<br>☺ | ½ A<br>1 |
| Plantains, green, boiled | piece<br>7.87oz/223g | ☺ | ¾<br>1¾ | ☺<br>☺ | ¼ FB<br>¾ |
| Plum, fresh | tbsp.<br>0.5ozfl/14.21ml | ☺ | ☺+ ×¼ unit<br>☺+ ×¼ unit | ☹<br>¾ | 21½ C<br>43 |
| Polenta | portion<br>8.47oz/240g | ½<br>+½ unit | ☺+ ×¼ unit<br>☺ | ☹<br>20¾ | 3¼ B<br>6¾ |
| Pomegranate juice | glass<br>8.4ozfl/240ml | ☺ | ¾<br>1½ | ☹<br>☹² | ☺<br>☺ |
| Pomegranate, fresh (arils-seed/juice sacs) | tbsp.<br>0.5ozfl/14.21ml | ☺ | ☺+ ×½ unit<br>☺+ ×¼ unit | ☹<br>2 | ☺<br>☺ |
| Poore Brothers® Potato Chips, Salt & Cracked Pepper | hand<br>0.75oz/21g | ☺ | 54<br>☺ | ☹<br>☺ | 10¾ A<br>21½ |
| Popcorn, store bought (prepopped), "buttered" | portion<br>1.06oz/30g | 36¾<br>+30¾ unit | ☺<br>☺ | ☺<br>☺ | ☺ CB<br>☺ |
| Popsicle | piece<br>1.84oz/52g | ☺ | ☺+ ×1¼ unit<br>☺+ ×½ unit | ☺<br>☺ | ☺<br>☺ |
| Popsicle, sugar free | piece<br>1.95oz/55g | ☺ | ☺<br>☺ | ☺<br>☺ | ☺<br>☺ |
| Pork cutlet (sirloin cutlet), visible fat eaten | portion<br>3oz/85g | ☺ | ☺<br>☺ | ☺<br>☺ | 1¼ A<br>2¾ |
| Port wine | glass<br>8.4ozfl/240ml | ☺ | ☹²<br>☹² | ☹<br>½ | ☺<br>☺ |

| KEYWORD INDEX | Unit | Lactose ᒼ + unit/ 💊 | Fructose* ᒼ Fructose* ᒼ | Sorbitol ᒼ Sorbitol ᒼ | FrucGalactans ᒼ FrucGalactans ᒼ 📖 |
|---|---|---|---|---|---|
| Portabella mushrooms, cooked from fresh | tbsp. 0.5ozfl/14.21ml | ☺ | ☺+ ×½ unit ☺+ ×¼ unit | ☹ ½ | 12¼ B 24½ |
| Potato bread | slice 1.2oz/34g | 6¼ +5¼ unit | ☺ ☺ | ☹ ☺ | 1½ A 3 |
| Potato chips, salted | hand 0.75oz/21g | ☺ | 41¾ 83½ | ☹ 79¼ | 10¾ A 21½ |
| Potato dumpling (Kartoffel-kloesse) | portion 4.94oz/140g | 45½ +37¾ unit | ☺+ ×¼ unit ☺ | ☹ 35½ | ☺ C ☺ |
| Potato gnocchi | portion 6.64oz/188g | 2½ +2 unit | ☺ ☺ | ☺ ☺ | 14 A 28¼ |
| Potato pancakes | portion 2.47oz/70g | ☺ | ☺+ ×½ unit ☺+ ×¼ unit | ☹ 12¾ | ☺ B ☺ |
| Potato salad, with egg, mayo dressing | portion 4.94oz/140g | ☺ | ☺+ ×½ unit ☺+ ×¼ unit | ☹ 2 | 1 CB 2 |
| Potato soup with broccoli and cheese | portion 8.65oz/245g | 29¾ +24¾ unit | ☺ ☺ | ☹ 13½ | ½ AC 1 |
| Potato sticks | hand 0.75oz/21g | ☺ | ☺ ☺ | ☹ 79¼ | 10¾ A 21½ |
| Potato, boiled, with skin | portion 3.89oz/110g | ☺ | ☺ ☺ | ☹ 45¼ | ☺ B ☺ |
| Potato, boiled, without skin | portion 3.89oz/110g | ☺ | ☺ ☺ | ☹ 45¼ | ☺ B ☺ |
| Power Bar® 20g Protein Plus, Chocolate Crisp | piece 2.16oz/61g | 3 +2½ unit | ☹¹ ¼ | ☹ ☹ | 4 G 8¼ |
| Power Bar® 20g Protein Plus, Chocolate Peanut Butter | piece 2.16oz/61g | 3 +2½ unit | ☹² ☹² | ☹ ☹ | 17 34¼ |
| Power Bar® 30g Protein Plus, Chocolate Brownie | piece 2.47oz/70g | 2 +1½ unit | ☺+ ×1½ unit ☺+ ×¾ unit | ☹ ☺ | 3¼ G 6½ |
| Power Bar® Harvest Energy®, Double Chocolate Crisp | piece 2.3oz/65g | 2¾ +2¼ unit | ☺+ ×5¾ unit ☺+ ×2¾ unit | ☹ 10¾ | ¼ AG ½ |
| Power Bar® Performance Energy®, Banana | piece 2.3oz/65g | ☺ | ¼ ¾ | ☹ ☺ | 10½ A 21 |

ᒼ *Level 0*: lactose measure ×½  
ᒼ *Level 1*: fructose measure ×2  
ᒼ *Level 2*: fructose-/sorbitol measure ×4. the rest ×2  
ᒼ *Level 3*: sorbitol measure ×7. the rest ×3  
📖: source of fruc/galactans data  

+ Unit/ 💊: added tolerated amount of unit per strong lactase capsule  
Fructose*: fructose, sorbitol adjusted  

☺+ ×[Amount] unit: Per unit consumed you can additionally tolerate up to [amount] × fructose(*)-unit of another product.  

☹: avoid;   ☹¹: ¼ at TL 1;   ☹²: ¼ at TL 2;   ☹³: ¼ at TL 3;   ☺: only contains traces;   ☺: is free from it

| Keyword Index | Unit | Lactose<br>+ unit/ | Fructose*<br>Fructose* | Sorbitol<br>Sorbitol | FrucGalactans<br>FrucGalactans |
|---|---|---|---|---|---|
| Power Bar® Performance Energy®, Chocolate | piece<br>2.3oz/65g | ☺ | ¼<br>¾ | ☹<br>76¾ | 3¼[AG]<br>6¾ |
| Power Bar® Performance Energy®, Cookie Dough | piece<br>2.3oz/65g | ☺ | ¼<br>¾ | ☹<br>☺ | 10½[A]<br>21 |
| Power Bar® Performance Energy®, Mixed Berry Blast | piece<br>2.3oz/65g | ☺ | ¼<br>¾ | ☹<br>19 | 10½[A]<br>21 |
| Power Bar® Performance Energy®, Vanilla Crisp | piece<br>2.3oz/65g | ☺ | ¼<br>¾ | ☹<br>☺ | 10½[A]<br>21 |
| Powerade®, all flavors | glass<br>8.4oz/240g | 7½<br>+6¼ unit | ☺+ ×1¼ unit<br>☺+ ×½ unit | ☺<br>☺ | 41½<br>83¼ |
| Pretzels, hard, unsalted, sticks | hand<br>0.75oz/21g | ☺ | ☺<br>☺ | ☺<br>☺ | 1½[A]<br>3¼ |
| Pringles® Light Fat Free Potato Crisps, Barbecue | hand<br>0.75oz/21g | ☺ | 37<br>74¼ | ☹<br>79¼ | 10¾[A]<br>21½ |
| Pringles® Potato Crisps, Loaded Baked Potato | hand<br>0.75oz/21g | ☺ | 41¾<br>83½ | ☹<br>79¼ | 10¾[A]<br>21½ |
| Pringles® Potato Crisps, Original | hand<br>0.75oz/21g | ☺ | 76¾<br>☺ | ☹<br>☺ | 10¾[A]<br>21½ |
| Pringles® Potato Crisps, Salt & Vinegar | hand<br>0.75oz/21g | ☺ | 41¾<br>83½ | ☹<br>79¼ | 10¾[A]<br>21½ |
| Pudding mix, other flavors, cooked type | portion<br>0.88oz/24.75g | ☺ | ☺<br>☺ | ☺<br>☺ | ☺<br>☺ |
| Pumpernickel roll | slice<br>1.49oz/42g | ☺ | ☺<br>☺ | ☺<br>☺ | ½[A]<br>1¼ |
| Pumpkin or squash seeds, shelled, unsalted | hand<br>1.06oz/30g | ☺ | ☺<br>☺ | ☺<br>☺ | 2¾[G]<br>5¾ |
| Pumpkin seed oil | portion<br>0.46oz/13g | ☺ | ☺<br>☺ | ☺<br>☺ | ☺<br>☺ |
| Purslane, raw | portion<br>3oz/85g | ☺ | 58¾<br>☺ | ☺<br>☺ | ☺<br>☺ |
| Quince, fresh | tbsp.<br>0.5ozfl/14.21ml | ☺ | 1¼<br>2¾ | ☺<br>☺ | ☺<br>☺ |
| Quinoa, cooked | portion<br>4.94oz/140g | ☺ | ☺+ ×1¾ unit<br>☺+ ×¾ unit | ☺<br>☺ | 2½[A]<br>5 |
| Radicchio, raw | portion<br>3oz/85g | ☺ | 2¼<br>4¾ | ☺<br>☺ | ¾<br>1½ |
| Radish, raw | portion<br>3oz/85g | ☺ | ☺+ ×½ unit<br>☺+ ×¼ unit | ☹<br>1 | ☺[C]<br>☺ |
| Raisins, uncooked | portion<br>1.42oz/40g | ☺ | ¼<br>1 | ☹<br>½ | 2[B]<br>4 |

| Keyword Index | Unit | Lactose ↳ + unit/ 💊 | Fructose* ↳ Fructose* ↳ | Sorbitol ↳ Sorbitol ↳ | FrucGalactans ↳ FrucGalactans ↳📖 |
|---|---|---|---|---|---|
| Rambutan, canned in syrup | portion 4.94oz/140g | ☺ | 1¼ 2¾ | ☺ ☺ | ¾ CB 1¾ |
| Raspberries, fresh, red | portion 4.94oz/140g | ☺ | ½ 1¼ | ☹ 1½ | 1 B 2¼ |
| Raspberry juice | glass 8.4ozfl/240ml | ☺ | ☹² ☹² | ☹ ☹² | ¾ B 1½ |
| Ratatouille | portion 3.89oz/110g | ☺ | ☺ ☺ | ☹ 1¼ | 4 B 8 |
| Red beans and rice soup mix, dry | portion 1.8oz/51g | ☺ | ¼ ¾ | ☹ ¼ | 1¼ AC 2¾ |
| Red Bull® Energy Drink | glass 8.4ozfl/240ml | ☺ | ☺+ ×7¾ unit ☺+ ×3¾ unit | ☺ ☺ | ☺ ☺ |
| Red Bull® Energy Drink Sugar Free | glass 8.4ozfl/240ml | ☺ | ☺ ☺ | ☺ ☺ | ☺ ☺ |
| Red pepper (cayenne), ground | pinch 0.04oz/1g | ☺ | 51 ☺ | ☺ ☺ | ☺ ☺ |
| Red wine vinegar | tbsp. 0.5ozfl/14.21ml | ☺ | ☺ ☺ | ☹ 20 | ☺ ☺ |
| Rhubarb pie, bottom crust only | piece 4.31oz/122g | ☺ | ☺ ☺ | ☺ ☺ | ¼ A ¾ |
| Rhubarb, fresh | portion 4.94oz/140g | ☺ | ☺ ☺ | ☺ ☺ | ☺ ☺ |
| Ribs, beef, spare, visible fat eaten | portion 3oz/85g | ☺ | ☺ ☺ | ☺ ☺ | ☺ ☺ |
| Rice bread | slice 1.49oz/42g | ☺ | ☺ ☺ | ☺ ☺ | ☺ A ☺ |
| Rice cake | piece 0.32oz/9g | ☺ | ☺ ☺ | ☺ ☺ | ☺ G ☺ |
| Rice Krispies® (Kellogg's®) | portion 1.06oz/30g | ☺ | ☺ ☺ | ☺ ☺ | 1½ A 3 |
| Rice milk, plain or original, unsweetened, enriched | glass 8.4oz/240g | ☺ | ☺+ ×¼ unit ☺ | ☺ ☺ | ☺ A ☺ |
| Rice noodles, fried | portion 0.89oz/25g | ☺ | ☺ ☺ | ☺ ☺ | ☺ A ☺ |

↳ *Level 0*: lactose measure ×½
↳ *Level 1*: fructose measure ×2
↳ *Level 2*: fructose-/sorbitol measure ×4. the rest ×2
↳ *Level 3*: sorbitol measure ×7. the rest ×3
📖: source of fruc/galactans data

+ Unit/💊: added tolerated amount of unit per strong lactase capsule
Fructose*: fructose, sorbitol adjusted

☺+ ×[Amount] unit: Per unit consumed you can additionally tolerate up to [amount] × fructose(*)-unit of another product.

☹: avoid;   ☹¹: ¼ at TL 1;   ☹²: ¼ at TL 2;   ☹³: ¼ at TL 3;   ☺: only contains traces;   ☺: is free from it

*LAXIBA*®   The Nutrition Navigator

| KEYWORD INDEX | Unit | Lactose 🠗 + unit/🍶 | Fructose* 🠗 Fructose* 🠗 | Sorbitol 🠗 Sorbitol 🠗 | FrucGalactans 🠗 FrucGalactans 🠗 📖 |
|---|---|---|---|---|---|
| Rice pudding (arroz con leche), coconut, raisins | piece 7.06oz/200g | ½ +¼ unit | 27¾ 55½ | ☹ 1¼ | 3¼ 6½ |
| Rice pudding (arroz con leche), plain | piece 7.06oz/200g | ½ +¼ unit | ☺+ ×½ unit ☺+ ×¼ unit | ☺ ☺ | 2¾ 5¾ |
| Rice pudding (arroz con leche), raisins | piece 7.06oz/200g | ½ +¼ unit | 3¾ 7½ | ☹ 1¼ | 3 6 |
| Ricotta cheese, part skim milk | portion 1.95oz/55g | 17½ +14½ unit | ☺ ☺ | ☺ ☺ | ☺ ☺ |
| Riesen® | piece 0.32oz/9g | 12¾ +10½ unit | ½ 1 | ☹ ☹³ | 71 ☺ |
| Riesling | glass 8.4ozfl/240ml | ☺ | 31¼ 62½ | ☹ ¾ | ☺ ☺ |
| Ritz Cracker (Nabisco®) | portion 1.06oz/30g | ☺ | ☺ ☺ | ☺ ☺ | ¼ A ½ |
| Rob Roy | glass 8.4ozfl/240ml | ☺ | ¼ ½ | ☹ 2½ | ☺ ☺ |
| Rocket (arugula), raw | portion 3oz/85g | ☺ | 4¾ 9¾ | ☺ ☺ | ☺ ☺ |
| Rockstar Original® | glass 8.4ozfl/240ml | ☺ | ☺+ ×2¾ unit ☺+ ×1¾ unit | ☹ 5 | ☺ ☺ |
| Rockstar Original® Sugar Free | glass 8.4ozfl/240ml | ☺ | ☺ ☺ | ☹ 5 | ☺ ☺ |
| Rompope (eggnog with alcohol) | glass 8.4ozfl/240ml | ¼ +¼ unit | ☺ ☺ | ☺ ☺ | 2¾ 5½ |
| Root beer | glass 8.4ozfl/240ml | ☺ | ½ 1¼ | ☺ ☺ | ☺ ☺ |
| Roquefort cheese | portion 1.06oz/30g | 5 +4 unit | ☺ ☺ | ☺ ☺ | 27¾ 55½ |
| Rose hips | portion 4.94oz/140g | ☺ | ☺+ ×½ unit ☺+ ×¼ unit | ☺ ☺ | ☺ ☺ |
| Rose wine, other types | glass 8.4ozfl/240ml | ☺ | ¾ 1¾ | ☺ ☺ | ☺ ☺ |
| Rosemary, dried | pinch 0.04oz/1g | ☺ | ☺ ☺ | ☺ ☺ | ☺ ☺ |
| Rum | glass 8.4ozfl/240ml | ☺ | ☺ ☺ | ☺ ☺ | ☺ ☺ |
| Rum and cola | glass 8.4ozfl/240ml | ☺ | 1 2 | ☺ ☺ | ☺ ☺ |
| Rusty nail | glass 8.4ozfl/240ml | ☺ | ☺+ ×1¾ unit ☺+ ×1 unit | ☹ ¾ | ☺ ☺ |

| Keyword Index | Unit<br>+ unit/💊 | Lactose ↓ | Fructose* ☿<br>Fructose* ↓ | Sorbitol ☿<br>Sorbitol ↓ | FrucGalactans ☿<br>FrucGalactans ↓ 📖 |
|---|---|---|---|---|---|
| Rutabaga, raw or blanched, marinated in oil mixture | portion<br>3oz/85g | ☺ | ☺+ ×1 unit<br>☺+ ×½ unit | ☺<br>☺ | ☺ CB<br>☺ |
| Rye bread | slice<br>1.49oz/42g | ☺ | ☺<br>☺ | ☺<br>☺ | ¾ A<br>1¾ |
| Rye flour, in recipes not containing yeast | portion<br>1.06oz/30g | ☺ | 27¾<br>55½ | ☺<br>☺ | 1¼ A<br>2½ |
| Rye roll | slice<br>1.49oz/42g | ☺ | ☺<br>☺ | ☺<br>☺ | ¾ A<br>1¾ |
| Safflower oil | portion<br>0.46oz/13g | ☺ | ☺<br>☺ | ☺<br>☺ | ☺<br>☺ |
| Sake | glass<br>8.4ozfl/240ml | ☺ | ☹²<br>☹² | ☹<br>½ | ☺<br>☺ |
| Salami, beer or beerwurst, beef | portion<br>1.95oz/55g | ☺ | ☺+ ×1 unit<br>☺+ ×½ unit | ☺<br>☺ | ☺<br>☺ |
| Salmon, red (sockeye), smoked | portion<br>1.95oz/55g | ☺ | ☺<br>☺ | ☺<br>☺ | ☺<br>☺ |
| Salsa, store bought | tbsp.<br>0.5ozfl/14.21ml | ☺ | 6¼<br>12½ | ☹<br>6¾ | 5½<br>11¼ |
| Sambuca | glass<br>8.4ozfl/240ml | ☺ | ☺+ ×4½ unit<br>☺+ ×2½ unit | ☹<br>¼ | ☺<br>☺ |
| Sandwich cookies, vanilla | piece<br>0.53oz/15g | 9<br>+7½ unit | ☺<br>☺ | ☺<br>☺ | 3 A<br>6¼ |
| Sangria | glass<br>8.4ozfl/240ml | ☺ | 7¾<br>15½ | ☹<br>¾ | ☺<br>☺ |
| Santa Claus melon | portion<br>4.94oz/140g | ☺ | 1¼<br>2½ | ☺<br>☺ | ☺<br>☺ |
| Sapodilla, fresh | portion<br>4.94oz/140g | ☺ | ☺+ ×3½ unit<br>☺+ ×1¾ unit | ☺<br>☺ | ☺<br>☺ |
| Sauerbraten | portion<br>5.61oz/159g | ☺ | 34¾<br>69¾ | ☺<br>☺ | ☺<br>☺ |
| Sauerkraut | tbsp.<br>0.5ozfl/14.21ml | ☺ | ☺<br>☺ | ☹<br>¾ | 7 B<br>14¼ |

☿ *Level 0*: lactose measure ×½  + Unit/💊: added tolerated amount of unit per strong lactase capsule
↓ *Level 1*: fructose measure ×2  Fructose*: fructose, sorbitol adjusted
☿ *Level 2*: fructose-/sorbitol measure ×4. the rest ×2  ☺+ ×[Amount] unit: Per unit consumed you can
☿ *Level 3*: sorbitol measure ×7. the rest ×3  additionally tolerate up to [amount] ×
📖: source of fruc/galactans data  fructose(*)-unit of another product.
☹: avoid;   ☹¹: ¼ at TL 1;   ☹²: ¼ at TL 2;   ☹³: ¼ at TL 3;   ☺: only contains traces;   ☺: is free from it

| Keyword Index | Unit + unit/ | Lactose ☻ | Fructose* ☻ Fructose* ☻ | Sorbitol ☻ Sorbitol ☻ | FrucGalactans ☻ FrucGalactans ☻ |
|---|---|---|---|---|---|
| Scallions or spring onions, raw or blanched, tops and bulbs, marinated in oil | piece 0.56oz/15.7g | ☻ | ☻+ ×¼ unit ☻ | ☹ 6 | ¼ G ¾ |
| Scallop squash | portion 3oz/85g | ☻ | 4 8¼ | ☻ ☻ | ☻ CB ☻ |
| Scallops | portion 3oz/85g | ☻ | ☻ ☻ | ☻ ☻ | ☻ ☻ |
| Schnapps, all flavors | glass 8.4ozfl/240ml | ☻ | ☻+ ×2¼ unit ☻+ ×1¼ unit | ☹ ½ | ☻ ☻ |
| Schweppes® Bitter Lemon | glass 8.4ozfl/240ml | ☻ | ☹² ☹² | ☻ ☻ | ☻ ☻ |
| Scotch and soda | glass 8.4ozfl/240ml | ☻ | ☻ ☻ | ☻ ☻ | ☻ ☻ |
| Scrambled egg with bacon | portion 3.89oz/110g | 2¼ +1¾ unit | ☻+ ×1¾ unit ☻+ ×¾ unit | ☻ ☻ | 12½ 25¼ |
| Screwdriver | glass 8.4ozfl/240ml | ☻ | 2 4¼ | ☹ ¼ | ☻ ☻ |
| Sea Pak® Seasoned Shrimp, Roasted Garlic | portion 3oz/85g | ☻ | ☻ ☻ | ☻ ☻ | ☻ ☻ |
| Sea Pak® Shrimp Scampi in Italian Parmesan Sauce | portion 3oz/85g | ☻ | ☻ ☻ | ☻ ☻ | ☻ ☻ |
| Seabreeze | glass 8.4ozfl/240ml | ☻ | ☻+ ×5¼ unit ☻+ ×2½ unit | ☹ 2½ | ☻ ☻ |
| Semolina flour | portion 1.06oz/30g | ☻ | ☻ ☻ | ☻ ☻ | 1¼ AD 2¾ |
| Sesame chicken | portion 8.89oz/252g | ☻ | ☻ ☻ | ☹ 3¾ | ☻ ☻ |
| Sesame sticks | hand 0.75oz/21g | ☻ | ☻ ☻ | ☹ ☻ | 1½ A 3¼ |
| Shallot, raw | tbsp. 0.5ozfl/14.21ml | ☻ | ☻ ☻ | ☻ ☻ | ¼ CB ½ |
| Shiitake mushrooms, cooked | tbsp. 0.5ozfl/14.21ml | ☻ | ☻+ ×1 unit ☻+ ×½ unit | ☹ ½ | ☻ ☻ |
| Singapore sling | glass 8.4ozfl/240ml | ☻ | ☻+ ×¼ unit ☻ | ☹ 4½ | ☻ ☻ |
| Slim-Fast® Easy to Digest, Vanilla, ready-to-drink can | glass 8.4oz/240g | 2½ +2 unit | ☻ ☻ | ☻ ☻ | 14¼ 28¾ |
| Sloe gin | glass 8.4ozfl/240ml | ☻ | ☻+ ×4½ unit ☻+ ×2½ unit | ☹ ¼ | ☻ ☻ |

| Keyword Index | Unit | Lactose ☹ + unit/💊 | Fructose* ☹ Fructose* ☹ | Sorbitol ☹ Sorbitol ☹ | FrucGalactans ☹ FrucGalactans ☹📖 |
|---|---|---|---|---|---|
| Sloe gin fizz | glass 8.4ozfl/240ml | ☺ | ☺+ ×¾ unit ☺+ ×¼ unit | ☹ 1½ | ☺ ☺ |
| Smart Balance® Light with Flax Oil Margarine, tub | portion 0.5oz/14g | 32¼ +27 unit | ☺ ☺ | ☺ ☺ | ☺ ☺ |
| Smart Balance® Margarine | portion 0.5oz/14g | 31 +25¾ unit | ☺ ☺ | ☺ ☺ | ☺ ☺ |
| Smarties® | hand 1.06oz/30g | ☺ | ☺+ ×55 unit ☺+ ×27½ unit | ☺ ☺ | ☺ ☺ |
| Snickers® | piece 2.08oz/58.7g | 1½ +1¼ unit | ☺+ ×7 unit ☺+ ×3½ unit | ☺ ☺ | 5¾ 11½ |
| Snickers®, Almond | piece 1.77oz/49.9g | 1¾ +1½ unit | ☺+ ×8¾ unit ☺+ ×4¼ unit | ☺ ☺ | 6½ G 13¼ |
| Snow peas (edible pea pods), cooked from fresh | portion 3oz/85g | ☺ | ☺+ ×3½ unit ☺+ ×1¾ unit | ☺ ☺ | ¾ B 1¾ |
| Sorbet, chocolate | portion 3.71oz/105g | ☺ | ☺+ ×3¼ unit ☺+ ×1½ unit | ☺ ☺ | 3 G 6¼ |
| Sorbet, coconut | portion 3.74oz/106g | 18¾ +15½ unit | ☺+ ×5 unit ☺+ ×2½ unit | ☺ ☺ | 3¼ 6½ |
| Sorbet, fruit | portion 3.74oz/106g | ☺ | ☺+ ×5½ unit ☺+ ×2¾ unit | ☺ ☺ | ☺ ☺ |
| Sorghum | portion 1.06oz/30g | ☺ | ☺ ☺ | ☺ ☺ | ☺ ☺ |
| Souffle, meat | portion 3.89oz/110g | 1¼ +1 unit | ☺+ ×½ unit ☺+ ×¼ unit | ☹ ☺ | 1¾ B 3¾ |
| Soup base | tbsp. 0.5ozfl/14.21ml | ☺ | 64 ☺ | ☹ 74 | ☺ ☺ |
| Sour cherries, fresh | tbsp. 0.5ozfl/14.21ml | ☺ | 10 20 | ☹ ½ | ☺ ☺ |
| Sour cream | portion 1.06oz/30g | 3¼ +2¾ unit | ☺ ☺ | ☺ ☺ | 19¼ 38½ |
| Sour pickles | portion 1.06oz/30g | ☺ | ☺+ ×¼ unit ☺ | ☹ 4¼ | 1 G 2¼ |

☹ *Level 0*: lactose measure ×½    + Unit/💊: added tolerated amount of unit per strong lactase capsule
☹ *Level 1*: fructose measure ×2    Fructose*: fructose, sorbitol adjusted
☹ *Level 2*: fructose-/sorbitol measure ×4. the rest ×2    ☺+ ×[Amount] unit: Per unit consumed you can
☹ *Level 3*: sorbitol measure ×7. the rest ×3    additionally tolerate up to [amount] ×
📖: source of fruc/galactans data    fructose(*)-unit of another product.
☹: avoid;    ☹[1]: ¼ at TL 1;    ☹[2]: ¼ at TL 2;    ☹[3]: ¼ at TL 3;    ☺: only contains traces;    ☺: is free from it

| Keyword Index | Unit | Lactose ↳ + unit/ 📖 | Fructose* ↯ Fructose* ↳ | Sorbitol ↯ Sorbitol ↳ | FrucGalactans ↯ FrucGalactans ↳ 📖 |
|---|---|---|---|---|---|
| Sourdough bread | slice 1.49oz/42g | ☺ | ☺ ☺ | ☺ ☺ | ¾ A 1½ |
| Soursop (guanabana), fresh | portion 4.94oz/140g | ☺ | 1¼ 2¾ | ☺ ☺ | ☺ ☺ |
| Southern Comfort® | glass 8.4ozfl/240ml | ☺ | ☺ ☺ | ☺ ☺ | ☺ ☺ |
| Soy bread | slice 1.49oz/42g | 3½ +3 unit | 11 22¼ | ☹ 2 | 1 A 2 |
| Soy chips | hand 0.75oz/21g | 5¼ +4¼ unit | 15 30 | ☹ 1 | 2 A 4 |
| Soy Kaas Fat Free, all flavors | portion 1.06oz/30g | 9 +7½ unit | 55½ ☺ | ☹ 18½ | 1¼ A 2¾ |
| Soy milk, chocolate, sweetened with sugar, not fortified | cup 5.2ozfl/150ml | ☺ | ☺ ☺ | ☹ 4¼ | ¼ A ½ |
| Soy milk, plain or original, sweetened with artificial sweetener | glass 8.4oz/240g | ☺ | 4¾ 9½ | ☹ 1½ | ☹ A ¼ |
| Soy milk, vanilla or other flavors, sweetened with sugar, fat free | glass 8.4oz/240g | ☺ | ☺+ ×¾ unit ☺+ ×¼ unit | ☹ 7 | ☹ A ¼ |
| Soy sauce | tbsp. 0.5ozfl/14.21ml | ☺ | ☺ ☺ | ☹ 4½ | 3 A 6 |
| Soybean oil, unhydrogenated | tbsp. 0.5ozfl/14.21ml | ☺ | ☺ ☺ | ☺ ☺ | ☺ ☺ |
| Soybean sprouts, raw | portion 3oz/85g | ☺ | ☺ ☺ | ☹ ½ | 3¾ CB 7½ |
| Soybeans, cooked from dried | tbsp. 0.5ozfl/14.21ml | ☺ | 9 18 | ☹ 3 | 3 A 6 |
| Spaetzle (spatzen) | portion 4.94oz/140g | 5¼ +4¼ unit | ☺+ ×¼ unit ☺ | ☺ ☺ | 1 A 2 |
| Spaghetti squash | portion 3oz/85g | ☺ | ☺+ ×¼ unit ☺ | ☺ ☺ | ☺ CB ☺ |
| Spaghetti, with carbonara sauce | portion 7.09oz/201g | 13½ +11¼ unit | ☺+ ×¾ unit ☺+ ×¼ unit | ☹ 6 | ½ A 1 |
| Spearmint tea | glass 8.4ozfl/240ml | ☺ | ☺ ☺ | ☺ ☺ | ☺ G ☺ |
| Special K® Blueberry cereal (Kellogg's®) | portion 1.06oz/30g | ☺ | ☺+ ×½ unit ☺+ ×¼ unit | ☹ 15 | ½ A 1¼ |
| Special K® Cinnamon Pecan cereal (Kellogg's®) | portion 1.06oz/30g | ☺ | ☺ ☺ | ☺ ☺ | ½ A 1¼ |

| Keyword Index | Unit | Lactose ⌇ + unit/ 🗨 | Fructose* ⌇ Fructose* ⌇ | Sorbitol ⌇ Sorbitol ⌇ | FrucGalactans ⌇ FrucGalactans ⌇ 📖 |
|---|---|---|---|---|---|
| Special K® Original cereal (Kellogg's®) | portion 1.06oz/30g | 13 +10¾ unit | ☺ ☺ | ☺ ☺ | ½ A 1¼ |
| Special K® Red Berries cereal (Kellogg's®) | portion 1.06oz/30g | ☺ | ☺ ☺ | ☹ 41½ | ½ A 1¼ |
| Spelt flour | portion 1.06oz/30g | ☺ | ☺+ ×¼ unit ☺ | ☺ ☺ | ☺ A ☺ |
| Spinach ravioli, with tomato sauce | portion 8.82oz/250g | 5½ +4½ unit | ☺+ ×¼ unit ☺ | ☹ ½ | ½ A 1 |
| Spinach, cooked from fresh | portion 3oz/85g | ☺ | ☺ ☺ | ☹ 13 | 4 CB 8¼ |
| Splenda® | portion 0oz/0g | ☺ | ☺ ☺ | ☺ ☺ | ☺ ☺ |
| Split pea sprouts, cooked | tbsp. 0.5ozfl/14.21ml | ☺ | ☺ ☺ | ☺ ☺ | 1¼ A 2½ |
| Spring roll | portion 4.94oz/140g | ☺ | 21 42 | ☹ 2¾ | ¼ ½ |
| Sprinkles Cookie Crisp® (General Mills®) | portion 1.06oz/30g | ☺ | ☺+ ×¼ unit ☺ | ☹ ☺ | ¾ A 1¾ |
| Sprite® | glass 8.4ozfl/240ml | ☺ | ☹² ☹² | ☺ ☺ | ☺ ☺ |
| Sprite® Zero | glass 8.4ozfl/240ml | ☺ | ☺ ☺ | ☺ ☺ | ☺ ☺ |
| Squash or pumpkin ravioli, with cream sauce | portion 8.82oz/250g | ½ +½ unit | ☺+ ×¼ unit ☺ | ☹ 40 | ½ A 1 |
| Starbucks® Hot Cocoa Double Chocolate, prepared | cup 5.2ozfl/150ml | ¼ +¼ unit | 37 74 | ☹ 66½ | 1¾ 3¾ |
| Starbucks® Hot Cocoa Salted Caramel, prepared | cup 5.2ozfl/150ml | ¼ +¼ unit | 33¼ 66½ | ☹ 66½ | 1¾ 3¾ |
| Starburst®, Original | piece 0.18oz/5g | ☺ | ☺+ ×½ unit ☺+ ×¼ unit | ☹ 30¼ | ☺ ☺ |
| Stewed green peas with sofrito | tbsp. 0.5oz.fl/14.8ml | ☺ +2¾ unit | ☺ ☺ | ☹ 5½ | 1¼ AB 2½ |

⌇ *Level 0*: lactose measure ×½  
⌇ *Level 1*: fructose measure ×2  
⌇ *Level 2*: fructose-/sorbitol measure ×4. the rest ×2  
⌇ *Level 3*: sorbitol measure ×7. the rest ×3  
📖: source of fruc/galactans data  
+ Unit/ 🗨: added tolerated amount of unit per strong lactase capsule  
Fructose*: fructose, sorbitol adjusted  
☺+ ×[Amount] unit: Per unit consumed you can additionally tolerate up to [amount] × fructose(*)-unit of another product.  

☹: avoid;   ☹¹: ¼ at TL 1;   ☹²: ¼ at TL 2;   ☹³: ¼ at TL 3;   ☺: only contains traces;   ☺: is free from it

| Keyword Index | Unit | Lactose ⓛ + unit/🥛 | Fructose* ☺ Fructose* ⓛ | Sorbitol ☺ Sorbitol ⓛ | FrucGalactans ☺ FrucGalactans ⓛ 📖 |
|---|---|---|---|---|---|
| Sticky bun | piece 2.51oz/71g | 8¾ +7¼ unit | ☺+ ×¾ unit ☺+ ×¼ unit | ☺ ☺ | ½ D 1 |
| Stonyfield® Oikos Greek Yogurt, Blueberry | piece 5.3oz/150g | ¼ +¼ unit | ☺+ ×1 unit ☺+ ×½ unit | ☺ ☺ | 1¾ 3½ |
| Stonyfield® Oikos Greek Yogurt, Caramel | piece 4.03oz/114g | ½ +½ unit | ☺+ ×½ unit ☺+ ×¼ unit | ☺ ☺ | 4 8 |
| Stonyfield® Oikos Greek Yogurt, Chocolate | piece 4.03oz/114g | ½ +¼ unit | 66½ ☺ | ☺ ☺ | 3 6¼ |
| Stonyfield® Oikos Greek Yogurt, Strawberry | piece 5.3oz/150g | ¼ +¼ unit | 4 8¼ | ☹ 2 | 1¾ 3½ |
| Straw mushrooms, canned, drained | portion 3oz/85g | ☺ | ☺ ☺ | ☹ ¼ | ☺ ☺ |
| Strawberries, fresh | portion 4.94oz/140g | ☺ | ½ 1¼ | ☹ ¼ | ☺ C ☺ |
| Strawberry milk, plain, prepared | glass 8.4oz/240g | ¼ +¼ unit | ☺ ☺ | ☺ ☺ | 1¾ 3½ |
| Strawberry pie, bottom crust only | piece 4.31oz/122g | ☺ | 1¾ 3¾ | ☹ ¾ | ¼ A ¾ |
| Streusel topping, crumb | portion 0.68oz/19g | 68¼ +57 unit | ☺ ☺ | ☺ ☺ | 2¾ A 5¾ |
| Subway® 9-grain Wheat bread | piece 2.76oz/78g | ☺ | 1 2 | ☺ ☺ | ¼ A ¾ |
| Subway® American cheese | portion 1.06oz/30g | 4½ +3¾ unit | ☺ ☺ | ☺ ☺ | 25¾ 51½ |
| Subway® bacon | portion 0.53oz/15g | ☺ | ☺ ☺ | ☺ ☺ | ☺ ☺ |
| Subway® cheddar cheese | portion 1.06oz/30g | 43¼ +36 unit | ☺ ☺ | ☺ ☺ | ☺ ☺ |
| Subway® chipotle southwest salad dressing | portion 1.06ozfl/30ml | 7¼ +6 unit | ☺ ☺ | ☺ ☺ | 40½ 81 |
| Subway® chocolate chip cookie | piece 1.59oz/45g | ☺ | ☺+ ×1 unit ☺+ ×½ unit | ☹ ☺ | ½ A 1 |
| Subway® chocolate chunk cookie | piece 1.59oz/45g | ☺ | ☺+ ×1 unit ☺+ ×½ unit | ☹ ☺ | ½ A 1 |
| Subway® Ham Sandwich with Veggies, no mayo | piece 7.73oz/219g | 12½ +10½ unit | ¾ 1¾ | ☹ 1¼ | ¼ A ½ |
| Subway® honey mustard salad dressing | portion 1.06oz/30g | ☺ | 4½ 9 | ☺ ☺ | ☺ ☺ |
| Subway® honey mustard sauce, fat free | portion 0.99oz/28g | ☺ | 4¾ 9½ | ☺ ☺ | ☺ ☺ |

| KEYWORD INDEX | Unit | Lactose ☽ + unit/ 💊 | Fructose* ☽ Fructose* ☾ | Sorbitol ☽ Sorbitol ☾ | FrucGalactans ☽ FrucGalactans ☾ 📖 |
|---|---|---|---|---|---|
| Subway® Honey Oat bread | piece 3.14oz/89g | ¾ +½ unit | 2½ 5¼ | ☹ 6½ | ¼ ¾ A |
| Subway® Italian BMT® Sandwich with Veggies, no mayo | piece 7.98oz/226g | 12½ +10½ unit | ¾ 1¾ | ☹ 1¼ | ¼ A ½ |
| Subway® M & M's® cookie | piece 1.59oz/45g | 9 +7½ unit | ☺+ ×½ unit ☺+ ×¼ unit | ☹ ☺ | ½ A 1 |
| Subway® mustard | portion 0.18oz/5g | ☺ | ☺ ☺ | ☺ ☺ | ☺ ☺ |
| Subway® Oven Roasted Chicken Sandwich with Veggies, no mayo | piece 8.22oz/233g | 12½ +10½ unit | 1¾ 3¾ | ☹ 1¼ | ☹ A ¼ |
| Subway® Parmesan Oregano bread | piece 2.65oz/75g | ☺ | ☺+ ×½ unit ☺+ ×¼ unit | ☺ ☺ | ¾ A 1½ |
| Subway® ranch salad dressing | portion 1.06ozfl/30ml | ☺ | ☺ ☺ | ☹ ☺ | ☺ ☺ |
| Subway® Roast Beef Sandwich with Veggies, no mayo | piece 8.22oz/233g | 12½ +10½ unit | ¾ 1¾ | ☹ 1¼ | ☹ A ¼ |
| Subway® Spicy Italian Sandwich with Veggies, no meat | piece 7.84oz/222g | 12½ +10½ unit | ¾ 1¾ | ☹ 1¼ | ¼ A ½ |
| Subway® Steak & Cheese Sandwich with Veggies, no mayo | piece 8.65oz/245g | ☺ | 1 2 | ☹ 1¼ | ☹ A ¼ |
| Subway® Sweet Onion Chicken Teriyaki Sandwich with Veggies, no mayo | piece 9.74oz/276g | 12½ +10½ unit | 22½ 45¼ | ☹ 1¼ | ☹ A ¼ |
| Subway® sweet onion salad dressing | portion 1.06ozfl/30ml | ☺ | ☺+ ×1 unit ☺+ ×½ unit | ☹ 55½ | ½ 1¼ |
| Subway® Tuna Sandwich with Veggies, no mayo | piece 8.22oz/233g | 12½ +10½ unit | ¾ 1¾ | ☹ 1¼ | ☹ A ¼ |
| Subway® Turkey Breast & Ham Sandwich with Veggies, no mayo | piece 7.73oz/219g | 12½ +10½ unit | ¾ 1¾ | ☹ 1¼ | ¼ A ½ |
| Subway® Turkey Breast Sandwich with Veggies, no mayo | piece 7.73oz/219g | 12½ +10½ unit | ¾ 1¾ | ☹ 1¼ | ¼ A ½ |

☽ *Level 0:* lactose measure ×½
☾ *Level 1:* fructose measure ×2
⚳ *Level 2:* fructose-/sorbitol measure ×4. the rest ×2
♃ *Level 3:* sorbitol measure ×7. the rest ×3
📖: source of fruc/galactans data

+ Unit/ 💊: added tolerated amount of unit per strong lactase capsule
Fructose*: fructose, sorbitol adjusted
☺+ ×[Amount] unit: Per unit consumed you can additionally tolerate up to [amount] × fructose(*)-unit of another product.

☹: avoid;   ☹[1]: ¼ at TL 1;   ☹[2]: ¼ at TL 2;   ☹[3]: ¼ at TL 3;   ☺: only contains traces;   ☺: is free from it

| Keyword Index | Unit | Lactose ↯ + unit/ 🥛 | Fructose* ↯ Fructose* ↯ | Sorbitol ↯ Sorbitol ↯ | FrucGalactans ↯ FrucGalactans ↯ 📖 |
|---|---|---|---|---|---|
| Subway® Veggie Delite Salad, no dressing | portion 3.53oz/100g | 34¼ +28½ unit | 83¼ ☺ | ☹ 2¼ | ☺ ☺ |
| Subway® Veggie Delite Sandwich, no mayo | piece 5.72oz/162g | 12½ +10½ unit | ¾ 1¾ | ☹ 1½ | ¼ A ½ |
| Subway® vinegar | portion 0.5ozfl/14ml | ☺ | ☺ ☺ | ☹ 20¼ | ☺ ☺ |
| Subway® white chip macadamia nut cookie | piece 1.59oz/45g | 6¾ +5½ unit | ☺ ☺ | ☺ ☺ | ½ A 1 |
| Subway® wrap bread | piece 3.64oz/103g | ☺ | ☺ ☺ | ☺ ☺ | ½ 1 A |
| Suckers®, sugar free | piece 0.5oz/14g | ☺ | ☹ ☹ | ☹ ☹ | ☺ ☺ |
| Sugar cookies, iced, store bought | piece 0.53oz/15g | ☺ | ☺ ☺ | ☺ ☺ | 3¼ A 6½ |
| Sugar, white granulated | tbsp. 0.5ozfl/14.21ml | ☺ | ☺ ☺ | ☺ ☺ | ☺ ☺ |
| Summer squash, cooked from fresh | portion 3oz/85g | ☺ | 2¼ 4¾ | ☺ ☺ | 2 CB 4 |
| Sunbelt Bakery® Chewy Granola Bar, Banana Harvest | piece 0.89oz/25g | 49 +40¾ unit | ☺+ ×½ unit ☺+ ×¼ unit | ☹ ¾ | ¾ A 1½ |
| Sunbelt Bakery® Chewy Granola Bar, Blueberry Harvest | piece 0.89oz/25g | 49 +40¾ unit | ☺+ ×½ unit ☺+ ×¼ unit | ☹ ¾ | ¾ A 1½ |
| Sunbelt Bakery® Chewy Granola Bar, Golden Almond | piece 0.99oz/28g | 4 +3¼ unit | 1½ 3¼ | ☹ ☹² | ½ A 1¼ |
| Sunbelt Bakery® Chewy Granola Bar, Low Fat Oatmeal Raisin | piece 1.06oz/30g | 11¾ +9¾ unit | ½ 1 | ☹ ☹² | ½ A 1¼ |
| Sunbelt Bakery® Chewy Granola Bar, Oats & Honey | piece 0.96oz/27g | 17½ +14¾ unit | 5¾ 11¾ | ☹ ☹² | ½ A 1¼ |
| Sunbelt Bakery® Fudge Dipped Chewy Granola Bar, Coconut | piece 1.03oz/29g | 17¼ +14½ unit | ¾ 1½ | ☹ ☹² | ½ A 1¼ |
| Sun-dried tomatoes, oil pack, drained | portion 1.06oz/30g | ☺ | ¼ ½ | ☹ ¼ | 4½ B 9¼ |
| Sunflower oil | tbsp. 0.5ozfl/14.21ml | ☺ | ☺ ☺ | ☺ ☺ | ☺ ☺ |
| Sunflower seeds, raw | hand 1.06oz/30g | ☺ | ☺ ☺ | ☺ ☺ | 2 G 4 |
| Sushi, with fish | portion 4.94oz/140g | ☺ | 10¼ 21 | ☹ 2½ | 📖 ☺ |

| Keyword Index | Unit | Lactose ↓ + unit/💊 | Fructose* ↓ Fructose* ↓ | Sorbitol ↓ Sorbitol ↓ | FrucGalactans ↓ FrucGalactans ↓ |
|---|---|---|---|---|---|
| Sushi, with fish and vegetables in seaweed | portion 4.94oz/140g | ☺ | ☺ ☺ | ☹ 2 | ☺ ☺ |
| Sushi, with vegetables in seaweed | portion 4.94oz/140g | ☺ | ☺ ☺ | ☹ 1½ | ☺ ☺ |
| Swedish Meatballs | portion 4.94oz/140g | 1½ +1¼ unit | ☺ ☺ | ☹ 71¼ | 9 18 |
| Sweet and sour chicken | tbsp. 0.5ozfl/14.21ml | ☺ | 2½ 5 | ☹ ☺ | ☺ ☺ |
| Sweet and sour sauce, store bought | tbsp. 0.5ozfl/14.21ml | ☺ | ½ 1¼ | ☹ 83¼ | ☺ ☺ |
| Sweet cherries, fresh | tbsp. 0.5ozfl/14.21ml | ☺ | 3¾ 7½ | ☹ ¼ | ☺ ☺ |
| Sweet potato bread | slice 1.49oz/42g | ☺ | ☺ ☺ | ☺ ☺ | 1½ A 3¼ |
| Sweetened condensed milk | portion 1.35ozfl/38ml | ½ +½ unit | ☺ ☺ | ☺ ☺ | 3¾ 7½ |
| Sweetened condensed milk, reduced fat | portion 1.38ozfl/39ml | ½ +½ unit | ☺ ☺ | ☺ ☺ | 3½ 7¼ |
| Swiss cheese, natural | portion 1.06oz/30g | ☺ | ☺+ ×¼ unit ☺ | ☺ ☺ | ☺ ☺ |
| Swiss cheese, natural, low sodium | portion 1.06oz/30g | ☺ | ☺+ ×¼ unit ☺ | ☺ ☺ | ☺ ☺ |
| Sylvaner | glass 8.4ozfl/240ml | ☺ | 31¼ 62½ | ☹ ¾ | ☺ ☺ |
| Tabasco® sauce | tbsp. 0.5ozfl/14.21ml | ☺ | ☺ ☺ | ☺ ☺ | ☺ ☺ |
| Taco Bell® 7-Layer Burrito | portion 4.94oz/140g | 25½ +21¼ unit | ☺ ☺ | ☹ 5¾ | ¼ A ¾ |
| Taco Bell® Crunchwrap Supreme | piece 8.65oz/245g | 4¼ +3½ unit | ☺ ☺ | ☹ 5 | ☹ A ¼ |
| Taco Bell® Mexican Pizza | piece 7.52oz/213g | 13¾ +11½ unit | 23¼ 46¾ | ☹ 1 | ¼ A ¾ |

♀ *Level 0*: lactose measure ×½  
↓ *Level 1*: fructose measure ×2  
↯ *Level 2*: fructose-/sorbitol measure ×4. the rest ×2  
↯ *Level 3*: sorbitol measure ×7. the rest ×3  
📖: source of fruc/galactans data  

+ Unit/💊: added tolerated amount of unit per strong lactase capsule  
Fructose*: fructose, sorbitol adjusted  

☺+ ×[Amount] unit: Per unit consumed you can additionally tolerate up to [amount] × fructose(*)-unit of another product.  

☹: avoid;   ☹¹: ¼ at TL 1;   ☹²: ¼ at TL 2;   ☹³: ¼ at TL 3;   ☺: only contains traces;   ☺: is free from it

| KEYWORD INDEX | Unit | Lactose ʇ + unit/ 🥛 | Fructose* ♀ʇ Fructose* ʇ | Sorbitol ♀ʇ Sorbitol ʇ | FrucGalactans ♀ʇ FrucGalactans ʇ 📖 |
|---|---|---|---|---|---|
| Taco Bell® Nachos Supreme | portion 4.94oz/140g | 6¼ +5¼ unit | ☺ ☺ | ☹ 7¾ | 35¾ [B] 71½ |
| Taco John's® nachos | hand 0.75oz/21g | 28 +23¼ unit | ☺ ☺ | ☹ ☺ | 10 [A] 20 |
| Taco sauce, red | portion 1.13oz/32g | ☺ | 2¾ 5¾ | ☹ 3 | 11 22 |
| Taco, soft corn shell, with beans, cheese | portion 4,94 oz/140g | ☺ +77 unit | 12¾ 25½ | ☺ 4¼ | ¼ [A] ½ |
| Taffy | piece 0.31oz/8.6g | ☺ | ☺+ ×4¼ unit ☺+ ×2 unit | ☺ ☺ | ☺ ☺ |
| Tahini (sesame butter) | portion 1.06oz/30g | ☺ | ☺ ☺ | ☺ ☺ | 1 [G] 2¼ |
| Tap water | glass 8.4ozfl/240ml | ☺ | ☺ ☺ | ☺ ☺ | ☺ ☺ |
| Tempeh | portion 3oz/85g | ☺ | 3¼ 6¾ | ☹ ½ | ½ [A] 1 |
| Tequila | glass 8.4ozfl/240ml | ☺ | ☺ ☺ | ☺ ☺ | ☺ ☺ |
| Tequila sunrise | glass 8.4ozfl/240ml | ☺ | ☺+ ×¼ unit ☺ | ☹ 3¼ | ☺ ☺ |
| Thyme, dried | pinch 0.04oz/1g | ☺ | ☺ ☺ | ☺ ☺ | ☺ ☺ |
| Tic Tacs® | 2 piece 0.05oz/1.15g | ☺ | ☺ ☺ | ☺ ☺ | ☺ ☺ |
| Tilsit cheese | portion 1.06oz/30g | 5¼ +4¼ unit | ☺ ☺ | ☺ ☺ | 29½ 59 |
| Tiramisu | portion 1.95oz/55g | 2½ +2 unit | ☺ ☺ | ☺ ☺ | 12 [A] 24 |
| Toast, cinnamon and sugar, whole wheat bread | slice 1.49oz/42g | 49½ +41¼ unit | 1½ 3¼ | ☺ ☺ | ¾ [A] 1¾ |
| Toast, wheat bread, with butter | slice 1.49oz/42g | 62½ +52 unit | 1¾ 3¾ | ☺ ☺ | 1¼ [A] 2½ |
| Toblerone® Swiss Dark Chocolate with Honey & Almond Nougat | piece 0.89oz/25g | 7¼ +6 unit | ☺ ☺ | ☹ 40 | 1½ 3¼ |
| Toblerone® Swiss Milk Chocolate with Honey & Almond Nougat | piece 0.89oz/25g | 1½ +1¼ unit | ☺ ☺ | ☺ ☺ | 1½ 3 |

| KEYWORD INDEX | Unit | Lactose ☹/ + unit/💊 | Fructose* ☹/ Fructose* ☺/ | Sorbitol ☹/ Sorbitol ☺/ | FrucGalactans ☹/ FrucGalactans ☺/ 📖 |
|---|---|---|---|---|---|
| Toblerone® Swiss White Confection with Honey & Almond Nougat | piece 0.89oz/25g | 1 +1 unit | ☺ ☺ | ☺ ☺ | 6¾ 13½ |
| Toffee | piece 0.25oz/7g | 40¾ +34 unit | ☺ ☺ | ☺ ☺ | ☺ ☺ |
| Toffifay® | piece 0.29oz/8.2g | 7½ +6¼ unit | ½ 1 | ☹ ☹² | 42¾ 85½ |
| Tofu, raw (not silken), cooked, low fat | portion 3oz/85g | ☺ | 2¼ 4¾ | ☹ ¾ | ½ ᴬ 1 |
| Tokaji Wine | glass 8.4ozfl/240ml | ☺ | ☹² ☹² | ☹ ½ | ☺ ☺ |
| Tom Collins | glass 8.4ozfl/240ml | ☺ | 31¼ 62½ | ☹ 16½ | ☺ ☺ |
| Tomato juice | glass 8.4ozfl/240ml | ☺ | 1¼ 2½ | ☹ ¼ | 2¾ ᴮ 5½ |
| Tomato relish | portion 0.53oz/15g | ☺ | ☺ ☺ | ☹ 5¼ | 33 66¼ |
| Tomato sauce | portion 2.12oz/60g | ☺ | ☺+ ×¾ unit ☺+ ×¼ unit | ☹ ¾ | 9¼ ᴮ 18½ |
| Tomato soup mix, dry | portion 1.2oz/34g | ¼ +0,24 unit | 13 26 | ☹ 2 | 1¼ ᴮ 2¾ |
| Tomato, cooked from fresh | portion 3oz/85g | ☺ | 4¼ 8½ | ☹ ¾ | 6½ ᴮ 13 |
| Tonic water | glass 8.4ozfl/240ml | ☺ | ☹² ☹² | ☺ ☺ | ☺ ☺ |
| Tonic water, diet | glass 8.4ozfl/240ml | ☺ | ☺ ☺ | ☺ ☺ | ☺ ☺ |
| Tootsie Pops® | piece 0.6oz/17g | ☺ | ☺+ ×2½ unit ☺+ ×1¼ unit | ☺ ☺ | ☺ ☺ |
| Tortilla, white, store bought, fried | piece 2.05oz/58g | ☺ | ☺ ☺ | ☺ ☺ | ¾ ᴬ 1¾ |
| Triple Sec | glass 8.4ozfl/240ml | ☺ | ☺+ ×4½ unit ☺+ ×2½ unit | ☹ ¼ | ☺ ☺ |

☹/ *Level 0*: lactose measure ×½    + Unit/💊: added tolerated amount of unit per strong lactase capsule
☹/ *Level 1*: fructose measure ×2    Fructose*: fructose, sorbitol adjusted
☹/ *Level 2*: fructose-/sorbitol measure ×4. the rest ×2    ☺+ ×[Amount] unit: Per unit consumed you can
☹/ *Level 3*: sorbitol measure ×7. the rest ×3    additionally tolerate up to [amount] ×
📖: source of fruc/galactans data    fructose(*)-unit of another product.
☹: avoid;    ☹¹: ¼ at TL 1;    ☹²: ¼ at TL 2;    ☹³: ¼ at TL 3;    ☺: only contains traces;    ☺: is free from it

| Keyword Index | Unit | Lactose ☺/ + unit/🥛 | Fructose* ☺/ Fructose* ☺/ | Sorbitol ☺/ Sorbitol ☺/ | FrucGalactans ☺/ FrucGalactans ☺/ 📖 |
|---|---|---|---|---|---|
| Triticale bread | slice 1.49oz/42g | ☺ | 2½ 5 | ☺ ☺ | 1 [A] 2 |
| Tuna, canned, light, oil pack, not drained | portion 1.95oz/55g | ☺ | ☺ ☺ | ☺ ☺ | ☺ ☺ |
| Turnip, cooked | portion 3oz/85g | ☺ | ☺+ ×½ unit ☺+ ×¼ unit | ☹ 2½ | ☺ [CB] ☺ |
| Twix® | piece 1.8oz/51g | 2 +1¾ unit | ☺+ ×1½ unit ☺+ ×¾ unit | ☺ ☺ | 1¾ [A] 3½ |
| Tzatziki sauce (yogurt and cucumber) | portion 1.06oz/30g | 4½ +3¾ unit | 38¾ 77½ | ☹ 9¼ | 11½ [FB] 23¼ |
| V-8® 100% A-C-E Vitamin Rich Vegetable Juice | glass 8.4ozfl/240ml | ☺ | ¼ ¾ | ☹ 3 | 2¾ [B] 5½ |
| Vanilla Coke® | glass 8.4ozfl/240ml | ☺ | ½ 1¼ | ☺ ☺ | ☺ ☺ |
| Vanilla sauce | tbsp. 0.5ozfl/14.21ml | ☺ | ☺ ☺ | ☺ ☺ | ☺ ☺ |
| Vegetable soup, condensed | portion 4.45oz/126g | ☺ | ☺+ ×¼ unit ☺ | ☹ 1 | 19¾ 39½ |
| Venison or deer, stewed | portion 3oz/85g | ☺ | ☺ ☺ | ☺ ☺ | ☺ ☺ |
| Veryfine Cranberry Raspberry | glass 8.4ozfl/240ml | ☺ | ☹[1] ¼ | ☹ ☹[2] | ¾ [B] 1½ |
| Vichyssoise soup | portion 8.65oz/245g | ¾ +½ unit | ☺+ ×¼ unit ☺ | ☹ 1¼ | 4¼ [AB] 8½ |
| Vodka | glass 8.4ozfl/240ml | ☺ | ☺ ☺ | ☺ ☺ | ☺ ☺ |
| Waffles, bran | piece 3.36oz/95g | ¾ +¾ unit | ☺+ ×¼ unit ☺ | ☺ ☺ | ¼ [A] ¾ |
| Waffles, whole wheat, from mix, add milk, fat and egg | piece 3.36oz/95g | 1 +¾ unit | ☺+ ×¼ unit ☺ | ☺ ☺ | ½ [A] 1 |
| Walnut oil | tbsp. 0.5ozfl/14.21ml | ☺ | ☺ ☺ | ☺ ☺ | ☺ ☺ |
| Walnuts | hand 1.06oz/30g | ☺ | ☺ ☺ | ☺ ☺ | 2¾ [G] 5¾ |
| Watercress, raw | pinch 0.04oz/1g | ☺ | ☺ ☺ | ☺ ☺ | ☺ ☺ |
| Watermelon, fresh | tbsp. 0.5ozfl/14.21ml | ☺ | 1¾ 3½ | ☹ ☺ | 10¼ [B] 20¾ |

| Keyword Index | Unit | Lactose ↯ + unit/💊 | Fructose* ↯ Fructose* ↯ | Sorbitol ↯ Sorbitol ↯ | FrucGalactans ↯ FrucGalactans ↯ 📖 |
|---|---|---|---|---|---|
| Wax beans (yellow beans), canned, drained | portion 3oz/85g | ☺ | ☺ ☺ | ☺ ☺ | ¼ ᴬ ¾ |
| Weetabix® Organic Crispy Flakes & Fiber (Barbara's Bakery®) | portion 1.95oz/55g | ☺ | ☺+ ×¾ unit ☺+ ×¾ unit | ☺ ☺ | ¼ ᴬ ¾ |
| Wendy's® Strawberry Shake | glass 8.4oz/240g | ¼ +¼ unit | ☺+ ×4¼ unit ☺+ ×2 unit | ☹ 3¼ | 1¾ 3¾ |
| Werther's® Original Caramel Coffee Hard Candies | piece 0.15oz/4g | 17¾ +14¾ unit | ☺+ ×½ unit ☺+ ×¼ unit | ☺ ☺ | ☺ ☺ |
| Wheat bran, unprocessed | tbsp. 0.5ozfl/14.21ml | ☺ | ☺ ☺ | ☺ ☺ | ½ ᴳ 1 |
| Wheaties® (General Mills®) | portion 1.06oz/30g | ☺ | 83¼ ☺ | ☺ ☺ | ½ ᴬ 1¼ |
| Whipped cream, aerosol | portion 0.25oz/7g | ☺ | ☺ ☺ | ☺ ☺ | ☺ ☺ |
| Whipped cream, aerosol, chocolate | portion 0.18oz/5g | 9¾ +8 unit | ☺ ☺ | ☹ ☺ | 54½ ☺ |
| Whipped cream, aerosol, fat free | portion 0.18oz/5g | 18¾ +15¾ unit | ☺+ ×¼ unit ☺ | ☺ ☺ | ☺ ☺ |
| Whiskey | glass 8.4ozfl/240ml | ☺ | ☺ ☺ | ☺ ☺ | ☺ ☺ |
| Whiskey sour | glass 8.4ozfl/240ml | ☺ | 9½ 19 | ☹ 6¼ | ☺ ☺ |
| whisky | glass 8ozfl/240mL | ☺ | ☺ ☺ | ☺ ☺ | ☺ ☺ |
| whisky sour | glass 8ozfl/240mL | ☺ | 9½ 19 | ☹ 6¼ | ☺ ☺ |
| White all-purpose flour, unenriched | portion 1.06oz/30g | ☺ | ☺ ☺ | ☺ ☺ | 1¼ ᴬ 2¾ |
| White bean stew with sofrito | tbsp. 0.5ozfl/14.21ml | ☺ | ☺ ☺ | ☹ ☺ | 3 ᴬᶜ 6 |
| White bread, store bought | slice 1.49oz/42g | ☺ | 1¼ 2¾ | ☺ ☺ | 1¼ ᴬ 2½ |

♀ Level 0: lactose measure ×½  
↯ Level 1: fructose measure ×2  
↯ Level 2: fructose-/sorbitol measure ×4. the rest ×2  
↯ Level 3: sorbitol measure ×7. the rest ×3  
📖: source of fruc/galactans data  

+ Unit/💊: added tolerated amount of unit per strong lactase capsule  
Fructose*: fructose, sorbitol adjusted  

☺+ ×[Amount] unit: Per unit consumed you can additionally tolerate up to [amount] × fructose(*)-unit of another product.  

☹: avoid;   ☹¹: ¼ at TL 1;   ☹²: ¼ at TL 2;   ☹³: ¼ at TL 3;   ☺: only contains traces;   ☺: is free from it

| Keyword Index | Unit | Lactose ↯<br>+ unit/🍞 | Fructose* ↯<br>Fructose* ↯ | Sorbitol ↯<br>Sorbitol ↯ | FrucGalactans ↯<br>FrucGalactans ↯📖 |
|---|---|---|---|---|---|
| White chocolate bar | piece<br>0.43ozfl/12g | 2½<br>+2 unit | ☺<br>☺ | ☺<br>☺ | 14<br>28¼ |
| White Russian | glass<br>8.4ozfl/240ml | 1½<br>+1¼ unit | ☺<br>☺ | ☹<br>8¼ | 9<br>18¼ |
| White sauce, store bought | tbsp.<br>0.5ozfl/14.21ml | 4<br>+3¼ unit | ☺<br>☺ | ☺<br>☺ | 22¼<br>44½ |
| White whole grain wheat bread | slice<br>1.49oz/42g | ☺ | ¾<br>1¾ | ☹<br>26¼ | ¾ [A]<br>1¾ |
| White whole wheat flour | portion<br>1.06oz/30g | ☺ | 33¼<br>66½ | ☺<br>☺ | 1¼ [AD]<br>2¾ |
| Whole wheat bread, store bought | slice<br>1.49oz/42g | ☺ | 1¼<br>2½ | ☺<br>☺ | 1 [A]<br>2¼ |
| Wild 'n Fruity Gummi Bears (Brach's®) | hand<br>1.06oz/30g | ☺ | ☺+ ×3½ unit<br>☺+ ×1¾ unit | ☹<br>☺ | ☺<br>☺ |
| Windmill cookies | piece<br>0.75oz/21g | ☺ | ☺<br>☺ | ☺<br>☺ | 6¼ [A]<br>12¾ |
| Wine spritzer | glass<br>8.4ozfl/240ml | ☺ | 27¾<br>55½ | ☹<br>1 | ☺<br>☺ |
| Winter (dark green or orange) squash, cooked | portion<br>4.59oz/130g | ☺ | 1¾<br>3¾ | ☺<br>☺ | ☺ [CB]<br>☺ |
| Winter melon (waxgourd or chinese preserving melon) | portion<br>3oz/85g | ☺ | ☺<br>☺ | ☺<br>☺ | ☺ [CB]<br>☺ |
| Wise Onion Flavored Rings | portion<br>1.06oz/30g | ☺ | ☺<br>☺ | ☹<br>☺ | 10¼ [AC]<br>20¾ |
| Yams, sweet potato type, boiled | portion<br>3.89oz/110g | ☺ | ☺<br>☺ | ☺<br>☺ | ☺ [B]<br>☺ |
| Yellow bell pepper, raw | portion<br>3oz/85g | ☺ | ½<br>1¼ | ☺<br>☺ | ☺ [CB]<br>☺ |
| Yellow tomato, raw | portion<br>3oz/85g | ☺ | 4½<br>9¼ | ☹<br>1 | 6½ [B]<br>13 |
| Yerba® Mate tea | glass<br>8.4ozfl/240ml | ☺ | ☺<br>☺ | ☺<br>☺ | ☺<br>☺ |
| Yogurt, chocolate or coffee flavors, nonfat, sweetened with aspartame | tbsp.<br>0.5ozfl/14.21ml | 4<br>+3¼ unit | ☺<br>☺ | ☺<br>☺ | 22½<br>45 |
| Yogurt, chocolate or coffee flavors, whole milk, sweetened with sucralose | piece<br>6.04oz/171g | ¼<br>+¼ unit | 40<br>80 | ☺<br>☺ | 1½<br>3¼ |
| Yogurt, fruited, whole milk | tbsp<br>0.5ozfl/14.21ml | 2¾<br>+2¼ unit | ¾<br>1½ | ☹<br>60½ | 16<br>32¼ |

| Keyword Index | Unit + unit/🗨 | Lactose 🝆 | Fructose* ⚯ Fructose* 🝆 | Sorbitol ⚯ Sorbitol 🝆 | FrucGalactans ⚯ FrucGalactans 🝆 📖 |
|---|---|---|---|---|---|
| Zsweet® | portion 0.18ozfl/5ml | ☺ | ☺ ☺ | ☹ ☹ | ☺ ☺ |

⚯ *Level 0:* lactose measure ×½    + Unit/🗨: added tolerated amount of unit per strong lactase capsule
🝆 *Level 1:* fructose measure ×2    Fructose*: fructose, sorbitol adjusted
🝆 *Level 2:* fructose-/sorbitol measure ×4. the rest ×2    ☺+ ×[Amount] unit: Per unit consumed you can
🝆 *Level 3:* sorbitol measure ×7. the rest ×3    additionally tolerate up to [amount] ×
📖: source of fruc/galactans data    fructose(*)-unit of another product.

☹: avoid;    ☹[1]: ¼ at TL 1;    ☹[2]: ¼ at TL 2;    ☹[3]: ¼ at TL 3;    ☺: only contains traces;    ☺: is free from it

# GLOSSARY

| Abbreviation | Meaning |
| --- | --- |
| Brick dragon | Metaphor for discomfort induced by the presence of quickly fermentable carbohydrates in an "irritable bowel". |
| Bricks | Carbohydrates that are quickly fermented in the intestine. To this group belong oligosaccharides (Fructose, Fructans and Galactans, Lactose) and sugar alcohols. |
| BTL | Basic tolerance level, i.e. as long as you consume less of a problematic brick than the stated maximum amount for this level, you are likely to be untroubled by symptoms from it. It only applies in case of intolerance or certain testphases and then refers to the lowest allowable portion sizes and holds at least until a level test has been taken. Note that if you consume the maximum (B)TL portion size for a food at a meal, you cannot eat any other foods that contain the brick at that meal. To combine two foods that contain a certain brick you have to reduce the stated portion sizes accordingly, e.g. by dividing both by two. |
| BTLs | Basic tolerance levels. |
| EFSA | European Food Safety Authority. |
| FDA | Food and Drug Administration. |
| Fructans | Quickly fermentable carbohydrates that are contained in grain products for example. In this book only inulin, kestose and nystose are attributed to this group. |
| Fructose | Oligosaccharide that is primarily contained in fruit. |
| Galactans | Quickly fermentable carbohydrates that are contained in beans, cabbage, lentils and peas for example. In this book only raffinose and stachyose are attributed to this group. |
| Interception shield | Metaphor for the normal bodily resorbtion of bricks. |

| Abbreviation | Meaning |
|---|---|
| Irritable bowel | Definition of this book: An irritable bowel is one that reacts much more intensely to indigestions than it is commonly the case. These indigestions are often caused by the presence of "bricks" in the intestine. |
| Lactose | Oligosaccharide that is primarily contained in dairy products. |
| Meal | A meal is defined as one of three mainmeals of a given day. The first meal happen at about 7 am, the second one at about 1pm and the third one at about 7 pm. Hence, between each meal there has to be a gap of about six hours in order to avoid overloading your "interception shield". The tolerable portion sizes are based on this definition of a meal. |
| NCC | Nutrition Coordination Center of the University of Minnesota. |
| Sorbitol | Sugar alcohol that also limits the "interception" of fructose. Besides, see "sugar alcohols". |
| Sugar alcohols | These are contained in some fruit, like apples. Moreover, they are part of many diabetic, dietary and light products as well as chewing gums and mints. They are not contained in stevia. Part of the group of sugar alcohols besides sorbitol are erythritol, inositol, isomalt, lactitol, maltitol, mannitol, pinitol and xylitol. |
| TL | Tolerance level. These are employed to differentiate the portion sizes stated in the food tables according to the amount of the respective brick that is tolerated by you per meal. There are four tolerance levels for any brick. TL 0 being the BTL and TL 1 to TL 3 representing higher tolerable amounts of a brick and thus larger portion sizes of the foods that contain it. You can determine the level that applies to you by taking the level test that is described in chapter 21.4. Please also read the BTL definition. |
| TLs | Tolerance levels. |

*This page has been intentionally left blank.*

# SOURCES

Ali, M., Rellos, P., & Cox, T. M. (1998). Heriditary fructose intolerance. *Journal of Medical Genetics*, 35(5), 353-365.

Barrett, J. S., Gearry, R. B., Muir, J. G., Irving, P. M., Rose, R., Rosella, O., ... & Gibson, P. R. (2010). Dietary poorly absorbed, short-chain carbohydrates increase delivery of water and fermentable substrates to the proximal colon. *Alimentary Pharmacology & Therapeutics*, 31(8), 874-882.

Balasubramanya, N. N., Sarwar, & Narayanan, K. M. (1993). Effect of stage of lactation on oligosaccharides level in milk. *Indian Journal of Dairy & Biosciences*, 4, 58-60. Abstract Retrieved from http://www.cabdirect.com (Record Number 19950401205)

Belitz, H.-D., Grosch, W., & Schieberle, P. (2008). *Lehrbuch der Lebensmittelchemie* (6th ed.), Berlin Heidelberg: Springer.

Berekoven, L., Eckert, W., Ellenrieder, P. (2009). Marktforschung: *Methodische Grundlagen und praktische Anwendung* (12th ed.). Wiesbaden: Gabler.

Biesiekierski, J. R., Rosella, O., Rose, R., Liels, K., Barrett, J. S., Shepherd, S. J., ... & Muir, J. G. (2011). Quantification of fructans, galacto-oligosacharides and other short-chain carbohydrates in processed grains and cereals. *Journal of Human Nutrition and Dietetics*, 24(2), 154-176.

Binnendijk, K. H., & Rijkers, G. T. (2013). What is a health benefit? an evaluation of EFSA opinions on health benefits with reference to probiotics. *Beneficial Microbes*, 4(3), 223-230.

Blumenthal, M. (1998). *The Complete German Commission E Monographs; Therapeutic Guide to Herbal Medicine*. Boston, MA: Integrative Medicine Communications.

Boehm, G., & Stahl, B. (2007). Oligosaccharides from milk. *The Journal of Nutrition*, 137(3), 847S-849S.

Bowden, P. (2011). *Telling It Like It Is*. Paul Bowden.

Briançon, S., Boini, S., Bertrais, S., Guillemin, F., Galan, P., & Hercberg, S. (2011). Long-term antioxidant supplementation has no effect on health-related quality of life: The randomized, double-blind, placebo-controlled, primary prevention SU.VI.MAX trial. *International Journal of Epidemiology*, 40(6), 1605-1616.

Campbell, J. M., Fahey, G. C., & Wolf, B. W. (1997). Selected indigestible oligosaccharides affect large bowel mass, cecal and fecal short-chain fatty acids, pH and microflora in rats. *The Journal of Nutrition*, 127(1), 130-136.

Chi, W. J., Chang, Y. K., & Hong, S. K. (2012). Agar degradation by microorganisms and agar-degrading enzymes. *Applied Microbiology and Biotechnology*, 94(4), 917-930.

Choi, Y. K; Johlin Jr., F. C.; Summers, R.W., Jackson, M., & Rao, S. S. C. (2003). Fructose intolerance: an under-recognized problem. *The American Journal of Gastroenterology*, 98(6) 2003, S. 1348-1353.

CIAA (n. d.). *CIAA agreed reference values for GDAs* [Table]. Retrieved from http://gda.fooddrinkeurope.eu/asp2/gdas_portions_rationale.asp?doc_id=127.

Connor, W. E. (2000). Importance of n−3 fatty acids in health and disease. *The American journal of clinical nutrition*, 71(1), 171S-175S.

Coraggio, L. (1990). *Deleterious Effects of Intermittent Interruptions on the Task Performance of Knowledge Workers: A Laboratory Investigation* (Doctoral Dissertation). Retrieved from http://arizona.openrepository.com.

Corazza, G. R., Strocchi, A., Rossi, R., Sirola, D., & Fasbarrini, G. (1988). Sorbitol malabsorption in normal volunteers and in patients with celiac disease. *Gut*, 29(1), 44-48.

Cummings, J. H. (1981). Short chain fatty acids in the human colon. *Gut*, 22(9), 763-779.

Cummings, J. H., & Macfarlane, G. T. (1997). Role of intestinal bacteria in nutrient metabolism. *Journal of Parental and Enteral Nutrition*, 21(6), 357-365.

DGE (2013). Vollwertig essen und trinken nach den 10 Regeln der DGE. 9th Edition, Bonn.

Diamond, J. (2005). *Collapse – How Societies Choose to Fail or to Survive*. New York: Viking Penguin.

Donker, G. A., Foets, M., & Spreeuwenberg, P. (1999). Patients with irritable bowel syndrome: health status and use of healthcare services. *British Journal of General Practice*, 49(447), 787-792.

Drossman, D. A., Li, Z., Andruzzi, E., Temple, R. D., Talley, N. J., Thompson, W. G. ...Corazziari, E. et al., (1993). US householder survey of functional gastrointestinal disorders: prevalence, sociodemography, and health impact. *Digestive Diseases and Sciences*, 38(9), 1569-1580.

Dukas, L., Willett, W. C., & Giovannucci, E. L. (2003). Association between physical activity, fiber intake, and other lifestyle variables and constipation in a study of women. *The American Journal of Gastroenterology*, 98(8), 1790-1796.

EFSA (2007). Opinion of the Scientific Panel on Dietetic Products, Nutrition and Allergies on a request from the Commission related to a notification from EPA on lactitol pursuant to Article 6, paragraph 11 of Directive 2000/13/EC- for permanent exemption from labeling. *The EFSA Journal*, 5(10), 565-570.

EFSA (2012a). Scientific Opinion on Dietary Reference Values for protein. *The EFSA Journal*, 10(2), 2557-2622.

EFSA (2012b). Scientific Opinion on the substantiation of health claims related to Lactobacillus casei DG CNCM I-1572 and decreasing potentially pathogenic gastro-intestinal microorganisms (ID 2949, 3061, further assessment) pursuant to Article 13(1) of Regulation (EC) No 1924/2006. *The EFSA Journal*, 10(6), 2723-2637.

EFSA (2012c). Scientific opinion on the tolerable upper intake level of eicosapentaenoic acid (epa), docosahexaenoic acid (dha) and docosapentaenoic acid (dpa). *The EFSA Journal*, 10(7), 2815-2862.

EFSA (2013). Scientific Opinion on the substantiation of a health claim related to Bimuno® GOS and reducing gastro-intestinal discomfort pursuant to Article 13(5) of Regulation (EC) No 1924/2006. *The EFSA Journal*, 11(6), 3259-3268.

Eisenführ, F., Weber, M., & Langer, T. (2010): *Rational Decision Making*, Heidelberg, Berlin: Springer.

Erdman, K., Tunnicliffe, J., Lun, V. M., & Reimer, R. A. (2013). Eating Patterns and Composition of Meals and Snacks in Elite Canadian Athletes. *International Journal Of Sport Nutrition & Exercise Metabolism*, 23(3), 210-219.

Falony, G., Verschaeren, A. De Bruycker, F., De Preter, V., Verbecke, F. L., & De Vuyst L. (2009b). In vitro kinetics of prebiotic inulin-type fructan fermentation by butyrate-producing colon bacteria: implementation of online gas chromatography for quantitative analysis of carbon dioxide and hydrogen gas production. *Applied Environmental Microbiology*, 75(18), 5884-5892.

FAO (2008). Fats and fatty acids in human nutrition. *FAO Food and Nutrition Paper*, 91, 9-20.

Farquhar, P. H., & Keller, L. R. (1989). Preference intensity measurement. *Annals of Operations Research*, 19(1), 205-217.

Farshchi, H. R., Taylor, M. A., & Macdonald, I. A. (2004). Regular meal frequency creates more appropriate insulin sensitivity and lipid profiles compared with irregular meal frequency in healthy lean women. *European Journal Of Clinical Nutrition*, 58(7), 1071-1077.

Fass, R., Fullerton, S., Naliboff, B., Hirsh, T., & Mayer, E. A. (1998). Sexual dysfunction in patients with irritable bowel syndrom and non-ulcer dyspepsia. *Digestion*, 59(1), 79-85.

Fernández-Bañares, F., Esteve-Pardo, M., de Leon, R., Humbert, P., Cabré, E., Llovet, J. M., & Gassull, M. A. (1993). Sugar malabsorption in functional bowel disease: clinical implications. *American Journal of Gastroenterology*, 88(12), 2044-2050.

Fox, K. (2013). N. t.. In Wells, V., Wyness, L., & Coe, S. (Eds.). The British Nutrition Foundation's 45th Anniversary Conference: Behaviour change in relation to healthier lifestyles. *Nutrition Bulletin*, 38(1), 100-107.

Gaby, A. R. (2005). Adverse effects of dietary fructose. *Alternative medicine review*, 10(4).

Gay-Crosier, F., Schreiber, G., & Hauser, C. (2000). Anaphylaxis from inulin in vegetables and processed food. *The New England Journal of Medicine*, 342(18), 1372.

German, J., Freeman, S., Lebrilla, C., & Mills, D. (2008). Human milk oligosaccharides: evolution, structures and bioselectivity as substrates for intestinal bacteria, *Nestlé Nutrition Workshop, Pediatric Program*, 62, 205-222.

Gibson, P. R., Newnham, E., Barrett, J. S., Shepherd, S. J., & Muir, J. G. (2007). Review article: Fructose malabsorption and the bigger picture. *Alimentary pharmacology & therapeutics*, 25(4), 349-363.

Gibson, P. R., & Shepherd, S. J. (2010). Evidence-based dietary management of functional gastrointestinal symptoms: the fodmap approach. Journal of *Gastroenterology and Hepatology*, 25(2), 252-258.

Gilbert, P. (2013). N. t.. In Wells, V., Wyness, L., & Coe, S. (Eds.). The British Nutrition Foundation's 45th Anniversary Conference: Behaviour change in relation to healthier lifestyles. *Nutrition Bulletin*, 38(1), 100-107.

Goldstein, R., Braverman, D., & Stankiewicz, H. (2000). Carbohydrate malabsorption and the effect of dietary restriction on symptoms of irritable bowel syndrome and functional bowel complaints. *Israel Medical Association Journal*, 2(8), 583-587.

Gralnek, I. M., Hays, R. D., Kilbourne, A., Naliboff, B., & Mayer, E. A. (2000). The impact of irritable bowel syndrome on health-related quality of life. *Gastroenterology*, 119(3), 654-660.

Hahn, B. A., Kirchdoerfer, L. J., Fullerton, S., & Mayer, S. (1997). Patient perceived severity of irritable bowel syndrome in relation to symptoms, health resource utilization and quality of life. *Alimentary Pharmacology and Therapeutics*, 11(3), 553-559.

Hawthorne, B., Lambert, S., Scott, D., & Scott, B. (1991). Food intolerance and the irritable bowel syndrome. *Journal of Human Nutrition and Dietetics*, 4(1), 19-23.

Hawking, S. (n. d.). Publications. Retrieved from http://www.hawking.org.uk/publications.html.

Hillson, M. (2013). N. t.. In Wells, V., Wyness, L., & Coe, S. (Eds.). The British Nutrition Foundation's 45th Anniversary Conference: Behaviour change in relation to healthier lifestyles. *Nutrition Bulletin*, 38(1), 100-107.

Hoekstra, J. H., van Kempen, A. A. M. W., & Kneepkens, C. M. F. (1993). Apple juice malabsorption: Fructose or sorbitol?. *Journal of Pediatric Gastroenterology and Nutrition*, 16(1), 39-42.

Huether, G. (Lecturer). (2014). Interview mit Prof. Dr. Gerald Hüther zu Angst & Berufung. Retrieved from http://www.coach-yourself.tv/Startseite/TV/InterviewmitProfDrH%C3%BCtherzuAngstBerufung/tabid/1341/Default.aspx

Hyams, J. S. (1983). Sorbitol intolerance: an unappreciated cause of functional gastrointestinal complaints. *Gastroenterology*, 84(1)1, 30-33.

Hyams, J. S., Etienne, N. L., Leichtner, A. M., & Theuer, R. C. (1988). Carbohydrate Malabsorption Following Fruit Juice Ingestion in Young Children. *Pediatrics*, 82(1), 64-68.

Jensen, R. G., Blanc, B., & Patton, S. (1995). Particulate Constituents in Human and Bovine Milks. In Jensen, R. G. (Ed.), *Handbook of Milk Composition* (pp. 51-62). San Diego: Academic Press.

Kennedy, E. (2004). Dietary diversity, diet quality, and body weight regulation. *Nutrition reviews*, 62(s2), S78-S81.

Kneepkens, C. M. F., Vonk, R. J., & Fernandes, J. (1984). Incomplete intestinal absorption of fructose. *Archives of Disease in Childhood*, 59(8), 735-738.

Kneepkens, C. M. F., Jakobs, C., & Douwes, A. C. (1989): Apple juice, fructose, and chronic nonspecific diarrhoea. *Pediatrics*, 148(6), 571-573.

Knudsen, B. K., & Hessov, I. (1995). Recovery of inulin from Jerusalem artichoke (Helianthus tuberosus L.) in the small intestine of man. *British Journal of Nutrition*, 74(01), 101-113.

Komericki, P., Akkilic-Materna, M., Strimitzer, T., Weyermair, K., Hammer, H. F., & Aberer, W. (2012). Oral xylose isomerase decreases breath hydrogen excretion and improves gastrointestinal symptoms in fructose malabsorption – a double-blind, placebo-controlled study. *Alimentary Pharmacology & Therapeutics*, 36(10), 980-987.

Kuhn, R., & Gauhe, A. (1965). Bestimmung der Bindungsstelle von Sialinsäureresten in Oligosacchariden mit Hilfe von Perjodat. *Chemische Berichte*, 98(2), 395-314.

Ladas, S. D., Grammenos, I., Tassios, P. S., & Raptis, S. A. (2000). Coincidental malabsorption of lactose, fructose, and sorbitol ingested at low doses is not common in normal adults. *Digestive Diseases and Sciences*, 45(12), 2357-2362.

Langkilde, A. M., Andersson, H., Schweizer, T. F., & Würsch, P. (1994). Digestion and absorption of sorbitol, maltitol and isomalt from the small bowel. A study in ileostomy subjects. *European Journal of Clinical Nutrition*, 48(11), 768-775.

Latulippe, M. E., & Skoog, S. M. (2011). Fructose malabsorption and intolerance: effects of fructose with and without simultaneous glucose ingestion. *Critical Reviews in Food Science and Nutrition*, 51(7), 583-592.

Le, A. S., & Mulderrig, K. B. (2001). *Sorbitol and mannitol*. Nabors, O'B. (Ed.). New York, NY: Marcel Dekker.

Ledochowski, M., Widner, B., Sperner-Unterweger, B., Probst, T., Vogel, W., & Fuchs, D. (2000). Carbohydrate malabsobtion syndromes and early signs of mental depression in females. *Digestive Diseases and Sciences*, 45(12), 1255-1259.

Ledochowski, M., Sperner-Unterweger, B., Widner, B., & Fuchs, D. (1998a). Fructose malabsorption is associated with early signs of mentral depression. *European Journal of Medical Research*, 3(6), 295-298.

Ledochowski, M., Sperner-Unterweger, B., & Fuchs, D. (1998b). Lactose malabsorption is associated with early signs of mental depression in females – a preliminary report. *Digestive Diseases and Sciences*, 43(11), 2513-2517.

Ledochowski, M., Überall, F., Propst, T., & Fuchs, D. (1999). Fructose malabsorption is associated with lower plasma folic acid concentrations in middle-aged subjects. *Clinical Chemistry*, 45(11), 2013-2014.

Ledochowski, M., Widner, B., Bair, H., Probst, T., & Fuchs, D. (2000a). Fructose-and sorbitol-reduced diet improves mood and gastrointestinal disturbances in fructose malabsorbers. *Scandinavian Journal of Gastroenterology*, 35(10), 1048-1052.

Ledochowski, M., Widner, B., Sperner-Unterweger, B., Probst, T., Vogel, W., & Fuchs, D. (2000b). Carbohydrate malabsobtion syndromes and early signs of mental depression in females. *Digestive Diseases and Sciences*, 45(12), 1255-1259.

Leinoel (n. d.). *Leinöl(Leinsamen)*. Retrieved from http://www.vitalstoff journal.de/vitalstoff-lexikon/l/leinoel-leinsamen/

Lewis, S. J., & Heaton, K. W. (1997). Stool form scale as a useful guide to intestinal transit time. *Scandinavian Journal of Gastroenterology*, 32(9), 920-924.

Lifschitz, C. H. (2000). Carbohydrate absorption from fruit juices in infants. *Pediatrics*, 105(1), e4.

Lombardi, D. A., Jin, K., Courtney, T. K., Arlinghaus, A., Folkard, S., Liang, Y., & Perry, M. J. (2014). The effects of rest breaks, work shift start time, and sleep on the onset of severe injury among workers in the People's Republic of China. *Scandinavian Journal of Work, Environment & Health*, 40(2), 146-155.

Lomer, M. C. E., Parkes, G. C., & Sanderson, J. D. (2008). Review article: Lactose intolerance in clinical practice – myths and realities. *Alimentary Pharmacology & Therapeutics*, 27(2), 93-103.

Longstreth, G. F., Thompson, W. G., Chey, W. D., Houghton, L. A., Mearin, F., & Spiller, R. C. (2006). Functional bowel disorders. *Gastroenterology*, 130(5), 1480-1491.

Maintz, L., & Novak, N. (2007). Histamine and histamine intolerance. *The American Journal of Clinical Nutrition*, 85(5), 1185-1196.

Makras, L., Van Acker, G., & De Vuyst, L. (2005). Lactobacillus paracasei subsp. paracasei 8700: 2 degrades inulin-type fructans exhibiting different degrees of polymerization. *Applied and Environmental Microbiology*, 71(11), 6531-6537.

McCoubrey, H., Parkes, G. C., Sanderson, J. D., & Lomer, M. C. E. (2008). Nutritional intakes in irritable bowel syndrome. *Journal of Human Nutrition and Dietetics*, 21(4), 396-397.

McKenzie, Y. A., Alder, A., Anderson, W. Goddard, L, Gulia, P., Jankovich, E. ...Lomer, M. C. E. (2012). British Dietic Association evidence-based guidelines for the dietary management of irritable bowel syndrome in adults. *Journal of Human Nutrition and Dietics*, 25(3), 260-274.

Meyrand, M., Dallas, D. C., Caillat, H., Bouvier, F., Martin, P., & Barile, D. (2013). Comparison of milk oligosaccharides between goats with and without the genetic ability to synthesize αs1-casein. *Small Ruminant Research*, 113(2), 411-420.

Michel, G., Nyval-Collen, P., Barbeyron, T., Czjzek, M., & Helbert, W. (2006). Bioconversion of red seaweed galactans: a focus on bacterial agarases and carrageenases. *Applied Microbiology and Biotechnology*, 71(1), 23-33.

Michie, S. (2013). N. t.. In Wells, V., Wyness, L., & Coe, S. (Eds.). The British Nutrition Foundation's 45th Anniversary Conference: Behaviour change in relation to healthier lifestyles. *Nutrition Bulletin*, 38(1), 100-107.

Mishkin, D., Sablauskas, L., Yalovsky, M., & Mishkin, S. (1997). Fructose and sorbitol malabsorption in ambulatory patients with functional dyspepsia: comparison with lactose maldigestion/malabsorption. *Digestive Diseases and Sciences*, 42(12), 2591-2598.

Montalto, M., Curigliano, V., Santoro, L., Vastola, M., Cammarota, G., Manna, R., ... & Gasbarrini, G. (2006). Management and treatment of lactose malabsorption. *World Journal of Gastroenterology*, 12(2), 187.

Molis, C., Flourié, B., Ouarne, F., Gailing, M. F., Lartigue, S., Guibert, A., Bornet, F., & Galmiche, F. P. (1996). Digestion, excretion, and energy value of fructooligosaccharides in healthy humans.*The American Society for Clinical Nutrition*, 64(3), 324-328.

*Mosby's Medical Dictionary* (8th ed.). St. Louis, MO: Mosby.

Monash University (2014). The Monash University Low Foodmap Diet [Software]. Available from http://www.med.monash.edu/cecs/gastro/fodmap/education.html

Moshfegh, A. J., James, E. F., Goldman, J. P., & Ahuja, J. L. C. (1999). Presence of inulin and oligofructose in the diets of Americans. *The Journal of Nutrition*, 129(7), 1407S-1411S.

Mount Sinai (n. d.). *Fiber Chart*. Retrieved from https://www.wehealny.org/healthinfo/dietaryfiber/fibercontentchart.html.

Mozaffarian, D., & Wu, J. H. (2011). Omega-3 fatty acids and cardiovascular disease effects on risk factors, molecular pathways, and clinical events. *Journal of the American College of Cardiology*, 58(20), 2047-2067.

Muir, J. G., Shepherd, S. J., Rosella, O., Rose, R., Barrett, J. S., & Gibson, P. R. (2007). Fructan and free fructose content of common Australian vegetables and fruit. *Journal of Agricultural and Food Chemistry*, 55(16), 6619-6627.

Muir, J. G., Rose, R., Rosella, O., Liels, K., Barrett, J. S., Shepherd, S. J., & Gibson, P. R. (2009). Measurement of short-chain carbohydrates in common Australian vegetables and fruits by high-performance liquid chromatography (HPLC). *Journal of Agricultural and Food Chemistry*, 57(2), 554-565.

Nanda, R., James, R., Smith, H., Dudley, C. R. K., & Jewell, D. P. (1989). Food intolerance and the irritable bowel syndrome. *Gut*, 30(8), 1099-1104.

Necas, J., Bartosikova, L. (2013). Carageenan: a review. *Veterinarni Medicina*, 58(4), 187-205.

Nelis, G. F., Vermeeren, M. A., & Jansen, W. (1990). Role of fructose-sorbitol malabsorbtion in the irritable bowel syndrome. *Gastroenterology*, 99(4), 10156-1020.

Newburg, D. S. & Neubauer, S. H. (1995). Carbohydrates in Milks: Analysis, Quantities, and Significance. In Jensen, R. G. (Ed.), *Handbook of Milk Composition* (pp. 273-349). San Diego: Academic Press.

NICNAS (2008). Multiple chemical sensitivity: identifying key research needs. *Scientific review report*.

Nucera, G., Gabrielli, M., Lupascu, A., Lauritano, E. C., Santoliquido, A., Cremonini, F., …Gasbarrini, A. (2005). Abnormal breath tests to lactose, fructose and sorbitol in irritable bowel syndrome may be explained by small intestinal bacterial overgrowth. *Alimentary Pharmacology & Therapeutics*, 21(11), 1391-1395.

O'Connell, S., & Walsh, G. (2006). Physicochemical characteristics of commercial lactases relevant to their application in the alleviation of lactose intolerance. *Applied Biochemistry and Biotechnology*, 134(2), 179-191.

Ong, D., Mitchell, S., Barrett, J., Shepherd, S., Irving, P., Biesiekierski, J., & … Muir, J. (2010). Manipulation of dietary short chain carbohydrates alters the pattern of gas production and genesis of symptoms in irritable bowel syndrome. *Journal of Gastroenterology & Hepatology*, 25(8), 1366-1373.

Park, Y. K., & Yetley, E. A. (1993). Intakes and food sources of fructose in the United States. *The American Journal of Clinical Nutrition*, 58(5), 737S-747S.

Parker, T. J., Naylor, S. J., Riordan, A. M., & Hunter, J. O. (1995). Management of patients with food intolerance in irritable bowel syndrome. The development and use of an exclusion diet. *Journal of Human Nutrition and Dietetics*, 8(3), 159-166.

Petitpierre, M., Gumowski, P., & Girard, J. P. (1985). Irritable bowel syndrome and hypersensitivity to food. *Annals of Allergy, Asthma & Immunology*, 54(6), 538-540.

Quigley, E., Fried, M., Gwee, K. A., Olano, C., Guarner, F., Khalif, I., … & Le Mair, A. W. (2009). Irritable bowel syndrome: a global perspective. *WGO Practice Guideline*.

Quigley, E., M., M., Hunt, R. H., Emmanuel, A., & Hungin, A. P. S. (2013). Irritable Bowel Syndrome (IBS): What is it, what causes it and can I do anything about it? Retrieved from http://client.blueskybroadcast.com/WGO/indeux.html

Raithel, M., Weidenhiller, M., Hagel, A.-F.-K., Hetterich, U., Neurath, M. F., & Konturek, P. C. (2013). The malabsorption of commonly occurring mono and disaccharides: levels of investigation and differential diagnoses. *Dtsch Arztebl Int*, 110(46), 775-782.

Riby, J. E., Fujisawa, T., & Kretchmer, N. (1993). Fructose absorption. *The American Journal of Clinical Nutrition*, 58(5), 748S-753S.

Ross, A. C., Manson, J. E., Abrams, S. A., Aloia, J. F., Brannon, P. M., Clinton, S. K., ... & Shapses, S. A. (2011). The 2011 report on dietary reference intakes for calcium and vitamin D from the Institute of Medicine: what clinicians need to know. *Journal of Clinical Endocrinology & Metabolism*, 96(1), 53-58.

Rumessen, J. J., & Gudmand-Høyer, E. (1986). Absorption capacity of fructose in healthy adults. Comparison with sucrose and its constituent monosaccharides. *Gut*, 27(10), 1161-1168.

Rumessen, J. J., & Gudmand-Høyer, E., (1987). Malabsoption of Fructose-sorbitol mixtures. Interactions causing abdominal distress. *Scandinavian Journal of Gastroenterology*, 22(4), 431-436.

Rumessen, J. J. (1992). Fructose and related food carbohydrates. sources, intake, absorbtion, and clinical implications. *Scandinavian Journal of Gastroenterology*, 27(10), 819-828.

Ruppin, H., Bar-Meir, S., Soergel, K. H., Wood, C. M., & Schmitt Jr, M. G. (1980). Absorption of short-chain fatty acids by the colon. *Gastroenterology*, 78(6), 1500-1507.

Rycroft, C. E., Jones, M. R., Gibson, G. R., & Rastall, R. A. (2001). A comparative in vitro evaluation of the fermentation properties of prebiotic oligosaccharides. *Journal of Applied Microbiology*, 91(5), 878-887.

Scientific Community on Food (2000). Opinion of the Scientific Committee on Food on the Tolerable Upper Intake Level of Folate.

Shepherd, S. J., & Gibson, P. R. (2006). Fructose malabsorption and symptoms of irritable bowel syndrome: guidelines for effective dietary management. *Journal of the American Dietetic Association*, 106(10), 1631-1639.

Shepherd, S. J., Parker, F. C., Muir, J. G., & Gibson, P. R. (2008). Dietary triggers of abdominal symptoms in patients with irritable bowel syndrome: randomized placebo-controlled evidence. *Clinical Gastroenterology and Hepatology*, 6(7), 765-771.

Silk, D. B. A., Davis, A., Vulevic, J., Tzortzis, G., & Gibson, G. R. (2009). Clinical trial: the effects of a trans-galactooligosaccharide prebiotic on faecal microbiota and symptoms in irritable bowel syndrome. *Alimentary pharmacology & therapeutics*, 29(5), 508-518.

Simopoulos, A. P. (1999). Essential fatty acids in health and chronic disease. *The American Journal of Clinical Nutrition*, 70(3), 560s-569s.

Speier, C., Vessey, I., & Valacich, J. S. (2003). The Effects of Interruptions, Task Complexity, and Information Presentation on Computer-Supported Decision-Making Performance. *Decision Sciences*, 34(4), 771-797.

Stefanini, G. F., Saggioro, A., Alvisi, V., Angelini, G., Capurso, L., Di, L. G., ...Melzi, G. (1995). Oral cromolyn sodium in comparison with elimination diet in the irritable bowel syndrome, diarrheic type. Multicenter study of 428 patients. *Scandinavian Journal of Gastroenterology*, 30(6), 535–541.

Stockwell, M. (n. d.). *Awards/Events*. Retrieved from http://www.melissastockwell.com/Melissa_Stockwell/Awards.html.

Stubbs, J. (2013). N. t.. In Wells, V., Wyness, L., & Coe, S. (Eds.). The British Nutrition Foundation's 45th Anniversary Conference: Behaviour change in relation to healthier lifestyles. *Nutrition Bulletin*, 38(1), 100-107.

Suarez, F. L., Savaiano, D. A., & Levitt, M. D. (1995). A comparison of symptoms after the consumption of milk or lactose-hydrolyzed milk by people with self-reported severe lactose intolerance. *New England Journal of Medicine*, 333(1), 1-4.

Suarez, F. L., Springfield, J., Furne, J. K., Lohrmann, T. T., Kerr, P. S., & Levitt, M. D. (1999). Gas production in humans ingesting a soybean flour derived from beans naturally low in oligosaccharides. *The American Journal of Clinical Nutrition*, 69(1), 135-139.

Tarpila, S., Tarpila, A., Grohn, P., Silvennoinen, T., & Lindberg, L. (2004). Efficacy of ground flaxseed on constipation in patients with irritable bowel syndrome. *Current Topics in Nutraceutical Research*, 2(2), 119–125.

Test (2008). Schneller, schöner, stärker. *test – Journal Gesundheit*, 43(02), 88-92.

Teuri, U., Vapaatalo, H., & Korpela, R. (1999). Fructooligosaccharides and lactulose cause more symptoms in lactose maldigesters and subjects with pseudohypolactasia than in control lactose digesters. *The American Journal of Clinical Nutrition*, 69(5), 973-979.

Thompson, Kyle (2006). Bristol Stool Chart [Graphical illustration]. Retrieved from http://commons.wikimedia.org/wiki/File:Bristol_Stool_Chart.png

Nanda, R., Shu, L. H., & Thomas, J. R. (2012). A fodmap diet update: craze or credible. *Practical Gastroenterology*, 10(12), 37-46.

Toschke, A. M., Thorsteinsdottir, K. H., & von Kries, R. (2009). Meal frequency, breakfast consumption and childhood obesity. *International Journal Of Pediatric Obesity*, 4(4), 242-248.

Tou, J. C., Chen, J., & Thompson, L. U. (1998). Flaxseed and its lignan precursor, secoisolariciresinol diglycoside, affect pregnancy outcome and reproductive development in rats. *The Journal of nutrition*, 128(11), 1861-1868.

Truswell, A. S., Seach, J. M., & Thorburn, A. W. (1988). Incomplete absorption of pure Fructose in healthy subjects and the facilitating effect of glucose. *The American Journal of Clinical Nutrition*, 48(6), 1424-1430.

U. S. Department of Agriculture and U. S. Department of Health and Human Services (2010). *Dietary Guidelines for Americans* (7th ed.). Washington, DC: U. S. Government Printing Office.

U. S. Department of Agriculture, Agricultural Research Service (2013). USDA National Nutrient Database for Standard Reference, Release 26. Nutrient Data Laboratory HomePage, http://www.ars.usda.gov/ba/bhnrc/ndl.

van Loo, J., Coussement, P., De Leenheer, L., Hoebregs, H., & Smits, G. (1995). On the presence of inulin and oligoFructose as natural ingredients in the western diet. *Critical Reviews in Food Science and Nutrition*, 35(6), 525–552.

Varea, V., de Carpi, J. M., Puig, C., Alda, J. A., Camacho, E., Ormazabal, A., ... & Gómez, L. (2005). Malabsorption of carbohydrates and depression in children and adolescents. *Journal of pediatric gastroenterology and nutrition*, 40(5), 561-565.

Verhoef, P., Stampfer, M. J., Buring, J. F., Gaziano, J. M., Allen, R. H., Stabler, S. P., ... & Willett, W. C. (1996). Homocysteine metabolism and risk of myocardial infarction: relation with vitamins B6, B12, and folate. *American Journal of Epidemiology*, 143(9), 845-859.

Vernia, P., Ricciardi, M. R., Frandina, C., Bilotta, T., & Frieri, G. (1995). Lactose malabsorption and irritable bowel syndrome. Effect of a long-term lactose-free diet. *The Italian Journal of Gastroenterology*, 27(3), 117-121.

Vesa, T. H., Korpela, R. A., & Sahi, T. (1996). Tolerance to small amounts of lactose in lactose maldigesters. *The American journal of clinical nutrition*, 64(2), 197-20.

Virtanen, S. M., Räsänen, L., Mäenpää, J., & Åkerblom, H. K. (1987). Dietary Survey of Finnish Adolescent Diabetics and Non-Diabetic Controls. *Acta Paediatrica*, 76(5), 801-808.

Vos, M. B., Kimmons, J. E., Gillespie, C., Welsh, J., & Blanck, H. M. (2008). Dietary Fructose consumption among US children and adults: the Third National Health and Nutrition Examination Survey. *The Medscape Journal of Medicine*, 10(7), 160.

Watson, B. D. (2008). Public health and carrageenan regulation : a review and analysis. *Journal of Applied Phycology*, 20(5), 505-513.

Webb, F. S., & Whitney, E. N. (2008). *Nutrition: Concepts and controversies* (11th ed.). Belmont, CA: Thomson/ Wadsworth.

Wells, N. E. J., Hahn, B. A., & Whorwell, P. J. (1997). Clinical economics review: irritable bowel syndrome. *Allimentary Pharmacology and Therapeutics*, 11, 1019-1030.

Winterfeldt, D. von, & Edwards, W. (1986). *Decision analysis and behavioral research*. Cambridge: Cambridge University Press.

--

**Sources regarding the prevalence of IBS:**

**England**

Jones, R., & Lydeard, S. (1992). Irritable bowel syndrom in the general population. *British Medical Journal*, 304(6819), 87-90.

**Japan and the Netherlands**

Schlemper, R. J., van der Werf, S. D. J., Vandenbroucke, J. P., Blemond, I., & Lamers, C. B. H. W. (1993). Peptic ulcer, non-ulcer dyspepsia and irritable bowel syndrom in the Netherlands and Japan. *Scandinavian Journal of Gastroenterology*, 28(200), 33-41.

**Nigeria**

Olubuykle, I. O., Olawuyl, F., & Fasanmade, A. A. (1995). A study of irritable bowel syndrom diagnosed by manning criteria in an african population. *Digestive Diseases and Sciences*, 40(5), 983-985.

**USA**

Longstreth, G. F., & Wolde-Tsadik, G. (1993). Irritable bowel-type symptoms in hmo examinees. *Digestive Diseases and Sciences*, 38(9), 1581-1589.

Talley, N. J., Zinsmeister, A. R., van Dyke, C., & Melton, L. J. (1991). Epidemiology of colonic symptoms and the irritable bowel syndrome. *Gastroenterology*, 101(4), 927-934.

O'Keefe, E. A., Talley, N. J., Zinsmeister, A. R., & Jacobsen, S. J. (1995). Bowel disorders impair functional status and quality of life in the elerdly: a population-based study. *Journal of Gastroenterology*, 50A, M184-M189.

--

Wilder-Smith, C. H., Materna, A., Wermelinger, C., & Schuler, J. (2013). Fruktose and Laktose intolerance and malabsorption testing: the relationship with symptoms in functional gastrointestinal disorders. *Alimentary Pharmacology and Therapeutics*, 37(11), 1074-1083.

Winterfeldt, D. von, & Edwards, W. (1986). *Decision analysis and behavioral research*. Cambridge: Cambridge University Press.

Zohar, D. (1999). When things go wrong: The effect of daily work hassles on effort, exertion and negative mood. *Journal of Occupational and Organizational Psychology*, 72(3), 265-283.

www.ingramcontent.com/pod-product-compliance
Lightning Source LLC
Chambersburg PA
CBHW081154020426
42333CB00020B/2504